"In these selected papers of Martin Bergmann, profound meditations are offered on love and death, the leap from hysteria to dream interpretation in Freud's intellectual development, the genetic roots of psychoanalysis in the creative clash between Enlightenment and Romantic ideas, old age as a clinical and theoretical phenomenon, the death instinct as clinical conundrum and controversy, and the interminable debate about termination in psychoanalysis and how to effect it. Crucial clinical and theoretical questions are constantly addressed and the challenges they pose cannot but engage and enlighten the reader. Bergmann is a philosopher of mind as much as he is a psychoanalyst and the range and scope of the ideas in these selected papers is impressive, instructive and illuminating."

– **Dr. Eugene Mahon**, training and supervising analyst, Columbia Psychoanalytic Center for Training and Research and member of the Center for Advanced Psychoanalytic Studies in Princeton.

"This collection of selected papers on the history of psychoanalysis, psychoanalytic technique, and on love convey the depth and breadth of Martin Bergmann's contributions to psychoanalysis. His clarity of thought, his creativity, his joy in learning, and his love of a good idea and their application in his seminars, which were ongoing for 35 years, inspired a generation of learning psychoanalytic work in the group."

– **Marilyn LaMonica**, MPS, NYS Licensed Psychoanalyst.

From the preface by Dr. Otto Kernberg: "The present volume provides the reader with a wide ranging, comprehensive set of contributions by Martin Bergmann to major aspects of psychoanalytic theory, technique, and applications. Major subject matters include psychoanalytic technique, the scientific and ideological aspects of psychoanalysis, and the study of love. In all these fields, Bergmann follows a general strategic approach: first, he masterfully synthesizes Freud's major contributions to a certain area, the origin and development of his thinking, the ramifications to present day psychoanalytic theory and practice, and, finally, Bergmann's explanation of the nature of still unresolved problems that require further work. It is an exciting intellectual journey that fosters the reader's confrontation with problems of actuality regarding theory, technique and application of psychoanalysis. The present volume is a rich, stimulating book that combines an historical analysis of Freud's contributions with Bergmann's analysis of the roots of present day controversies and unresolved challenges for the psychoanalytic community. It is relevant for clinicians, theoreticians, and, hopefully, a new generation of researchers as well."

– **Otto F. Kernberg**, Director, Personality Disorders Institute, New York Presbyterian Hospital, Westchester Division; Professor of Psychiatry, Weill Medical College of Cornell University; Training and Supervising Analyst, Columbia University Center for Psychoanalytic Training and Research.

The Origins and Organization of Unconscious Conflict

The Origins and Organization of Unconscious Conflict provides a comprehensive set of contributions by Martin S. Bergmann to psychoanalytic theory, technique, and its applications. Following a general approach, Bergmann synthesizes Freud's major contributions, the development of his thinking, the ramifications to present day psychoanalytic theory and practice, and, finally, discusses unresolved problems requiring further work.

In these selected papers, profound meditations are offered on love and death, the leap from hysteria to dream interpretation in Freud's intellectual development, the genetic roots of psychoanalysis in the creative clash between Enlightenment and Romantic ideas, old age as a clinical and theoretical phenomenon, the death instinct as clinical controversy, and the interminable debate about termination in psychoanalysis and how to effect it. Crucial clinical and theoretical questions are constantly addressed and the challenges they pose will engage and enlighten the reader. Bergmann was a philosopher of mind as much as a psychoanalyst, and the range and scope of the ideas in these selected papers is impressive, instructive and illuminating.

Bergmann deals with psychoanalysis as a science, and with an ideology – referring to psychoanalysis as a "*Weltanschauung*," a philosophical basis for psychoanalytic theory. He presented empirical research for validation from other sciences, attempting to clarify his own observations about irrational forces that constitute major motivators of human life, and require taking an existential position regarding their implications: the search for the meaning of one's existence.

The Origins and Organization of Unconscious Conflict is an exciting intellectual journey of the scientific and ideological aspects of psychoanalysis and the study of love. It will appeal to psychoanalysts, psychologists, philosophers and both undergraduate and postgraduate students studying in these fields, as well as anyone with an interest in mental health and human behaviour.

Martin S. Bergmann (1913–2014) was a Freudian psychoanalyst, author and educator. For many years he taught a course on the history of psychoanalysis in the postdoctoral program on psychoanalysis and psychotherapy at New York University and in private seminars. He was an honorary member of the American Psychoanalytic Association, an honorary fellow of the Post-Graduate Center for Mental Health, and a member of the International Psychoanalytic Association.

World Library of Mental Health

The *World Library of Mental Health* celebrates the important contributions to mental health made by leading experts in their individual fields. Each author has compiled a career-long collection of what they consider to be their finest pieces: extracts from books, journals, articles, major theoretical and practical contributions, and salient research findings.

For the first time ever the work of each contributor is presented in a single volume so readers can follow the themes and progress of their work and identify the contributions made to, and the development of, the fields themselves.

Each book in the series features a specially written introduction by the contributor giving an overview of their career, contextualizing their selection within the development of the field, and showing how their own thinking developed over time.

Titles in this series:

Passions, Persons, Psychotherapy, Politics: The selected works of Andrew Samuels
By Andrew Samuels

Towards a Radical Redefinition of Psychology: The selected works of Miller Mair
Edited by David Winter and Nick Reed

Living Archetypes: The selected works of Anthony Stevens
By Anthony Stevens

Soul: Treatment and Recovery: The selected works of Murray Stein
By Murray Stein

A Developmentalist's Approach to Research, Theory, and Therapy: The selected works of Joseph Lichtenberg
By Joseph D. Lichtenberg

Existential Psychotherapy and Counselling after Postmodernism: The selected works of Del Loewenthal
By Del Loewenthal

Love the Wild Swan: The selected works of Judith Edwards
By Judith Edwards

Conscience and Critic: The selected works of Keith Tudor
By Keith Tudor

The Origins and Organization of Unconscious Conflict

The selected works of Martin S. Bergmann

Martin S. Bergmann

Routledge
Taylor & Francis Group
LONDON AND NEW YORK

First published 2017
by Routledge
2 Park Square, Milton Park, Abingdon, Oxon OX14 4RN

and by Routledge
711 Third Avenue, New York, NY 10017

Routledge is an imprint of the Taylor & Francis Group, an informa business

British Library Cataloguing in Publication Data
A catalogue record for this book is available from the British Library

Library of Congress Cataloguing in Publication Data
Names: Bergmann, Martin S., 1913–2014, author.
Title: The origins and organization of unconscious conflict:
the selected works of Martin S. Bergmann / Martin S. Bergmann.
Description: Abingdon, Oxon; New York, NY : Routledge, 2017. |
Series: World library of mental health; v. 14 |
Includes bibliographical references and index.
Identifiers: LCCN 2016011556| ISBN 9781138938649 (hardback : alk. paper) |
ISBN 9781315672625 (e-book : alk. paper) |
ISBN 9781138941939 (pbk. : alk. paper)
Subjects: LCSH: Psychoanalysis. | Psychiatry.
Classification: LCC RC504 .B325 2017 | DDC 616.89/17–dc23
LC record available at https://lccn.loc.gov/2016011556

ISBN: 978-1-138-93864-9 (hbk)
ISBN: 978-1-315-67262-5 (ebk)

Typeset in Sabon
by Out of House Publishing

MIX
Paper from responsible sources
FSC www.fsc.org FSC® C013604

Printed and bound by CPI Group (UK) Ltd, Croydon, CR0 4YY

CONTENTS

ACKNOWLEDGMENTS

This group of papers was selected for publication by Martin S. Bergmann.

My thanks to Dr. Otto F. Kernberg, whose interest in these papers shepherded this book; Ms. Jill Delaney, for my initial contact with my publisher; and to Ms. Karen Duda, who assisted with typing this manuscript.

Maria V. Bergmann

PREFACE

The present volume provides the reader with a wide ranging, comprehensive set of contributions by Martin Bergmann to major aspects of psychoanalytic theory, technique, and applications. Major subject matters include psychoanalytic technique, the scientific and ideological aspects of psychoanalysis, and the study of love. In all these fields, Bergmann follows a general strategic approach: first, he masterfully synthesizes Freud's major contributions to a certain area, the origin and development of his thinking, the ramifications to present day psychoanalytic theory and practice, and, finally, Bergmann's explanation of the nature of still unresolved problems that require further work. It is an exciting intellectual journey that fosters the reader's confrontation with problems of actuality regarding theory, technique and application of psychoanalysis.

Regarding the area of psychoanalytic technique, Bergmann describes how significant creative leaps permitted Freud to discover the essentials of psychoanalytic technique. The leap from his *Studies on Hysteria* to *The Interpretation of Dreams* included Freud's discovery of free association, the basic contribution of the patient to the collaborative work with the analyst, complemented by the analyst's free floating attention. This method facilitated the discovery of the Dynamic Unconscious, and continues, to this day, to be the cornerstone of clinical psychoanalytic exploration. This method has been expanded by Bion's recommendation to enter each session "without memory nor desire," and continues to be an essential aspect not only of psychoanalytic technique, but of all derived psychoanalytic psychotherapies.

The discovery of the Dynamic Unconscious was complemented, Bergmann goes on, by Freud's description of the very nature of primary process functioning and its impact on preconscious thinking, humor, fantasy, and distortions of language. The analysis of the Dynamic Unconscious led to the fundamental importance of infantile sexuality and the oedipal constellation. The next step was the discovery of the unconscious repetition in the "here and now" of unresolved conflicts of the past; i.e., transference, leading to transference analysis as an essential technique of contemporary psychoanalytic treatment.

Bergmann then describes the second great leap in Freud's development, the formulation of the structural theory, the discovery of super ego functions and super ego pathology, clarifying, in the process, depression and masochism, and leading to the discovery of the importance of severe, primary aggression directed against self and others, Freud's formulation of the concept of the death drive. Today we assume that both love and aggression originate in biologically determined positive and negative affect systems that, from birth on, determine the infant's interactions with mother and with the expanding social world, and are expressed in the dynamics of unconscious conflict in all areas of development and psychic experience.

In the analysis of the nature of passionate love, Bergmann points to the combination of the unconscious search for the oedipally beloved or ambivalently loved object, but he also stresses the importance of the symbiotic longing for the original encounter with mother that has been highlighted in the study of early infant-mother relations. Nowadays, we consider attachment, eroticism and play-bonding as those primary positive affect systems that come together in what Freud denominated libido; in contrast to the death drive, that may be considered derived from the negative affect systems of "fight-flight" and "separation panic."

Bergmann stresses the parallel development of Freud's exploration of the unconscious life of his patients and of his own life experience as an ongoing task during his lifetime. Freud used the analysis of his own dreams, by means of free association, to explore his own unconscious; and Bergmann raises the question to what extent free association and dream analysis still continue to be the essential tools for investigating the deeper layers of the mind. While transference analysis has become the dominant focus of psychoanalytic technique, dream analysis is still a "royal road" to the unconscious. The importance of dream analysis continues to haunt psychoanalytic technique: recent developments of the neo-Bionian approach consider the patient's free associations as similar to the manifest contents of dreams, so that patients' descriptions of their emotional reality and their fantasies are treated as manifest contents of deeper unconscious developments that may be captured, in turn, by the analyst's "reverie."

Bergmann presents a penetrating analysis of the unresolved issue of analytic goals. He points to the fact that, in many cases, the aspired freedom from neurotic conflicts and pathological inhibitions to be achieved by psychoanalysis remains an unattained goal. This has become a growing concern for the profession, and has led to a sophisticated analysis of cases that do not respond to psychoanalysis proper but may respond to modified treatments: psychoanalytic psychotherapies. Bergmann points to the initial reluctance within psychoanalysis to engage in such modified treatments and, appropriately I believe, reaches the conclusion that psychoanalytic psychotherapy is an important area to explore and develop in order to help a much larger patient population than those responding to standard psychoanalysis. We already have solid empirical research that psychoanalytic psychotherapies have demonstrated their effectiveness. The discussion of the goals of psychoanalysis leads Bergmann to explore the differentiation between treatment goals and life goals, and the importance of setting up realistic indications and outcome expectations.

The analysis of erotic transference and countertransference is one of the richest contributions of this book. Bergmann points to Freud's discovery of the importance of erotic countertransference and its challenge to technical neutrality, on the one hand; and the question of whether transference love is "real love" or a form of "neurotic" love. Bergmann convincingly shows how the characteristics of erotic transference correspond to those of a real, passionate love experience; but, insofar as it is directed to an unavailable object, it also acquires the nature of the oedipal situation. In contrast to the original oedipal situation, it now may be explored in the treatment – and, under optimal circumstances, resolved in a mourning reaction – that permits the transfer of the capacity for love to an available object in the patient's real life. Bergmann wisely analyzes limitations to this optimal development and the risk that the relationship with the analyst, at times, is so much better than anything the patient has found in life before that it becomes difficult to resolve this transference.

Bergmann points to important contemporary developments in countertransference awareness, and the gradual shift of the analytic attitude from considering countertransference as an obstacle to the view of countertransference as crucial information regarding transference developments. He also discusses countertransference in connection with complications in the termination of treatment. Bergmann candidly discusses the difficulty of the analyst, as well as of the patient, in ending a relationship that has been so uniquely helpful, and, in fact, that may have been the most positive relationship that some patients have had in their entire life! Here the working through of termination becomes complex, and the mourning over the end of the analysis may become a major source of conflict and disappointment. Bergmann illustrates these conflicts with numerous clinical examples that reveal the subtlety and creativity of his approach to individual cases, his stepping outside the conventional assumptions regarding the effects of psychoanalytic technique, and his openness to unexpected and surprising developments in the analytic relationship. This openness also applies to Bergmann's observations regarding the developments of analysis during old age. The discussion of the loss of the dimension of the future in old age, the objective risks of loneliness and lack of support, the traumatic death of a spouse of many years, and patients' concerns over the possibility of the death of an aging analyst, are amongst the most interesting reflections of this volume.

A major part of the book deals with psychoanalysis as a science, and with what I have called an ideology – referring to psychoanalysis as a "*Weltanschauung*," a philosophical basis for psychoanalytic theory. Bergmann presents an original, penetrating analysis of Freud's inner struggle, throughout his entire life, between the consideration of analysis as a science, to be submitted to empirical research and validation and related to other sciences; and, alternatively, analysis as the discovery of the deep, irrational forces that constitute major motivators of human life, and require taking an existential position regarding their implications: the search for the meaning of one's existence in this dramatic context.

Bergmann classifies major contributors to psychoanalytic thinking as heretics, modifiers and extenders. Heretics separated their thinking from that of Freud. Historically, the most important were Adler, Stekel, Jung, Rank and Wilhelm Reich. Bergmann states that during Freud's lifetime there were only heretics; extenders and modifiers appeared after Freud's death, when no one could lay claim to being the only heir to Freud's legacy. Modifiers significantly recast psychoanalytic theory and technique, but maintain themselves in the psychoanalytic mainstream. The most important early modifiers were Ferenczi and Federn, later ones included Hartmann, Melanie Klein, Winnicott, Lacan and Kohut. Bergmann proposes that extenders usually expanded psychoanalysis into new areas, but their findings did not demand modification. Among them, he refers to Karl Abraham, Hermann Nunberg, Robert Waelder and Otto Fenichel; interestingly enough, all of them (except Abraham) are linked with ego psychology. One might add that modifiers who remained within the psychoanalytic fold in turn gave origin to extenders, such as, for example, Bion, Rosenfeld and Meltzer as extenders of Kleinian theory. While relational psychoanalysis probably has not originated any major modifiers, it does constitute, as a group, a significant constellation of extenders in the development of object relations theory and technique. In any case, as Bergmann points out, the examination of the total field of modifiers and extenders indicates that there exist some major controversies in psychoanalysis that have not been resolved and are expressed in different theoretical and technical approaches that create an ongoing dynamic and problematic question about their resolution.

Bergmann points out that the essential controversy may be between those who see psychoanalysis as a scientific approach to the study of the unconscious and the resolution of neurotic conflict by resolving unconscious conflicts – following, in this regard, Freud's major traditional approach – and a radical opposite position, implying that what is therapeutic is not only the interpretation of unconscious conflicts, but the very relationship that the patient establishes with the analyst. Ferenczi, Balint and Winnicot moved in that direction, and the entire contemporary relationist school has pointed to the fundamental importance of the reliving, in the analytic situation, of past traumatic experiences of etiological importance in the patient suffering. Whether what dominates in the cure are interpretations or a new relationship is a major question that separates ego psychologists, Kleinians, British Independent, and French analysts from the relationist school with its various facets of intersubjectivity, relational analysis, interpersonal analysis and self psychology.

Bergmann points to the difficulty of resolving this controversy on the basis of simply comparing clinical experiences that tend to be colored by the theoretical and clinical biases of the psychoanalyst. He proposes that these questions will have to be resolved by means of empirical research – an endeavor the psychoanalytic establishment has been so reluctant to embrace. In fact, I believe that the traditional reluctance – and even animosity against – empirical research has harmed psychoanalysis. It has isolated it from the university and academia, and slowed down the new applications to psychoanalytic psychotherapies.

Again, Bergmann points out how, behind this controversy, lurks the bigger one between psychoanalysis as a science or an ideology, a *Weltanschauung*. This, he observes, already became evident in the struggle between Freud and Jung – with Freud's insistence on the scientific nature of psychoanalysis; while Jung pointed to the obscure and primitive nature of the unconscious forces affecting the human being in a manner that reflected the profound spiritual currents of German romanticist philosophy.

Bergmann convincingly illustrates this struggle between science and ideology in the three chapters dedicated to Freud's conflict between enlightenment and romantic philosophy, involving the impact of Freud's death drive theory, and the Jewish and German roots of psychoanalysis. In the process, Bergmann describes the fundamental influence of German philosophy on Freud, on the one hand, and, on the other, the uncompromising scientific attitude of Brücke, whose assistant he had been at one point.

Freud the scientist had demonstrated his deep knowledge of the neurology of his time in his book on Aphasia. When he abandoned his efforts to base his psychological theories on neurobiology, he did so because he realized that the neurobiology of his time was not yet at the level that permitted him to do that. In this connection, I have no doubt that if Freud were alive today his views would be profoundly influenced by the new developments in our neurobiological understanding – very much in contrast to psychoanalysts who hang on to ideas that clearly reflect Freud's dependency on the neurobiology of the past.

But then, in the 1920s, the effects of the First World War and Freud's discovery of the profound influence of unconscious aggression and their self-destructive effects under the disguise of the moral constellation of the super ego, led him to become aware of the dark sight of existence, the thin layer of rational adaptation to social reality. This finding moved him again into the direction of ideology, a *Weltanschauung*, without explicitly stating that position. The very concept of the death drive implied an existential view of the fundamental struggle between love, happiness, and the drive to relate, on the one hand; and to aggression, turned inward toward the self or in the outward expression of violence toward others on a massive scale, on the other ... Freud's analysis of the psychology of regressive mass movements, and their relationship to a leader, predicted with frightening accuracy the horrible mass destruction movements of the 1930s and 1940s, and, again, what we now perceive in the primitive destructiveness of political Islam.

Bergmann describes the controversy generated in the psychoanalytic establishment by Freud's structural theory, and his new theory of libido and the death drive, and how it remains one of the major divisive themes that agitates the psychoanalytic community. Ego psychology and the relationalist approach tend to reject the concept of the death drive, while Kleinian analysis and French analysis accept the theory of the death drive to this day.

In my view, we do have solid evidence that inborn negative affect systems – the "fight-flight" system and the "panic-separation" system – originate the potential for aggressive behavior that, under conditions of environmental traumatization may expand, become dominant, and be structurally built into the individual's character structure and superego, or else remain as repressed forces that may be triggered at moments of regression. André Green's proposal that narcissism represents not only the libidinal investment in the self, but also expresses the combined investment of libido and aggression in the self, is convincing to me. Under normal circumstances, the overcoming of the paranoid-schizoid position, the integration that is reflected in the depressive position, permits the modulation of aggression: love dominates and modulates and tones down aggression. Under pathological circumstances, with an excessive development of aggressive drive, severe splits of the personality may remain, giving rise to borderline personality organization. Under these circumstances aggression also may invade a pathological grandiose self, giving rise to malignant narcissism and to personality structures in which aggression becomes the dominant motivation of the individual.

In his book *On the Future of an Illusion*, Freud expressed his conviction that religion reflects the remnants of an infantile search for a protective, powerful benign father figure. He expressed his hope that in the long run rationality will prevail and make religion unnecessary. Bergmann agrees, and takes the side of a scientific approach. To me, Freud's affirmation, however, seems more an ideological hopefulness than a scientific observation. Psychoanalysis has much to say about religiosity and the development of the capability for a spiritual realm of existence, but cannot make decisions about the truth values of theological affirmation. Here Martin Bergmann and I diverge, because Martin, in a proud gesture, was prone to say: "The buck stops here."

The final section of the book contains a major contribution to our understanding of passionate love. Here Bergmann draws on his own work, but also considers the limited psychoanalytic literature about the subject and, of course, Freud's contributions to the subject. Freud described the essential function of the oedipal constellation in determining one's search for a lost love object. Mother is the first love object: after the intensity of longing for her related to the oedipal phase of development, and the decrease of the intensity of this relation during the latent period, the search for a refinding of this first love object re-emerges in adolescence. Now both erotic feelings and tenderness combine in the search for an object that unconsciously represents mother and, by the same token – in the case of women – the idealized father of the oedipal period. Opposed to this search is the unconscious guilt over oedipal longings, with the potential of defensive splitting between tender feelings and sexual feelings, the various types of sexual pathology that include impotence, sexual inhibitions, masochistic approaches to love, or aggressive efforts to exact revenge for oedipal disappointments. Bergmann stresses, in combination with these major determinants, the development of narcissistic features – in the sense of the idealization of the love object that is internalized as the ego ideal – and then reprojected outside in order to find, in external reality, the person that symbolically will reflect one's own ego ideal. And underneath these features, Bergmann stresses the wish for fusion with the symbiotic mother of earliest development.

The fact that mother unconsciously induces a capability for erotic desire in the infant, in correspondence with the activation of a neurobiological erotic affect disposition of the infant, is one of the major new developments in psychoanalytic understanding. Martin Bergmann stresses the importance of the search for an ecstatic primary erotic union in adulthood. At the same time, he emphasizes the developing human capacity for idealization in the developing ego idea and the development of oedipal love, which together determine the capacity for a passionate love engagement. This general concept is beautifully illustrated in clinical manifestations of these desires. Bergmann describes, among the pathology of love relations, the repetition compulsion of traumatic past relationships that are unconsciously reactivated in new love relations. These dynamics are expressed, for example, in the selection of an object totally opposite to the maternal one, the development of intolerance of separation as part of love relations, the reactivation of conflicts of separation individuation, and the many difficulties in integrating developmentally the various currents that determine the capacity for passionate love.

Bergmann attempts, through a historical review of the development of our knowledge of sexuality, to synthesize what we now know about it, and points to what we still have to learn regarding the ultimate integration of erotic desire, emotional tenderness, idealizing relations and the intense search for fusion in love relations. He implies that we know more about the pathology of love relations than about the characteristics of mature love.

In the last chapter of this section Bergmann once again comes back to the relationship between transference love and love in real life. Bergmann concludes that love may be repetitive in terms of the refinding of the primary love object, but it also has an element of novelty derived from real life. He states that transference love is not adaptive by itself, and that it is only the sublimation of transference love with the aid of the analyst that makes it adaptive for the purposes of cure when serious love problems affected the patient before the treatment. Oedipal love necessarily leads to disillusionment, which fosters the building up of defenses against loving. The working through of transference love liberates the capacity for love, that now can be invested in a new object – but the first new object will necessarily be the analyst himself. The mechanism of sublimation will permit the renunciation and transfer of this newly learned capacity. Transference love, therefore, is a "special hot house variety of love."

The present volume is a rich, stimulating book that combines an historical analysis of Freud's contributions with Bergmann's analysis of the roots of present day controversies and unresolved challenges for the psychoanalytic community. It is relevant for clinicians, theoreticians, and, hopefully, a new generation of researchers as well.

Otto F. Kernberg, M.D.
May 14, 2015
*Director, Personality Disorders Institute,
New York Presbyterian Hospital, Westchester Division
Professor of Psychiatry, Weill Medical College of Cornell University
Training and Supervising Analyst, Columbia University Center for
Psychoanalytic Training and Research

PART I

THEORY

CHAPTER 1

PSYCHOANALYTIC OBSERVATIONS ON THE CAPACITY TO LOVE[1]

From the Greek tragedians and the Roman poets, the Western world has inherited the idea that love is an overwhelming and dangerous emotion that reduces the mind to a state of inconstancy and childishness. The destructive power of love is described with particular force by Euripides in *Hippolytus*. That play, it will be recalled, records the gradual disintegration of Queen Phaedra's superego and ego under the impact of her love for her stepson. Euripides lets the nurse say to Phaedra, "The love queen's onset in her might is more than man can bear," and the chorus implores Aphrodite: "O never in evil mood appear to me, nor out of time and tune approach" (Coleridge translation). Sophocles lets the chorus in *Antigone* sing:

> Love, unconquered in the fight, Love, who makest havoc of wealth, who keepest thy vigil on the soft cheek of a maiden; thou roamest over the sea, and among the homes of dwellers in the wilds; no immortal can escape thee, nor any among men whose life is for a day; and he to whom thou hast come is mad.
> The just themselves have their minds warped by thee to wrong, for their ruin ...
>
> (Oates and O'Neil 1938, p. 445)

In a similar vein, Menander treats love as a sickness, and Plutarch regards love as a form of madness. With the notable exception of Ovid, the poets of antiquity feared love because it induced regression; and they were dimly aware of a relationship between love and infancy.

By contrast, Shakespeare's dominant attitude toward love is ambivalence:

> The bitter-sweet character of the food of love is emphasised by Shakespeare as by no one else. It is luscious and bitter, sweet and sour, delicious and loathsome, "a choking gall and a preserving sweet."
>
> (Spurgeon 1958, p. 147)

The metaphors with which Shakespeare expresses love are strikingly oral: "Love surfeit not. Lust like a glutton dies." And of Cleopatra it is said, "other women cloy the appetite they feed, but she makes hungry." And Juliet, the heroine who embodies love as few of his heroines do, declared, "My bounty is as boundless as the sea. My love as deep." Plato expressed the ambivalent feelings toward love by a myth. Eros is described in the *Symposium* (p. 203) as the Son of Plenty (Poros) and Poverty (Penia). From his father he has inherited the sense of plenty that accompanies love; and from his mother, the distress that lovers feel.

Finally, there is a third group of poets and philsophers who affirm love without reservation. Bertrand Russell (1930) once quoted an anonymous poet who wrote that "Love" was greatly wronged by those who called its sweetness bitter, when in fact the richness of its fruit was such that nothing could surpass its sweetness. And he himself adds:

> not only is love a source of delight, but its absence is a source of pain ... it enhances all the best pleasures, such as music, and sunrise in mountains, and the sea under the full moon. A man who has never enjoyed beautiful things in the company of a woman whom he loved has not experienced to the full the magic power of which such things are capable.
>
> (p. 40)

The three basic attitudes have in common the conviction that love is an overwhelming emotion which fundamentally affects the mental stability and the outlook on life of the person who is "in love." We intuitively recognize that a relationship is not love when a radical change in mood has not taken place or when the beloved is painlessly exchanged for another.

We speak of selecting a mate as we speak of choosing an occupation, and we know that both decisions are the result of a complex interaction between conscious reality-oriented considerations and unconscious wishes. However, when the mate is chosen on the basis of realistic considerations, we suspect prudence rather than love. We speak of "falling in love," and earlier writers spoke of being smitten by love, and evoked the mythological image of the blindfolded Amor. Other languages maintain a similar distinction, as the German distinction between "*lieben*" and "*sich verlieben*." In the vocabulary that Federn developed, we may say that love can be experienced with active or passive ego feelings (Bergmann 1963). Thus, Robert Browning:

> How say you? Let us, O my dove,
> Let us be unashamed of soul,
> As earth lies bare to heaven above!
> How is it under our control
> To love or not to love?
>
> (*Two in the Campagna*)

In keeping with these passive feelings, lovers are prone to stress the accidental and unpremeditated nature of their meetings. Love, however, cannot simply be equated with a selection of a mate based on unconscious rather than utilitarian reasons. Psychoanalytic experience demonstrates that it is possible to have a relationship which is monogamous and tenaciously adhered to, and yet devoid of the experience of love. Such mates often stand for parental figures that were more hated than loved, or for repudiated aspects of themselves.

Before Freud, love was the domain of philosophers and poets. Freud drew heavily upon this Western tradition, but these philosophers and poets did not have a genetic psychology at their disposal. They therefore could not discern how one form of love could be related to another, nor could they gain insight into the psychic forces that promote or retard the development of the capacity to love. By contrast, Freud approached the mystery of love through a path that had never been tried before – infantile sexuality. From this vantage point, psychoanalysis could make its unique contribution to the understanding of the origin of the capacity to love. I hope to show that today we can go further than Freud did in this understanding, since we have at our disposal not only his insights but also the findings of Mahler and her co-workers, observations that I believe have special relevance to the genesis of the capacity to love.

On the subject of love, classical thought from Hesiod to Lucretius remained firmly rooted in the mythopoetic point of view. Hesiod saw Eros not only as the god of sensuous love, but also as the power that binds the separate elements of the world. This view was taken over by the pre-Socratic philosophers. To Parmenides (fragment 13), love was the force that made men live and thrive. To Democritus (fragment 78), it was the desire for all beautiful things (Bowra 1957, p. 196).

Freud (1937a) acknowledged his indebtedness to one of the pre-Socratic philosophers, Empedocles, when he said:

> I can never be certain, in view of the wide extent of my reading in early years, whether what I took for a new creation might not be an effect of cryptomnesia.
> (p. 245)

Freud (1925a) acknowledged his indebtedness to Plato, at least indirectly, when he said:

> what psycho-analysis called sexuality was by no means identical with the impulsion towards a union of the two sexes or towards producing a pleasurable sensation in the genitals; it had far more resemblance to the all-inclusive and all-preserving Eros of Plato's *Symposium*.
> (p. 218)

It is possible that Freud was also influenced by other Greek philosophers, since we know (Eissler 1951) that Gomperz's *Greek Thinkers* was one of Freud's ten favorite books.

In keeping with the mythopoetic view, love and hate were to Empedocles quasi-natural and quasi-mythological forces.

> when the elements combine to form animals or plants, men say these are born, and when they scatter again men call it death ... Never will boundless time be emptied of these two [fragment 16].
>
> In Anger all are diverse and sundered, but in Love they come together and are desired of each other. For out of these are born whatever was and is and will be – trees, men, women, beasts, birds and water-feeding fishes, yea and long-lived gods highest in honours [fragment 21].

To Empedocles, Aphrodite was not only a goddess residing on Olympus, but she literally entered men.

> she it is who is acknowledged to be implanted in the limbs of mortals, whereby they think kindly thoughts and do peaceful works, calling her Joy by name and Aphrodite.
> (fragment 17 [Guthrie 1962])

I have quoted the Greek philosophers at some length because I wish to stress that the Greek concept of love was indeed a broad one, and Freud's idea of sublimation is at least implicit in their writings. It becomes explicit in the writings of Plato, who believed that all arts and sciences sprang from some longing or desire and therefore had their origin in Eros. "Touched by love, every one becomes a poet even though he had no music in him before." Not only the "melody of the muses" but also "the arts of medicine," the "metallurgy of Hephaestus," and the "weaving of Athena" are inspired by Eros (*Symposium*, p. 197). I have shown elsewhere (Bergmann 1966) that Plato also anticipated Freud's topographic division when he described the emergence of oedipal wishes in dreams, "when the mild and rational soul is asleep." To Eros, Plato assigned the task of bringing together the two natures of man, the divine self and the tethered beast in him (Dodds 1951).

Aristotle quoted with approval Euripedes' statement, "Parched earth loves the rain and stately heaven, when filled with rain, yearns on the earth to fall" (*The Nichomachean Ethics*, Book 8). Browning, in the poem quoted earlier, used the same language, but to him the embrace of heaven and earth was a poetic metaphor, while to Aristotle it was a scientific explanation that illuminated the deeper origins of love.

This mythopoetic view of love as a cosmic force is beautifully expressed by Lucretius in his evocation of Venus (*Lucretius de Rerum Natura*, English translation, W.H.D. Rouse, Book 1, Verse 1–50).

> O goddess, from thee, the winds flee away, the clouds of heaven from thee and thy coming; for thee the wonder-working earth puts forth sweet flowers, for thee the wide stretches of ocean laugh, and heaven grown peaceful glows with outpoured light.
>
> ... the herds go wild and dance over the rich pastures and swim across rapid rivers, so greedily does each one follow thee, held captive by their charm ...
>
> For thou alone canst delight mortals with quiet peace, since Mars mighty in battle rules the savage works of war, who often casts himself upon thy lap wholly vanquished by the ever-living would of love ...

The image evoked by Lucretius became popular in the Renaissance in the many paintings depicting Venus as holding the sleeping Mars in her arms and thus assuring peace. Freud's idea of taming aggression by fusion with libido leans upon a long mythopoetic tradition. Greek philosophers also raised a number of the questions which Freud (1914d) dealt with in his study of narcissism. They wondered whether love arose from the need for an unlike complement or whether like was attracted by like. Aristotle even asked whether it was possible for a man to "feel friendship for himself." He went on to add, "devoted attachment to someone else comes to resemble love for oneself" (*The Nichomachean Ethics*, Book 9, chapter 4).

In the context of this essay, it is of interest to note that Aristotle defined love as an intensification of friendship, "an emotion of such high intensity that it can be felt only for one person at a time" (*The Nichomachean Ethics*, Book 9; see also Hazo 1967). Freud (1930) derived aim-inhibited love from sensual love (p. 103). Aristotle also recognized their affinity but, unlike Freud, derived love from friendship. Here I will be concerned only with love as defined by Aristotle and leave aside the manifestations of aim-inhibited libido.

Plato intuitively comprehended an aspect of love that psychoanalysis learned to appreciate only after Mahler illuminated the significance of the symbiotic phase in human development.

In the well-known myth told in the *Symposium*, man was originally a double. As punishment for his rebellion against the gods, he was cut in half, and the two halves forever yearn to be reunited.

> For the intense yearning which each of them has towards the other does not appear to be the desire of lover's intercourse, but of something else which the soul of either evidently desires and cannot tell, and of which she has only a dark and doubtful presentiment. Suppose Hephaestus, with his instruments, to come to the pair who are lying side by side ... and said to them ... "Do you desire to be wholly one always day and night to be in one another's company? for if this is what you desire, I am ready to melt you into one and let you grow together ..." there is not a man of them who when he heard the proposal would deny that this meeting and melting into one another, this becoming one instead of two, was the very expression of his ancient need.
>
> (*Symposium* 192, Jowell translation)

Two-and-a-half millennia have passed since these lines were written, but only our recently gained knowledge of the intensity of the mother-infant relationship enables us to understand fully what Plato meant by the term "ancient need."

Freud's interest in this myth is worth noting. He knew of its existence at least as early as 1905, when he referred to it (1905b, p. 136) without mentioning Plato by name, calling it a poetic fable. He returned to it fifteen years later (1920, pp. 57, 58). He was then interested enough in this myth to ask Gomperz about its origin, and learned that it went back to the Upanishads, and even further back to Babylonian times. Freud was intrigued by this myth because it supported his hypothesis that the drives have "a need to restore an earlier state of things" (1920, p. 57).

Mahler's discovery of the symbiotic phase offers a plausible explanation and enables us to substantiate a demonstrable psychological phase for a biological speculation that even Freud accepted with reservations. He made the pertinent observation that, "At the height of being in love the boundary between ego and object threatens to melt away. Against all the evidence of his senses, a man who is in love declares 'I' and 'you' are one, and is prepared to behave as if it were a fact" (1930, p. 66).

In the Bible, too, we find an awareness of the significance of symbiotic elements in love: "Therefore shall a man leave his father and his mother, and shall cleave unto his wife: and they shall be one flesh" (Genesis 2: 24).

In a fascinating study, Panofsky (1939) traced the motif of the blind cupid. We are so accustomed to the portrayal of the god of love as blindfolded that it comes as a surprise that Greek and Roman art never portrayed him as such. He appears blindfolded for the first time in the *Trecento*. "Blind cupid," says Panofsky, "started his career in a rather terrifying company. He belonged to night, synagogue, infidelity and death" (p. 112). The allegorical interpretation was most unflattering. "Cupid is nude and blind because he deprives men of their garments, their possessions, their good sense, and their wisdom" (p. 107).

Freud reversed the blind cupid metaphor. It is not Eros who is blind, but we who do not dare look at him. There were at least two reasons why Freud could look at love in a way it had never been looked at before. I have already mentioned that he looked for its origin in the formerly unsuspected area of infantile sexuality. Another reason was that love entered unbidden into his consultation room in the form of transference. It is fascinating to follow Freud's struggle against the acceptance of transference as a legitimate therapeutic tool. Breuer and Freud (1893–1895) referred to transference as a *mésalliance*, and called it "an external obstacle arising from a false connection" (pp. 301–304). After the turn of the century, Freud's understanding of transference had deepened:

> What are the transferences? They are new editions or facsimiles of the impulses and phantasies which are aroused and made conscious during the progress of analysis; but they have this peculiarity, which is characteristic for their species, that they replace some earlier person by the person of the physician.
>
> (Freud 1905a, p. 116)

For the next ten years, Freud maintained a line of demarcation between transference and love. However, in 1915, speaking of transference love, Freud concluded:

> It is true that the love consists of new editions of old traits and that it repeats infantile reactions. But this is the essential character of every state of being in love. There is no such state which does not reproduce infantile prototypes. It is precisely from this infantile determination that it receives its compulsive character, verging as it does on the pathological. Transference-love has perhaps a degree less of freedom than the love which appears in ordinary life and is called normal; it displays its dependence on the infantile pattern more clearly and is less adaptable and capable of modification; but that is all, and not what is essential.
>
> (1915b, p. 168)

Fromm (1956) accused Freud of failing to understand the nature of mature love. This I regard as a misunderstanding. A careful reading of the quotation above shows that, even in 1915, Freud was aware of the role of the ego in transforming or moderating the power of the infantile prototypes and adapting their demands to reality. However, in the context in which Freud was writing, this process was of secondary consequence, for the significant discovery was that love derives its power from the reawakening and the refinding of early relationships. It was this insight that enables Freud to throw new light on the nature of love.

Apart from transference, references to love appear in Freud's writings as early as 1894, when he communicated to Fliess:

> Quite particularly often melancholics have been anaesthetic. They have no need for coitus. But they have a great longing for love in its psychical form.
>
> (Freud 1892–99, p. 192)

Although this early analysis of melancholia was still crude, if we compare it to Freud's paper on *Mourning and Melancholia* (1917) we find that he had already made the significant observation, amply confirmed in subsequent psychoanalytic literature, that depressives have a particularly strong need to be loved.

Freud made two contributions to the understanding of love at two different periods in his life. The first extends from 1905 to 1912; the second has its origin in the discovery of narcissism and extends from 1914 to 1921. The basic discoveries of the first period can be summarized by two statements: "Every state of being in love reproduces infantile prototypes," and "The finding of an object is in fact a refinding" (Freud 1905b, p. 222). This formulation echoes Plato's famous dictum, "All cognition is recognition." However, Plato believed that we recognize what we knew before birth, while Freud stressed that we refind what we once experienced as infants. At times, the resemblance to the infantile prototype may be no more than a similarity in facial features, bodily build, character traits, or even name. At other times, the whole state of being in love reproduces an infantile mode of feeling or an early ego state.

Freud has now formed an outline for a theory of adult love: love becomes possible after puberty by the fusion of "two currents of libido." The first, "affective current" goes back to infancy and to the parental prototypes; while the second, the "sensual current," has its origin in puberty. A failure to fuse the two currents into one can result in neurosis (Freud 1912a, p. 180).

The inclusion of the infantile prototype in adult love does not by itself lead to neurosis. It is conducive to a neurosis only under specific conditions. Freud (1910a, 1912a) describes the neurotic nature of certain infantile prototypes in detail, calling them "necessary conditions for loving."

> In normal love only a few characteristics survive which reveal unmistakably the maternal prototype of the object-choice, as, for instance, the preference shown by young men for maturer women; the detachment of libido from the mother has been effected relatively swiftly. In our type, on the other hand, the libido has remained attached to the mother for so long, even after the onset of puberty, that the maternal characteristics remain stamped on the love objects that are chosen later, and all these turn into easily recognizable mother-surrogates (Freud 1910a, p. 169).

Examples of such conditions or preconditions for loving may be found in the compulsive need of some men to fall in love with women who belong to other men, with promiscuous women, or with women who are or appear to be in need of rescue. Freud demonstrated that all these preconditions are techniques by which the primary process converts the woman into a mother substitute. They are "consequences of the fixation on the mother."

Neurotic women may suffer from similar preconditions. They are frigid in marital relationships and lose their frigidity only when love is secret or forbidden. Freud (1912a) commented:

> Where they love, they do not desire, and where they desire, they cannot love. They seek objects which they do not love in order to keep their sensuality away from the object they love.
>
> (p. 183)

This was written before Freud established the role of aggression in mental development, and fixations are described only in libidinal terms. Today, we know that hostility toward the original object is more important in the maintenance of such a fixation than the magnitude of infantile love.

Freud's papers on love were written only a decade or so after the discovery of the Oedipus complex as the nucleus of neurosis. During this period, he saw all difficulties in love as stemming from an arrest caused by the Oedipus complex. That the inability to love may reach further back into preoedipal periods was as yet unknown. It should be noted also that these papers deal more with psychic impotence than with the inability to love.

In 1905, Freud (1905b) saw impotence as an infrequent problem. Later, he became more critical of civilization:

> I shall put forward the view that psychical impotence is much more widespread than is supposed, and that a certain amount of this behavior does in fact characterize the love of civilized man.
>
> (Freud 1912a p. 184)

Freud came close to advocating psychoanalysis as the only remedy for a nearly universal psychic impotence.

> yet it must nevertheless be said that anyone who is to be really free and happy in love must have surmounted his respect for women and have come to terms with the idea of incest with his mother or sister.
>
> (1912a, p. 186)

It is possible to surmount what Freud called "respect for women" even without psychoanalysis, but it is difficult to imagine that anybody can, by his own efforts, overcome the horror of incest.

The discovery of narcissism opened the second period of Freud's insight into the nature of love. The concept of narcissism enabled him to differentiate two sources of love. According to the narcissistic model, a person may love what he himself is, what he was, what he would like to be, or someone who was once part of himself. According to the anaclitic model, a person may love the woman who feeds or the man who protects (Freud 1914d, pp. 88–101). Both forms of love will pose difficulties in the course of development. Narcissistic love is unstable. Any disappointment in the perfection of the love object endangers it and it is easily withdrawn back to the self. Anaclitic love is passive in its orientation. When it predominates, the active phallic wishes in a man and the corresponding wishes in a woman to share the burden of life with her mate remain underdeveloped.

It is not unusual to find that patients seek analysis after the collapse of a love relationship. Here, important differences can be seen. When love is primarily based on object libido, the disappointment leads to mourning, but if the love relationship is primarily narcissistic, the desertion takes on the characteristic of a depressive constellation in the sense in which Bibring (1953) described it. It is then usually associated with rage, humiliation and the collapse of self-esteem.

The concept of narcissism enabled Freud to gain a new understanding of the sense of bliss associated with loving: "Real happy love corresponds to the original condition in which object libido and ego libido cannot be distinguished" (Freud 1914d p. 100). When large quantities of libido are withdrawn from the self to the object, there often can arise a feeling of impoverishment. This is the metapsychological reason why so many lovers feel humble and only when their love is returned is the narcissistic balance restored (p. 98). The feeling of impoverishment associated with love that Freud speaks of is reminiscent of Plato's myth that Eros is the son of Poverty. In one of his later papers, Freud added, "The difference between an ordinary erotic object cathexis and the state of being in love is that in the latter, incomparably more cathexis passes over to the object and the ego empties itself as it were in favor of the object" (1927b, pp. 164–165). But why must man love at all? This question was answered by Freud in quantitative terms:

> A strong egoism is a protection against falling ill, but in the last resort we must begin to love in order not to fall ill, and we are bound to fall ill if, in consequence of frustration, we are unable to love.
>
> (Freud 1914d, p. 85)

Narcissism also enabled Freud to understand one of the puzzling features of love, namely idealization:

> The tendency which falsifies judgment in this respect is that of *idealization* … We see that the object is being treated in the same way as our own ego, so that when we are in love a considerable amount of narcissistic libido overflows on to the object. It is even obvious, in many forms of love-choice, that the object serves as a substitute for some unattained ego ideal of our own. We love it on account of the perfections which we have striven to reach for our own ego, and which we should now like to procure in this roundabout way as a means of satisfying our narcissism.
>
> (1921, p. 113)

Freud's belief in the close connection between love and idealization is supported by Goethe's famous, posthumously published love poem (Eissler 1963a p. 181). There, Goethe mournfully complains that only he and his beloved had been denied the eternal bliss of loving without knowing each other; that is, without seeing in the other what he never was.

Among psychoanalytic writers, Reik (1944) was particularly influenced by this view of Freud, and made it into the cornerstone of his own theory of love. Reik believed that a person who is about to fall in love suffers from a sense of discomfort and feels acutely aware that he has fallen short of his own ego ideal. Love offers an escape from this inner discontent. Reik (1944) quotes a statement by Goethe in *Wilhelm Meister's Apprenticeship* (1795): "There are no means of safety against superior qualities of another person but to love him." This view of love also goes back to Plato's *Symposium*, when Socrates traps Agathon, who has just delivered a hymn in the praise of love, into admitting that love is inferior because it wants what it does not possess.

Reik abandoned the hard-won connection between love and infantile sexuality. Like so many pre-Freudian philosophers, he draws an absolute distinction between lust and love. Lust is selfish, biological, and lacks constancy. Love is artificially fostered by culture and only one person can be loved at a time.

Idealization, as Freud had observed, constitutes an essential component of the capacity to love. Those who can idealize can establish a positive transference. However, I have often observed that the transformation of such a proneness for idealization into a capacity to love can be an exceedingly difficult psychoanalytic task.

Annie Reich (1953) described women who live in a subservient relationship with men whom they consider admirable, and without whom they believe they cannot exist. The partner, Reich suggests, "represents the personification of a very early phallic ego-ideal. These phallic features overshadow the individual traits of the father" (p. 27). These women exemplify Freud's statement, quoted earlier, that "the object has taken the place of the Ego Ideal."

Following Freud's formulations (1921), Reich emphasizes that these women suffer from an intolerable conflict between ego and ego ideal which has remained megalomanic. Failure to desexualize the paternal phallus is the main reason why the real characteristics of the father are unimportant in the selection of the mate. In other spheres of their lives, such women have a well-integrated personality and maintain a critical self-evaluation and good reality testing. Unlike the typical borderline and psychotic – whose ego functions, as well as the libidinal relationships, undergo regression – these women illustrate that ego functions can be maintained on a high level, but the selection of the love object is in the service of a reliving of an early ego state.

Jacobson (1967) described a homosexual relationship almost opposite to that described by Reich. In her case, the lover retained for himself the prerogatives of the ego ideal and the rescuer, while he projected his id wishes on the partner. When these efforts to reform and rescue the love object failed, not only the relationship but also the inner stability of the patient was endangered.

That projective mechanisms can be important in the selection of a mate without involving the ego ideal was demonstrated by a case reported by Ritvo (1966). A young man who was phobic as a child and compulsive as an adult, married, in the middle of his analysis, a phobic woman who, like him, had suffered from separation anxiety as a child. The marriage to a phobic woman enabled the patient to become the reassuring object. The marriage could also be used as a defense against the danger of regression to a phobic state.

In the cases described by Reich, Jacobson and Ritvo, we can speak of the selection of a mate based on unconscious needs; but the question remains whether the emotion of love is experienced in such relationships.

While the writings of Balint (1948), Hitschmann (1952), and more recently Eissler (1963a) show that psychoanalysts have never lost their interest in the subject of love, one must also admit that little new ground has been broken since Freud's contributions. Examination of the psychoanalytic literature reveals that very few contributions have been made specifically on the subject of love. I believe that this decline in interest goes back to Abraham, who equated love with genitality. In his classical table (Abraham 1924a, p. 496), he divided the libidinal stages of organization into six, beginning with the early oral stage and ending with the final genital stage. Corresponding to the stages of libidinal organization were six stages of object love beginning with auto-eroticism and ending with object love. In the course of this development, object relationships were said to develop from preambivalent to ambivalent and postambivalent. The genital stage was conceptualized as postambivalent. Although this classification was made in 1924, it was not yet based on the dual instinct theory. Derivatives of the aggressive drive are treated as belonging to the pregenital stages. Therefore, the genital stage could be conceptualized as devoid of aggression and hence synonymous with love (Abraham 1924a). Freud's demands were less exacting:

> We cannot go so far as to assert that the ambivalence of emotional cathexes is a universally valid law, and that it is absolutely impossible to feel great love for a person without its being accompanied by a hatred that is perhaps equally great, or vice versa. Normal adults do undoubtedly succeed in separating those two attitudes from each other, and do not find themselves obliged to hate their love-objects and to love their enemy as well as hate him. But this seems to be the result of later developments. In the first phases of erotic life, ambivalence is evidently the rule. Many people retain this archaic trait all through their lives.
>
> (Freud 1931b, p. 235)

Abraham's table was incorporated without modification by Fenichel, and it served until recently as the basis for psychoanalytic nosology. Fenichel's fomulations can be taken as representing the psychoanalytic view up to the end of the Second World War.

> children frequently are in love with themselves (secondary narcissism). They are capable of distinguishing objects and of loving objects as long as the objects procure satisfaction ...
>
> (Fenichel 1945, p. 84)

It is evident that Fenichel believed that children do not pass beyond the stage of need gratification. That children are capable of reaching the stage of object constancy is knowledge which has been acquired only after the Second World War. Fenichel went on to say:

> One can speak of love only when consideration of the object goes so far that one's own satisfaction is impossible without satisfying the object, too ... in love, it must be a kind of partial and temporary identification for empathic purposes which either exists alongside the object relationship or alternates with it in short intervals. We know nothing about the specific nature of this identification.
>
> (p. 84)

Under the influence of Wilhelm Reich, Fenichel added: "Persons in whom the genital primacy is lacking, that is, orgastically impotent persons, are also incapable of love" (pp. 84–85).

What matters most for our purposes is Abraham's and Fenichel's seemingly self-evident equation of genitality with a postambivalent attitude, and hence with love.

Anna Freud's concept of developmental lines has modified, and in many ways replaced, Abraham's classical table in current psychoanalytic thinking. She does not speak of a capacity to love, but only of "genital supremacy with libidinal cathexis transferred to objects of the opposite sex outside the family" (A. Freud 1965b, p. 248).

This historical survey has led me to conclude that psychoanalytic theory in its classical phase – that is, up to the end of the Second World War – had not developed a coherent theory on the subject of love. It did, however, formulate three basic ideas: (1) love becomes possible by the rediscovery in a new person of some aspects of the early love object; (2) love represents the transformation of narcissistic libido into object libido and a concomitant projection of the ego ideal on the beloved; (3) love becomes possible only when the genital phase has been reached. These ideas cannot easily be amalgamated into a coherent theory of love, for the first links love to a genetic sequence of events, the second conceptualizes love as a quantitative flow of libido from self to object, while the third sees love as an automatic byproduct of the last psychosexual phase of development.

Eissler, in his biography of Goethe, further expanded the second; that is, the economic point of view on love. He noted that lovers never tire of repeating their vows of love. They behave in a way reminiscent of mourning:

> But while the mourner is at a loss as to where to put his libido, the lover cannot obtain enough libido. Any libido that becomes disposable finds a set of images

> ready to be invested. The more he loves, the more he regrets that he does not have more libido to bestow.
>
> (1963a, Vol. 1, p. 660)

Furthermore, Eissler noticed that in a state of love, the flow of libido is not diminished by sexual gratification. These observations tally well with the quotations of Shakespeare that I have presented at the opening of this paper. Eissler is of the opinion that these repetitious declarations of love are attempts not only to overcome ambivalence, but also to facilitate the withdrawal of the libido from the infantile objects. Thus, Goethe could love only when he developed an inhibition against writing to his sister.

In Eissler's analysis, love does not come after the resolution of the oedipal and other incestual ties, but is itself the process in which these ties are resolved. Whether this is true for love in general, or only for the love of Goethe, is a matter that would require further investigation. Like Freud, Eissler saw the roots of the ability to love in the oedipal and other incestuous relationships. I believe that due to the contributions of Mahler and her co-workers, it is now possible to go further and seek the roots of the capacity to love in an earlier period of life.

According to Mahler's findings, after a brief, normal autistic phase, the infant enters into the symbiotic phase. Mahler writes:

> The essential feature of symbiosis is hallucinatory or delusional, somatopsychic, omnipotent fusion with the representation of the mother and, in particular, delusion of common boundary of the two actually and physically separate Individuals ...
>
> (Mahler 1967, p. 742)

I have earlier quoted Freud (1914d, 1930) to the effect that love breaks down the barrier between self and object, and between narcissistic and object libido. We may conclude therefore that love revives, if not direct memories, then feelings and archaic ego states that were once active in the symbiotic phase.

In the great love stories, *Tristan and Isolde* or *Romeo and Juliet*, the *Liebestod* is chosen in preference to separation. It represents a poetic rendering of the emotions that belong to the symbiotic phase where separation means death. In real life, as Plato so beautifully described in the *Symposium*, lovers use such a language, but fortunately they speak in metaphors. When this feeling is experienced as an entirely real one, we are no longer dealing with mature love but with a dangerous regression to the symbiotic phase. Because love revives emotions that once belonged to the symbiotic phase, it is often feared as endangering the boundary of the self. If I am right in the assumption that love has its origin in the symbiotic phase, then it becomes easier to understand why so many poets, notably Shakespeare, speak of love in terms of food. It is also more understandable why those who fear love so often employ the vocabulary of the oral triad (Lewin 1950) and express the fear of being devoured by the love object.

> The specific smiling response at the peak of the symbiotic phase predicates that the infant is responding to the symbiotic partner in a manner different from that in which he responds to other human beings. In the second half of the first year, the symbiotic partner is no longer interchangeable ...
>
> (Mahler 1967, p. 745)

Robert Browning, in "My Last Duchess," has given us a poetic description of the innocence of a woman who had not yet reached the stage of object constancy and therefore could not love:

> She had
> A heart – how shall I say? – too soon made glad,
> Too easily impressed; she liked whate'er
> She looked on, and her looks went everywhere. ...
> She smiled, no doubt,
> Whene'er I passed her; but who passed without
> Much the same smile?

Although the partner is no longer interchangeable in the symbiotic phase, it is only in the fourth subphase of separation-individuation (Mahler 1966) that a degree of object constancy is attained that makes the representation of the mother intrapsychically available to the child, even in her absence.

In the sixth of the *Sonnets from the Portuguese*, Elizabeth Browning drew upon emotions that had their origin in the symbiotic phase, together with the security that comes from the attainment of object constancy.

> Go from me. Yet I feel that I shall stand
> Henceforeward in thy shadow. Nevermore
> Alone upon the threshold of my door
> Of individual life, ...
> The widest land
> Doom takes to part us, leaves thy heart in mine
> With pulses that beat double. What I do
> And what I dream include thee, as the wine
> Must taste of its own grapes. And when I sue
> God for myself, He hears that name of thine,
> And sees within my eyes the tears of two.

The separation-individuation phase has its contribution to make to the capacity for love. It is during this phase that the child first learns to be separate in the presence of the mother. Winnicott (1958) calls this capacity ego-relatedness, but he contrasts this ability to be alone in the presence of another object with love, which he calls an id relationship. My own observations have led me to different conclusions. Those who cannot love also cannot be alone with the love object. They need entertainment and socialization and prefer short sexual encounters. They often dread the time when they will be alone with their partners. Analysis shows that the mothers of such people were either excessively intrusive or so detached that they could not maintain contact with the child, and yet let him be on his own or allow the child to be alone in their presence. In transference, this state may manifest itself in a wish to be with the analyst but not be forced to talk. Such patients experience, intensely, a seemingly paradoxical wish that the analyst remain available to them but refrain from intruding. This wish can easily be mistaken for a form of resistance, but it represents a new kind of relating and may be the forerunner for the capacity to love.

The relevance of object constancy to the capacity to love was not always appreciated in the psychoanalytic literature. For example, Hitschmann wrote:

> I once knew a man ... who used to fall in love with every young mother he met who held a child in her arms. He was motivated by the repressed memory of his mother with his younger brother in her arms.
>
> (1952, p. 423)

Hitschmann, who here made full use of Freud's concept of the prototype, did not explain why this repressed memory evoked love when we would expect it to evoke jealousy or anger. One could argue, of course, that this falling in love represented a reaction formation against the aggressive wishes evoked by the sight of the young mother holding a child. However, I do not believe that it is desirable to speak of love when it is evoked by a category of women rather than by one woman. If Hitschmann's patient were neurotic, he could have fallen in love with one woman because he saw her holding a child. But this link to infancy would have undergone repression and would not be transferable to every woman holding a child. If the wish remains conscious, we are dealing with a special type of Don Juanism; that is, with a compulsive need to possess every woman with a young child, but not with love.

George Bernard Shaw is quoted by Hitschmann (1952) as having said, "Being in love means greatly exaggerating the difference between one woman and another." Following Mahler, we can say that it is the symbiotic phase and its successful resolution in the individuation-separation phase which makes it possible for some to exaggerate the difference between one human being and another, and hence enables them to love.

Shaw's remarks can be contrasted with Russell's dedication in his autobiography (1951). It is a poem of an old man oriented toward death rather than that of a man seeking a life partner. Nevertheless, or perhaps even because it is a poem of old age, it has captured an essential feature of love. It speaks of the peacefulness and ecstasy that the old man has obtained from knowing, after so many years of loneliness, what love and life can be; he is able to sleep with fulfillment.

Russell asks for the difficult combination of ecstasy and peace, and love has to transform for him the fear of death into the fulfilled sleep of the satiated infant (Lewin 1950). Many men have experienced genital pleasure including regard, tenderness, and empathy for their partner, and yet they have not known the experience Russell has described.

I would like now to add a number of probabilistic statements which I regard as likely to be true, but which will require further study before they can be definitely confirmed.

If we agree that the term "love" should be confined to the feeling that one person, and that person alone, can assure happiness, then those children who were reared by a series of rapidly changing nurses, or in institutions that did not permit a strong relationship to develop toward one person during the symbiotic phase, should, like Shaw, be unable to exaggerate the difference between one person and another and therefore be incapable of loving. Children whose parents were divorced and remarried before a stable object representation was established will have difficulty in loving. We often learn from patients that they had two fathers or two mothers, that maternal functions were divided between the mother and an older sibling, the mother and grandmother, or mother and nurse, and even mother and father. In the absence of one significant person during infancy, the integrative functions of the ego have a difficult task to perform. When such a child grows up, in order to love he must find in another person characteristics taken from many objects and integrate them into one. He often fails in this task and, as a result, every relationship represents for him only one aspect of an early significant love object. Sometimes the best that can be attained in such a case is a rotation of objects or the finding of an object that satisfies only one aspect of the unconscious need.

Particular difficulties are encountered when the father assumed maternal functions early in the infant's life; that is, when he bathed, fed, and otherwise cared for the infant. The difficulty is augmented when the father showed more tenderness than the mother.

When the original object was disappointing, the selection of the new object is based not on refinding but on a compulsive avoidance of the original object. On the model of counteridentification, I would like to call such a selection "counter-refinding." Such relationships can at times be stable and may lead to important corrective emotional experiences, but they lack the ardor of the relationsips which are based on the refinding of the original object. In some cases, I have noticed that the selection on such a basis leaves a sense of estrangment; that is, the person cannot understand why he selected his partner. Genitality may have been reached, but something crucial is missing. In such cases, psychoanalytic therapy can be helpful. When the attachment to the original object is made conscious and the patient realizes that the selection was made on the basis of counter-refinding, mourning for the lost original object can take place. When the libido is detached from the unsatisfactory object, new capacities for love become available. However, it must be admitted that when the mother-child relationship has been pathological, the urge to refind a similar pathological relationship and then to attempt to reform the partner is often overwhelming.

Children whose relationship to the mother had reached adequate intensity, but where the mother was either ambivalent or hating, also experience a special difficulty in loving. They can establish stable relationships and can even love, but since they themselves do not believe that they are lovable, assurances to the contrary are to no avail. They tend to provoke their mates to demonstrate that they are not loved. This is the pattern which Berliner (1958) has found to be typical of masochistic relationships. I have observed that women who were hated by their mothers and loved by their fathers can love, but do not believe that they are lovable.

Abandonment by the mother, or her substitute, during infancy or early childhood severely impairs the capacity to love. Nevertheless, some find unique ways of reliving the trauma in a restorative way, as the following case will illustrate.

Until the third year of life, Mr. A. was reared exclusively by a nurse, who with the advent of the war had to flee the country without even saying goodbye to him. The nurse seems to have been a cold, demanding and meticulous person. She dressed the child carefully, kept him clean, quiet, and away from the company of other children. When the patient came to treatment, he was meticulously dressed and made a scrubbed impression. To himself, as well as to his family, he was a puzzle. He was devoid of ambition, he seldom worked, he had cronies but no friends. There was nothing that he could tell one person that he could not, just as easily, communicate to another. He lacked any capacity for intimacy. Sexuality was limited to compulsive masturbation, and he had to prove to himself time and again that he was not injured by this masturbation. As one would expect, his relationship to the therapist was positive, but lacked any discernible intensity. He enjoyed coming and talking, but claimed that the analysis only helped him to fill empty hours. During summer vacations, he insisted that he never missed the analyst or gave the analysis any thought. His character structure and behavior in the analysis fitted well into the category that Gitelson (1958) described as ego defects.

During the third year of treatment, a nephew was born. Almost immediately, the patient identified with this nephew, and the relationship to the baby was the first in which I could discern any warmth. He displayed an unusual interest in the baby's welfare. He babysat, played with him, and even invented stories for him. When the boy reached the age at which the patient's nurse had left him, he fell in love with that boy's nurse, and thus established the first heterosexual relationship.

Perhaps because the disturbance was so great, the refinding process in this case had to take an almost uncanny concrete form. It also seems, probably, that a period of identification with the infant had to precede the renewal of the capacity to refind the lost object. It is not easy to determine whether treatment here facilitated this refinding, or whether the great similarity between the infantile and adult situation would by itself have created the preconditions for loving.

If the line of reasoning here pursued should prove to be correct, then the capacity to love presupposes a symbiotic experience which was allowed to proceed without traumatic interruption, and an individuation-separation phase in which the mother did not attempt to rebind the child to herself. The question still remains open whether the successful passage of these two phases by itself guarantees the capacity to love, or whether it is only a necessary, but not necessarily sufficient, condition for it. Clinical experience has shown that some lovers have successfully transferred character traits from the original oedipal parent to the new love object only to discover that they were repeating the unhappy relationship they had experienced as children. Such patients have reached the oedipal phase and have been successful in the displacement of their oedipal wishes upon new objects; yet this refinding was not conducive to happiness, but merely recapitulated the infantile situation. We must, therefore, assume that in order to be able to love, the early object representations must be benign and cathected more with libido than with aggression to make a happy displacement possible.

Love is experienced subjectively as an utterly unexpected event and often as a miracle. It is suggested that the sense of the miraculous results from a dim presentiment that many psychic events have taken place simultaneously, quickly, and without conscious awareness. Furthermore, the psychopathology of love teaches us that love can take place only if every psychic event does not exceed a certain limit.

Freud had stressed that every finding must be a refinding, but this refinding must take place without reawakening the incest taboo. Later, Freud assumed that narcissistic libido must be transformed into object libido, but that this transformation must take place without impoverishing the self. I have stressed further that feelings belonging to the symbiotic phase of development must be awakened but without bringing with them a dangerous ego regression. It should be added that certain ego functions must be temporarily suspended; for example, reality testing must be given up if the necessary idealization is to take place and yet, paradoxically, this very ego function must simultaneously make possible the selection of a good mate.

That so much can take place in a short time and end well in spite of the many pitfalls constitutes the unending fascination of love. As a result of these interactions, love presents us with a paradox. On the one hand, it is experienced as a unique, unexpected, and even unbelievable event. Lovers often express astonishment that they are capable of such bliss and such a weather of emotions. On the other hand, the examination of love relationships often reveals that they represent, unconsciously, the resumption of significant relationships that were interrupted long ago. It would not be correct to assert that all lovers experience the emotions which we assume to be active in the symbiotic phase, but frequently love revives such feelings. We are thus led to the conclusion that when the symbiotic phase gives way to further development, it leaves as a residue a longing which remains ungratified until love comes into adult life.

Note

1 Originally published as Bergmann, M., *Psychoanalytic Observations on the Capacity to Love* in *Separation-Individuation: Essays in Honor of Margaret S. Mahler*, ed. J. McDevitt (International Universities Press, 1971).

References

Abraham, K. (1924a) A Short Study of the Development of the Libido, Viewed in the Light of Mental Disorders. In *Karl Abraham, Selected Papers* (Vol. 1: Selected Papers on Psychoanalysis). New York: Basic Books, 1953, pp. 418–501.

Balint, M. (1947) On Genital Love. *International Journal of Psychoanalysis* 29: 34–40.

Bergmann, M.S. (1963) The Place of Paul Federn's Ego Psychology in Psychoanalytic Metapsychology. *Journal of the American Psychoanalytic Association* 11: 97–116.

Bergmann, M.S. (1966) The Intrapsychic and Communicative Aspects of the Dream – Their Role in Psycho-Analysis and Psychotherapy. *International Journal of Psychoanalysis* 47: 356–363.

Berliner, B. (1958) The Role of Object Relations in Moral Masochism. *Psychoanalytic Quarterly* 27: 38–56.

Bibring, E. (1953) The Mechanism of Depression. In *Affective Disorders*, ed. P. Greenacre. New York: International Universities Press, pp. 13–48.

Bowra, C.M. (1957) *The Greek Experience*. New York: World Publishing Co.

Dodds, E.R. (1951) *The Greeks and the Irrational*. Berkeley, CA: University of California Press.

Eissler, K. (1963a) *Goethe: A Psychoanalytic Study*, Vols 1 & 2. Detroit: Wayne State University Press.

Eissler, K.R. (1951) An Unknown Autobiographical Letter by Freud and a Short Comment. *International Journal of Psychoanalysis* 32: 319–324.

Fenichel, O. (1945) *The Psychoanalytic Theory of Neurosis*. New York: W.W. Norton & Co., Inc.

Freud, A. (1965a) The Concept of Developmental Lines. *The Psychoanalytic Study of the Child* 18: 245–265. New York: International Universities Press.

Freud, S. (1892–99) Extracts from the Fliess papers. S.E. 1: 175–280.

Freud, S. (1905a) Fragment of an Analysis of a Case of Hysteria. S.E. 7: 3–124.

Freud, S. (1905b) Three Essays on the Theory of Sexuality. S.E. 7: 135–245.

Freud, S. (1910a) Five Lectures of Psycho-Analysis. SE 11: 1–5.

Freud, S. (1912a) On the Universal Tendency to Debasement in the Sphere of Love. S.E. 11: 177–190.

Freud, S. (1914d) On Narcissism: An Introduction. S.E. 14: 73–102.

Freud, S. (1915b) Observations on Transference-Love: Technique of Psycho-Analysis. S.E. 12: 159–171.

Freud, S. (1920) Beyond the Pleasure Principle. S.E. 18: 7–64.

Freud, S. (1921) Group Psychology and the Analysis of the Ego. S.E. 18: 69–143.

Freud, S. (1925a) Resistance to Psychoanalysis. S.E. 19: 212–222.

Freud, S. (1927b) Humour. S.E. 21: 161–166.

Freud, S. (1930) Civilization and its Discontents. S.E. 21: 57–145.
Freud, S. (1931b) Female Sexuality. S.E. 21: 223–243.
Freud, S. (1937a) Analysis, Terminable and Interminable. S.E. 23: 211–253.
Fromm, E. (1956) *The Art of Loving*. New York: Harper & Row.
Gitelson, M. (1958) On Ego Distortion. *International Journal of Psychoanalysis* 19: 245–257.
Guthrie, W.K. (1962) *The History of Greek Philosophy* (2 vols). Cambridge, England: Cambridge University Press.
Hazo, R.G. (1967) *The Idea of Love*. New York: Praeger.
Hitschmann, E. (1952). Freud's Conception of Love. *International Journal of Psychoanalysis* 33: 421–428.
Jacobson, E. (1967) *Psychotic Conflict and Reality*. New York: International Universities Press.
Lewin, B.D. (1950) *The Psychoanalysis of Elation*. New York: Norton.
Mahler, M.S. (1966) Notes on the Development of Basic Moods: The Depressive Affect. In *Psychoanalysis – a General Psychology: Essays in Honor of Heinz Hartmann*, eds R.M. Loewenstein, L.M. Newman, M. Schur and A.J. Solnit. New York: International Universities Press, 152–168.
Mahler, M.S. (1967) On Human Symbiosis and the Vicissitudes of Individuation. *Journal of the American Psychoanalytic Association* 15: 740–763.
Oates, W.J. and O'Neil, E. Jr., eds (1938) *The Complete Greek Drama*, trans. R.C. Jebb, New York: Random House.
Panofsky, E. (1939) Blind Cupid. In *Studies in Iconology*. New York: Harper Torch Books, 1962.
Reich, A. (1953) Narcissistic Object Choice in Women. *Journal of the American Psychoanalytic Association* 1: 22–44.
Reik, T. (1944) *A Psychologist Looks at Love*. New York: Farrar & Rinehart.
Ritvo, S. (1966) Correlation of a Childhood and Adult Neurosis. *International Journal of Psychoanalysis* 47: 130–131.
Russell, B. (1930) *The Conquest of Happiness*. London: Allen & Unwin.
Spurgeon, C. (1958) *Shakespeare's Imagery*. Boston: Beacon Press.
Winnicott, D.W. (1958) The Capacity to be Alone. *International Journal of Psychoanalysis* 39: 416–420.

CHAPTER 2

THE LEAP FROM THE *STUDIES ON HYSTERIA* TO *THE INTERPRETATION OF DREAMS*[1]

Only five years stand between the publication of Breuer and Freud's *Studies on Hysteria*, published in 1895, and Freud's *Interpretation of Dreams*, which appeared in 1900. The history of thought does not offer many examples of so profound a change taking place in one man's thinking within such a short span of time. *Studies on Hysteria* is a book written by two neurologists, addressed to fellow physicians who treat patients suffering from hysteria. The book takes its place comfortably beside the works of other physicians, such as Charcot, Janet and Bernheim.

By contrast, *The Interpretation of Dreams* (1900) is one of those seminal works that differentiate the twentieth century from the nineteenth. It contains the first three of Freud's great discoveries: the discovery that dreams have meaning, and that this meaning can be discovered through the technique of free association, and that all civilized men and women carry within them repressed unconscious thoughts and wishes that influence their lives without being known to them. Man is not rational, not a master in his own house, but subject – to varying degrees – to forces within him that are unknown to him. As a result of these insights the absolute demarcation line between normal and neurotic lost much of its validity. It was the loss of this demarcation line that proved to have momentous consequences. The unconscious will be of interest not only to the neurotically ill, but also to all those who wish to know themselves.

Noteworthy in view of subsequent developments was the confidence Breuer and Freud (1895) had in the results of their work:

> For we found to our great surprise at first, that each individual hysterical symptom immediately and permanently disappeared when we had succeeded in bringing clearly to light the memory of the event by which it was provoked and in arousing its accompanying affect and when the patient had described that even in the greatest possible detail and had put the affect into words.
>
> (p. 6)

What is still admirable in *Studies on Hysteria* is the complete harmony between theory and technique, a harmony that psychoanalysis will try in vain to recapture in its subsequent development. The theory postulated that hysterics suffer from reminiscences of a repressed psychic trauma inflicted upon them as children by the imposed sexuality of adults. Hysterics as children were victims of sexual abuse; as adults they suffer from strangulated affect that cannot find discharge. Breuer and

Freud offer a remedy. The hysterical patient can be hypnotized and under hypnosis abreact their memories. Their painful memories can heal once a cathartic method is used, allowing these repressed and sequestered memories to emerge into consciousness with the full quantum of affect with which they were originally repressed. I wish to draw attention to the way Freud conceptualized repressed reminiscences. These reminiscences, while not consciously available to the patient, nevertheless can be recalled under hypnosis. No reconstructions are necessary.

The term *catharsis* was taken over from Aristotle's statement that tragedy on the stage evokes terror and pity and thus purges the emotions (catharsis). The application of the Greek term to the therapeutic procedure was not altogether felicitous for, as Jonathan Lear (1990) observed, in literature the spectator remains aware of the guilt that separates his life from that of the dramatic hero. The identification is temporary and imaginative. Catharsis takes place within a fine balance of sympathy and distance. The hysteric lacks this balance (p. 54).

The major change that Breuer and Freud demanded from the physician was that he listen to the patient. To convert an autocratic physician into a person who had to learn the biography of each patient, and discover something new in every case in which treatment was undertaken, was a major step forward. We should also note that unlike Charcot's hospitalized patients, who came from inarticulate farming and labor classes, the patients that Breuer and Freud treated were middle and upper class, urban and well-educated, mostly Jewish, and possessed a capacity to articulate what ailed them.

When in 1908 a second edition of *Studies on Hysteria* came out, Breuer and Freud could no longer combine their views in a preface. Breuer stressed: "As I personally am concerned, I have since the time had no active dealings with the subject; I have had no part in its important development and I could add nothing fresh to what was written in 1895" (p. xxxi).

Freud, on the other hand, said:

> Even to-day I regard [my initial views] not as errors but as valuable first approximations to the knowledge which could only be fully acquired after long and continuous efforts ... I can give no better advice to anyone interested in the development of catharsis into psychoanalysis than to begin with *Studies on Hysteria* and thus follow that path that I myself have trodden.
>
> (p. xxxi)

In the nineteenth century, hysteria was not at the center of medical interest. It was, as Freud memorably stated in 1910, a rather despised branch of medicine.

> Thus the recognition of the illness as hysteria makes little difference to the patient; but to the doctor quite the reverse. It is noticeable that his attitude towards hysterical patients is quite other than towards sufferers of organic diseases. He does not have the same sympathy for the former as for the latter.
>
> (p. 11)

Goldstein (1982) and McGrath (1992) have made us aware that the topic of hysteria was not, politically speaking, a neutral one. For, throughout history, or at least since the twelfth century when St. Francis of Assisi showed his stigmata, many men and women in *imitatio Christi* have bled from hands and feet in a state of trance. The Church has taken these manifestations as proof of its teaching. To unmask them as hysteria, and, worse, to be able to replicate them under hypnosis, was in the religious debate of the nineteenth century a highly charged subject.

Ellenberger (1970) surveyed the contemporary literature as to how the *Studies on Hysteria* was received. He noted that on the whole, the reviews were highly favorable, although some expressed concern over the right of physicians to inquire into the most detailed sexual affairs of their patients. Others were not so sure that what emerges in hypnosis is the historical truth rather than buried fantasies. The contemporary controversy between historical and narrative truth is already present at the very birth of psychoanalysis. We may conclude, using Kuhn's (1962) language, that *Studies on Hysteria* was a contribution to normal science, and that the authors received the expected rewards that come to those who contribute within the confines of normal science.

The shift from *Studies on Hysteria* to psychoanalysis proper entailed two major changes. Freud slowly replaced the hypnotic method by the technique of free association. The seduction theory as the cause of hysteria slowly gave way to the recognition of the role of infantile sexuality that culminated in the Oedipus complex. In *The Interpretation of Dreams*, Freud said:

> Being in love with one parent and hating the other are among the essential constituents of the stock of psychical impulses which is formed at that time and which is of such importance in determining the symptoms of later neurosis. It is not my belief, however, that psycho-neurotics differ sharply in this respect from other human beings who remain normal.
>
> (pp. 260–261)

If we ask ourselves how Freud managed to bring about so substantial a change in his theory within such a short span of years, we will find the answer in his self-analysis.

Freud's self-analysis became possible when he replaced hypnosis by free association. Systematically, Freud wrote down his dreams and wrote down every association to every item in the dream. He continued to do so until the dream yielded a meaning. Only after different schools of psychoanalysis emerged did it become clear that finding a meaning in a dream, or even in a symptom, does not guarantee that we have found the meaning. Different schools can discover different meanings in any dream reported in a psychoanalytic session. When a meaning emerged, Freud felt he had arrived at the latent content of the dream.

Freud's self-analysis enabled him to overcome the inhibition of visiting Rome (Bergmann 1976). It also enabled him to overcome his idealization of Fliess and to free himself from the bondage to him. Above all, in 1899 Freud was able to begin writing his *Interpretation of Dreams*. Freud's self-analysis continued throughout his life. There is considerable evidence, as Grubrich-Simitis (1991) has pointed out, that Freud's last book, *Moses and Monotheism* (1939) becomes intelligible if we understand Freud's preoccupation with Moses as a continuation of his own self-analysis. There are two ways of looking at Freud's self-analysis. Ernst Jones (1953), Freud's authorized biographer, described it thus:

> In the summer of 1897 the spell began to break, and Freud undertook his most heroic feat – an analysis of his own unconscious. It is hard for us nowadays to imagine how momentous this achievement was, that difficulty being but the fate of most pioneering exploits. Yet the uniqueness of the feat remains.

> Once done it is done forever. For no one again can be the first to explore those depths.
>
> (p. 319)

Eissler (1971) has added:

> Freud discovered, from the analysis of one of his own dreams, that he was harboring a death wish toward his oldest son, who had been at the front but who was missing at that time. We can get some inkling of the shock and agitation to which his psychic apparatus was at times exposed. The courage it took to publish that dream along with its interpretation, is hardly imaginable.
>
> (p. 307)

Outside of psychoanalysis, Freud's self-analysis was not regarded with the same awe. Ellenberger (1970) classified Freud's self-analysis as a form of creative illness:

> A creative illness succeeds a period of intense preoccupation with an idea and search for a certain truth. It is a polymorphous condition that can take the shape of depression, neurosis, psychosomatic ailments, or even psychosis. Whatever the symptoms, they are felt as painful, if not agonizing by the subject, with alternating periods of alleviation and worsening. Throughout the illness the subject never loses the threat of his dominating preoccupation. It is often compatible with normal professional activity and family life. But even if he keeps to his social activities, he is almost entirely absorbed with himself. He suffers from feelings of utter isolation, even when he has a mentor who guides him through the ordeal (like the shaman apprentice with his master). The termination is often rapid, marked by a phase of exhilaration. The subject emerges from his ordeal with a permanent transformation in his personality and the conviction that he has discovered a great truth or a new spiritual world.
>
> (pp. 447–448)

In Ellenberger's view, Fechner, Nietzsche and Jung, in addition to Freud, went through such a creative illness. Freud can be compared with the other three only if we believe that he emerged from his self-analysis in possession of a personal truth only. If he discovered, as psychoanalysis claims, hitherto inaccessible objective truths, then his endeavor cannot be compared with the other three. This event is unparalleled in the history of science. That introspective work of the scientist himself can bring about a substantial change in an already reasonably well-established scientific procedure is a unique feature in the history of psychoanalysis. Among Freud's contemporaries, Marcel Proust can be singled out as one who underwent an analogous "creative illness," but in his case the outcome was an entirely new type of novel: *Remembrance of Things Past*. That book, like Freud's work, contributed to giving to the twentieth century its intellectual climate.

The Interpretation of Dreams laid the foundation for the study of culture, for now not only were hysterics suffering from excessive repression, but the culture as a whole could be seen as demanding so high a degree of instinctual renunciation as to make most of its members – particularly those not strong enough to defy its restrictions – neurotic. This insight is not as yet explicit in *The Interpretation of Dreams*, but it is expressed in *"Civilized" Sexual Morality and Modern Nervous*

Illness (Freud 1908a). Freud and those who followed him were attempting not only to cure neurotic patients, but also to become critics of Western civilization.

Three further questions have to be addressed: (1) Was Freud himself aware of the magnitude of the change between the two books? (2) Did Freud in his thinking really break with the ideas he had expressed in *Studies on Hysteria*, or did they serve as a substratum for his psychoanalytic point of view? (3) To what extent was Freud himself aware of the role of his self-analysis in bringing about the change in his therapeutic technique and therapeutic philosophy?

As to the significant role of self-analysis, in the preface to the second edition to *The Interpretation of Dreams*, written in 1908, Freud said:

> For this book has a further subjective significance for me personally – a significance which I only grasped after I had completed it. It was, I found, a portion of my own self-analysis, my reaction to my father's death – that is to say, to the most important event, the most poignant loss, of man's life. Having discovered that this was so, I felt unable to obliterate the traces of the experience. To my readers, however, it will be a matter of indifference upon what particular material they learn to appreciate the importance of dreams and how I interpret them.
>
> (p. xxvi)

In the last remark, Freud could not have been more wrong. A whole literature has grown around Freud's self-analysis and the analysis of his dreams. His readers, far from being indifferent to the material upon which Freud built his dream interpretation, have studied these dreams and his memories from many points of view, including the limitations beyond which his self-analysis did not go.

As to the questions of whether Freud was aware of the jump that took place between the two works, the answer is yes, but not immediately.

In the opening paragraph of the case of Dora (Freud 1905a), we read with some astonishment:

> In 1895 and 1896 I put forward certain views upon the pathogenesis of hysterical symptoms and upon the mental processes occurring in hysteria. Since that time, several years have passed. In now proposing, therefore, to substantiate those views by giving a detailed report of the history of a case and its treatment I cannot avoid making a few introductory remarks ...
>
> (p. 7)

As late as 1905, Freud understood his work with Dora not as a new beginning, but as a confirmation of what Breuer and he had discovered.

The way Dora was interrogated and treated also shows that Freud as a therapist had not moved very far from the way patients were treated in *Studies on Hysteria*:

[*Freud*] I will explain that to you presently. Does nothing else occur to you in connection with the jewel-case? So far you have only talked about jewelry and said nothing about a case.

[*Dora*] Yes, Herr K. had made me a present of an expensive jewel-case a little time before.

[*Freud*] Then a return-present would have been very appropriate. Perhaps you do not know that "jewel-case" ... is a favorite expression ... for the female genitals.

[*Dora*] I knew you would say that.
[*Freud*] That is to say you knew that it ***was*** so. – The meaning of the dream is now becoming even clearer. You said to yourself: "This man is persecuting me; he wants to force his way into my room. My "jewel-case" is in danger and if anything happens it will be Father's fault."

(p. 69)

We learn from this exchange – as well as from many others – that, while Dora is no longer under hypnosis, she is still very far from a free-associating analysand.

Even in his Clark University lectures, delivered in 1909 (Freud 1910a), we will note that the leap I am referring to has not yet been understood by Freud. The first two lectures summarize the work with Breuer; the third begins with the recognition of the power of resistance that was discernible only after hypnosis was given up. The chapter deals with the analysis of jokes and dreams and the mechanism of repression. There is no sharply discernible demarcation line between the two.

Even in the *Introductory Lectures* (Freud 1916–17) we find the following statement: "An introduction to psycho-analysis is provided by the study of parapraxis and dreams; the theory of neurosis is psychoanalysis itself" (p. 379). We are entitled to conclude that up to the end of the First World War psychoanalysis was, to Freud, primarily a theory of neurosis. By 1926 a major shift had taken place:

> There is no reason for surprise, that psycho-analysis, which was originally no more than an attempt at explaining pathological mental phenomena, should have developed into a psychology of normal mental life. The justifications for this arose with the discovery that the dreams and mistakes ("parapraxes" such as slips of the tongue, etc.) of normal men have the same mechanism as neurotic symptoms.
>
> (Freud 1926, pp. 266–267)

The major step took place in 1900, but the full significance of this step became conscious to Freud only in 1926. In the *New Introductory Lectures* (1933) the emphasis is even sharper:

> We should turn our attention first to the position of the theory of dreams. It occupies a special place in the history of psycho-analysis and marks the turning point; it was with it that analysis took the step from being a psychotherapeutic procedure to being a depth psychology.
>
> (p. 7).

It is evident that it took a long time for Freud to understand the full meaning of his own development. It was only after he had published a number of books dealing with the general problems of mankind that it dawned upon him that psychoanalysis contains with it two significantly different lines of development. The first is concerned primarily with the process of cure that can be brought about by Freud's technique. The other attempts to understand the profound implications that the Freudian point of view has brought about in our understanding of human culture and human nature.

On the basis of Freud's published writings, we probably would not have been able to reconstruct the transition from *Studies on Hysteria* to *The Interpretation of*

Dreams. It was only because the Princess Bonaparte refused to obey Freud's wishes and destroy the letters to his friend Fliess (Freud 1887–1904) that it is at all possible for us to learn how Freud made the transition between the two books, and the enormous role that his self-analysis played in this process.

The correspondence shows that Freud's self-analysis was reported to Fliess on August 18, 1897, two years after the publication of *Studies on Hysteria*:

> The chief patient I am preoccupied with is myself. My little hysteria, though greatly accentuated by my work, has resolved itself a bit further. The rest is still at a standstill. That is what my mood primarily depends on. The analysis is more difficult than any other. It is, in fact, what paralyzes my psychic strength for describing and communicating what I have known so far. Still I believe it must be done and is a necessary intermediate stage of my work.
>
> (Freud 1887–1904, p. 261)

The self-analysis becomes the main focus of interest in the correspondence of October 3, 1897, where Freud reports actually having succeeded in lifting some of his childhood amnesia as he recalled having seen his mother nude between the ages of two and two-and-a-half years old. On October 15 of that year, Freud writes:

> My self-analysis is in fact the most essential thing I have at present and promises to become of greatest value to me if it reaches its end. In the middle of it, it suddenly ceased for three days during which I had the feeling of being tied up inside (which patients complain of so much) and I was really disconsolate.
>
> (p. 270)

It was in the same letter that Freud communicates to Fliess the discovery of the Oedipus complex as the universal phenomenon of childhood: "I have found in my own case too being in love with my mother and jealous of my father, and I now consider it a universal event in early childhood" (p. 272).

We should note that in his self-analysis, Freud discovered only being in love with his mother and jealousy toward the father; that is, mild and acceptable derivatives of the Oedipus complex. That Freud ever experienced in his self-analysis the full impact of his sexual desire for his mother and the full measure of murderous hatred for his father is doubtful. What probably facilitated the discovery of the Oedipus complex was Freud's reading of Sophocles' tragedy as an adolescent when he fell in love with Gisela Fluss. I consider this as a remarkable transmission of insight across two thousand years. At this crucial juncture in the history of psychoanalysis Freud's familiarity with the Western literary tradition came to his aid. The discovery of the Oedipus complex was based on the recall of some childhood memories, but to these was added a major reconstruction that was possible because Freud had retained his preconscious memory of *Oedipus Rex* and *Hamlet*. This may very well be why reconstruction continued to be so central to his thinking and analyzing. Freud goes on to say:

> We can understand the gripping power of Oedipus Rex ... Everyone in the audience was once a budding Oedipus in fantasy and each recoils in horror from the dream fulfillment here transplanted into reality, with the full quantity of repression which separates his infantile state from his present one.
>
> (p. 272)

Everyone may have once been a budding Oedipus, and Sophocles must have aroused in his audience some of the anxiety associated with the oedipal wish, but like every great writer, Sophocles also saw to it that this arousal turned to pity rather than anxiety. Only one man, living more than two thousand years later, grasped the nature of the universal component that makes this tragedy so arresting, and he was able to do so only because, in his self-analysis, he took the preliminary steps that made it possible to unravel the tragedy's secrets.

Freud often wondered why a world that accepted the Sophoclean tragedy offered such resistance to his proclamation that the Oedipus complex is the kernel of neurosis. In a paper entitled "Creative Writers and Day-Dreaming" (Freud 1908b), he himself supplied the answer. Sophocles, being a creative writer, employs a number of strategies to make Oedipus acceptable to his audience, describing him as a highly conscientious monarch who appeals to us because he is such a relentless seeker of the truth, even if it leads to his downfall. Furthermore, strictly speaking, Oedipus is not guilty of the murder of his father and the marriage to his mother, since he killed the father and married the mother unknowingly. Add to this the fact that he owed his parents no filial devotion – since they exposed him to die on the wilderness of the mountain. Finally, whatever punitive needs are evoked in the audience, Sophocles satisfies them by letting Oedipus blind himself. But above all, Sophocles describes the fate of one man, whereas Freud proclaims the universality of the oedipal wishes.

Freud repeats the content of the letter to Fliess almost verbatim in *The Interpretation of Dreams*. But he is obviously not yet aware of the magnitude of the discovery of the Oedipus complex, for he hides it inconspicuously in a chapter called "Typical dreams" (Freud 1900, p. 262–266), adding an optimistic note:

> King Oedipus, who slew his father Laius and married his mother Jocasta, clearly shows us the fulfillment of our childhood wishes, but more fortunate than he, we have meanwhile succeeded insofar as we have not become psychoneurotic, in detaching our sexual impulses from our mothers and forgetting our jealousies of our fathers.
>
> (p. 262)

It will take another ten years for Freud to understand that this detachment of the libido in so-called normal has only rarely been achieved as successfully as he believed in 1900, and that the Oedipus complex remains a psychic constellation against which most people struggle throughout their lives.

> Fleetingly the thought passed through my head that the same thing might be at the bottom of Hamlet as well. I am not thinking of Shakespeare's conscious intention, but believe rather that a real event stimulated the poet to his representation, in that his unconscious understood the unconscious of his hero. How does Hamlet the hysteric justify the words, "Thus conscience doth makes cowards of us all"?
>
> (Freud 1887–1904, p. 272)

Unlike Oedipus, Hamlet had not killed his father or married his mother. How are we to understand the phrase "fleetingly the thought occurred to me"? The expression itself suggests some ambivalence. In *The Interpretation of Dreams*, Freud writes:

> Another of the great creations of tragic poetry, Shakespeare's *Hamlet*, has its roots in the same soil as *Oedipus Rex*. But the changed treatment of the same material reveals the whole difference in the mental life of these widely separated epochs of civilization: the secular advance of repression in the emotional life of mankind. In the *Oedipus*, the child's wishful fantasy that underlies it is brought to the open and realized as it would be in a dream. In *Hamlet* it remains repressed; and – just as in the case of neurosis – we only learn of its existence from its inhibiting consequences.
>
> (Freud 1900, p. 264)

In *Hamlet*, Freud was able to deduce the paralyzing effects of the Oedipus complex from Hamlet's symptom: the hesitation over the fulfillment of the task of revenge. It is noteworthy that before Freud, no adequate explanation of Hamlet's hesitation had been offered. I would like to add that Hamlet finally commits the murder only when he himself is about to die. Oedipus pays with blindness for the parricide, even though he did not know that he was killing his father. Hamlet pays with his own death for the murder of a father substitute, the man who, according to Freud, carried out Hamlet's own parricidal wishes. The oedipal wish is more subtly presented in *Hamlet* and much better disguised than in *Oedipus Rex*. Freud attributes to Hamlet only oedipal wishes, but these wishes are strong enough to awaken in him a sense of guilt that paralyzes his actions. Freud admires the capacity of great writers to compel their readers to accept ideas they would otherwise reject as immoral.

In an earlier letter, written on October 5, 1897, Freud recalls a memory of an old woman who was his teacher in sexual matters and who "complained because I was clumsy and unable to do anything" (Freud 1887–1904, p. 268). This was a standard type of memory that patients produced under hypnosis during the Breuer period. Freud recalls further memories that the same woman washed him in reddish water, in which she had previously washed herself. He returns to the subject of his nurse in the letter of October 15, in which he reports to Fliess that he did what many analysands would do after him: ask his mother to verify his memories. The mother reported that indeed there was such an old woman who stole *kreuzers* (pennies) from him as a child. Her theft was discovered and she was given ten months in jail. On the basis of this communication from his mother, Freud understood for the first time a puzzling scene from his childhood – in which he had asked his 20-year-old brother to unlock a cupboard, expecting that his mother was locked inside it. Disappointed, the young Sigmund had cried, and eventually his mother reappeared. Freud understood that he had heard that this nurse was "boxed-up" – slang for incarcerated – and he now looked for the incarcerated mother in the cupboard. It was immediately after this recollection that Freud described to Fliess the Oedipus complex.

In the chapter, "Childhood and concealing memories," Freud (1901) retells the same incident, but adds the following:

> I suspected that my naughty brother had done the same thing to her that he had done to the nurse and I forced him to open the cupboard [*kasten*] for me. I now understand, too, why in the translation of this visual childhood scene my mother's slimness was emphasized: it must have struck me as just having been restored to her. I am two and a half years older than the sister who was born at the time, and when I was three years old my half brother and I ceased living in the same place.
>
> (p. 51)

In 1924, he added another footnote of considerable significance:

> The child of not yet three had understood that the little sister who had recently arrived had grown inside his mother. He was very far from approving of this addition to the family, and was full of mistrust and anxiety that his mother's inside might conceal still more children. The wardrobe or cupboard was a symbol for him for his mother's inside, so he insisted in looking into this cupboard and turned for this to his big brother who (as is clear from other material) had taken his father's place as the child's rival.
>
> (p. 51)

Freud now recognized that he as a child had wanted to enter and destroy the babies inside his mother's womb, a trend of thought we usually associate with the work of Melanie Klein. We learn from these two additions to the early memory that Freud's self-analysis was a continuous process.

Today, we surmise that the nurse must have been far more important to the child Freud than he discovered in his self-analysis. Object loss in infancy was reported without having been fully experienced. A memory of the loss of an important figure in Freud's childhood thus remained hidden behind the discovery of the Oedipus complex. Was one discovery made at the expense of the other?

In retrospect, Freud made two separate, highly significant discoveries. He discovered the Oedipus complex and almost discovered the role of the early attachment between infant and caretaker, including the traumatic effect of an early separation from that caretaker. The first finding was acknowledged, and as a result the Oedipus complex was regarded as the nucleus of neurosis. The full significance of the second discovery was not articulated and was discovered a generation later by other analysts: Winnicott, Margaret Mahler, Anna Freud and Melanie Klein. What matters in this historical context is that another investigator traveling the same road could have failed to discover the Oedipus complex but highlighted the significance of separation trauma. We would then have had a very different history of psychoanalysis. At this historical juncture, more than one possibility existed and another self-analyzer, undertaking the same journey that Freud did, would have come up with other conclusions. That discoveries occur at crossroads remains a permanent feature in the history of psychoanalysis. It is also repeated in every individual analysis. Indeed, it must be so when the unconscious is explored through rational means. I consider this to be a major reason why it is so difficult to convert explanations of the unconscious into a scientific discipline.

Freud was a lonely self-analyzer; ultimately the balance of inner forces determined the direction that his self-analysis took. It is even conceivable that had he not read *Oedipus Rex* or *Hamlet* he would have more easily discovered the role of object loss in early childhood rather than the Oedipus complex. In a regular analysis, at a similar juncture, the analysand is not as free as Freud was, for it will all too often happen that the therapist's philosophy and his understanding of infancy will be decisive in the direction that the associations of the analysands will take. Had Freud's wish to burn the Fliess letters succeeded, we would never have known the crucial role his self-analysis played in the sequence of what he discovered, and what he failed to discover.

Note

1 Originally published as Bergmann, M.S., "The Leap from the 'Studies on Hysteria' to the 'Interpretation of Dreams' (pp. 343–358). In Dinen and Harris, eds, *Storms in Her Head: Freud and the Construction of Hysteria* (New York: Other Press, 2001). All reasonable effort and due diligence has been made by both Routledge and Maria S. Bergmann to obtain permission to reprint this chapter from Other Press, LLC.

References

Bergmann, M.S. (1976) Moses and the Evolution of Freud's Jewish Identity. In *Judaism and Psychoanalysis*, ed. M. Ostow. New York: Ktav Publishing House, 1982, pp. 115–141.
Breuer, J. and Freud, S. (1895) Studies on Hysteria. S.E. 2: 1–335.
Eissler, K.R. (1971) *Talent and Genius: The Fictitious Case of Tausk Contra Freud*. New York: Quadrangle.
Ellenberger, H. (1970) *The Discovery of the Unconscious: The History and Evolution of Dynamic Psychiatry*. New York: Basic Books.
Freud, S. (1887–1904) *The Complete Letters of Sigmund Freud to Wilhelm Fliess, 1887–1904*, ed. and trans. J.M. Masson. Cambridge, MA: Harvard University Press, 1985.
Freud, S. (1900) The Interpretation of Dreams, Part I and Part II. S.E. 4–5: 1–625.
Freud, S. (1901) The Psychopathology of Everyday Life. S.E. 6: 1–336.
Freud, S. (1905a) Fragment of an Analysis of a Case of Hysteria. S.E. 7: 3–124.
Freud, S. (1908a) "Civilized" Sexual Morality and Modern Nervous Illness. S.E. 9: 177–204.
Freud, S. (1910a) Five Lectures of Psycho-Analysis. SE 11: 1–5.
Freud, S. (1916–17a) Introductory Lectures on Psychoanalysis, Parts I and II. SE 15: 9–239.
Freud, S. (1916–17b) Introductory Lectures on Psychoanalysis, Part III. SE 16: 243–463.
Freud, S. (1926) The Question of Lay Analysis. S.E. 20: 177–250.
Freud, S. (1933) New Introductory Lectures on Psycho-Analysis. S.E. 22: 1–182.
Goldstein, J. (1982) The Hysteria Diagnosis and the Politics of Anticlericalism in Late Nineteenth-Century France. *Journal of Modern History* 54: 209–239.
Grubrich-Simitis, I. (1991) *Freud's Moses-Studie als Tagtraum*. Weinheim: Verlag Internationale Psychanalyse.
Jones, E. (1953) *The Life and Work of Sigmund Freud, Vol. I: The Formative Years and the Great Discoveries, 1856–1900*. New York: Basic Books.
Kuhn, T. (1962) *The Structures of Scientific Revolutions*. Chicago, IL: University of Chicago Press.
Lear, J. (1990) *Love and its Place in Nature: A Philosophical Interpretations of Freudian Psychoanalysis*. New York: Farrar, Straus & Giroux.
McGrath, W.J. (1992) Freud and the Force of History. In *Freud and the History of Psychoanalysis*, eds T. Gelfands and J. Kerr, Hillsdale, NJ: Analytic Press, 79–97.

PART II

TECHNIQUE

CHAPTER 3

LIFE GOALS AND PSYCHOANALYTIC GOALS FROM A HISTORICAL PERSPECTIVE[1]

Ernst Ticho introduced the difference between life goals and treatment goals in the psychoanalytic process.

In medicine, the goal of treatment is to undo the deleterious effect of the disease, to bring back the status quo before the disease disturbs the equilibrium. In traumatic neurosis, a similar aim can be pursued, but even there, if psychoanalysis has not failed, something new that was never there before emerges.

Because psychoanalysis aims at more than restoration, the issue of its goals is both interesting and controversial. In the present climate of opinion, psychoanalysis is pressed to demonstrate its cost effectiveness against other therapies. The outcome of that controversy is still in doubt, but what remains certain is that if the value of "know thyself" – first articulated in the city of Delphi in Ancient Greece – is still important, psychoanalysis has no rival among other forms of psychotherapy.

The first historical phase

When Freud exchanged the hypnotic method for free associations around the turn of the century, he moved from the highly authoritarian stance of a hypnotist who gives orders to a hypnotized patient, to that of a therapist who must listen carefully to the associations of an analysand and make sense of them to make an interpretation. Freud expressed the difference between the analyst and the hypnotist in a beautiful metaphor taken from Leonardo da Vinci. Leonardo wrote that a painter adds substance to the canvas in the form of paint, whereas the sculptor works by removing blocks of stone from the statue that he is freeing from imprisonment within the stone. As he put it, the painter works via *di porre*, while the sculptor works via *di levare* (Freud 1905c, p. 260). The psychoanalyst shall take the sculptor as his or her ideal.

In 1914, Freud noted that this very significant step was not the result of a deliberate process of thought, but rather of following a "dim presentiment" (1914c, p. 19). Logical thinking (secondary process) is by its very nature goal directed. Freud's goal of making the unconscious conscious rested on a basic belief that the fragile ego of the child has no choice but to repress, while the adult undergoing psychoanalysis can tolerate the derivatives of what has had to be repressed, ultimately confronting the unconscious in a way the child could not. This optimism, which Freud inherited from the era of Enlightenment, did not always prove to be true. Many adults repress as much as children do, and many adults are more afraid of their unconscious than children are.

According to Freud, the analyst should follow free associations. In 1912, he put it thus:

> The technique, however, is a very simple one. As we shall see, it rejects the use of any special expedient (even that of taking notes). It consists simply in not directing one's notice to anything in particular and in maintaining the same "evenly-suspended attention" (as I have called it) in the face of all that one hears. In this way we spare ourselves a strain on our attention which could not in any case be kept up for several hours daily, and we avoid a danger which is inseparable from the exercise of deliberate attention.
>
> (Freud 1912c, pp. 111–112)

If both analyst and analysand try to follow their respective roles, the analytic process will be set into motion. Freud noted that when his patients tried to remember their childhoods, gaps appeared in their memories, chronology became confused, and causal connections were broken; the free association lost coherence. When that happened, Freud understood that resistance to the analytic process had set in. Once childhood amnesia was overcome, symptoms tended to lose their grip on the patient.

Freud believed that during analysis, the increased understanding of oneself goes hand in hand with the process of cure. He continuously warned his disciples against the excessive zeal to cure. Rather, they should enable the analysand to obtain a conscious grasp of unconscious wishes. The attainment of this goal represented a major triumph for the rationality of the Enlightenment. Freud could claim that he had found a method to subjugate the inner life of man to the scientific demands of natural science. As Fenichel would later put it in 1945, there are many ways of curing psychoneurosis, but only one way to understand it, and that was Freud's way. In the same spirit, Freud published his papers on technique (1912). He carefully called them "recommendations."

Among Freud's disciples, those who knew him face to face, Theodor Reik reacted with enthusiasm to the technique in which both analyst and analysand relinquish all aims except to let their unconscious minds speak. In a book published only in German, *Der Überraschte Psychologe* (1935), Reik suggested that, as the analyst listens to the patient, the analyst moves from guessing to understanding. However, this technique, Reik believed, cannot be taught but can only be experienced. After his immigration to the United States, Reik was not accepted as a member of the American Psychoanalytic Association, and his ideas were no longer included in the official psychoanalytic curriculum. Identifying himself with a younger Freud during "his splendid isolation" (Freud 1914c, p. 22), Reik began to publish a series of books addressed to the general reader, and gradually assembled his own group of disciples; he was a very popular writer for a time. In 1948 *Listening with the Third Ear: The Inner Experience of the Analyst* appeared. This book was followed in 1949 by *Fragment of a Great Confession: A Psychoanalytic Autobiography.*

In 1967, Bion made recommendations about the analyst's attitude which were similar to Freud's, when he wrote:

> Psychoanalytic observation is concerned neither with what has happened nor with what is going to happen, but rather with what is happening ... Every session attended by the psychoanalyst must have no history and no future ... Do not remember past sessions. The greater the impulse to remember what has been said or done, the more the need to resist it.
>
> (Bion 1967, p. 272)

Fenichel, in his 1941 book on technique, warned of two dangers at opposite ends of a spectrum:

> Psychoanalytic technique is a complicated task. Its tool is the unconscious of the analyst which intuitively comprehends the unconscious of the patient. Its aim is to lift this comprehension out of intuition into scientific clarity.
>
> (Fenichel 1941, p. 12)

It is Green's (1999) belief that the 1912 concept has not lost its vitality.

> I hear the analysand's communication from two points of view at once. That is to say, on the one hand, I try to perceive the internal conflicts that **inhibit** it and, on the other, I consider it from the point of view of something addressed, implicitly or explicitly, to me.
>
> (p. 278)

The second phase

In his 1914(a) paper on technique, Freud introduced new goals. These included analyzing screen memories. Screen memories were equivalent to the manifest content of dreams, and could be made to reveal hidden latent content (p. 148). The next task was to transform what the analytic patient tended to act out in memories. Freud realized that a neurotic illness is not something that happened in the past, but rather is "a present day force" (p. 151). Freud believed that the most important technical tool he had originated was the intensification of the transference, such that the analysand's neurosis is transformed into a transference neurosis, in which every important aspect of the patient's past is relived in the relationship to the analyst.

Freud's emphasis on making the unconscious conscious was consistent with his early topographical point of view, which could easily incorporate his idea that the analyst should pursue no specific goals. In contrast, the structural point of view, introduced in 1923, in which Freud divided the psychic apparatus into superego, ego and id, created new aims for psychoanalysis beyond the early idea of making the unconscious conscious. In the 1923 formulation, only when the ego is strong enough to hold in check both id and superego does a person approach mental health. In delinquency and perversion, the id overrules the ego, and in depression and melancholia it is the superego that has acquired dominance. Within this structural point of view, the aim of psychoanalysis became the strengthening of the ego against the other two institutions and helping the ego free itself from the power of some of its own defense mechanisms, which cripple the ego's freedom of movement. The aim of psychoanalysis became the achievement of a more favorable kind of intrapsychic compromise formation.

Developments after Freud

During the teens of the twentieth century, Freud's voice alone determined the course psychoanalysis would take, but beginning with the 1920s, other voices, not always in agreement with his, began to influence the development of psychoanalysis. In 1924, Ferenczi and Rank jointly published a book, which – at least in the original German edition – had the word "goals" in its very title, *Entwicklungsziele der Psychoanalyse*. (The English translation, published in 1925, was entitled *The Development of Psychoanalysis*.) In their view, the psychoanalytic situation exposes the patient to early infantile traumatic situations. A parental *imago* is offered with whom the patient can relive early libidinal emotions and early traumatic experiences. Many patients feel cured when they have happily fallen in love with their analysts; but the analyst cannot stop at such a point, for analysis aims at weaning the analysand through insight; the analysand must understand that psychoanalysis reawakened infantile wishes contradicted by current reality and the adult's ego ideal.

In *The Trauma of Birth* (1924), Rank made the abreaction to the "birth trauma" the final aim of psychoanalytic psychotherapy. Ferenczi, in a book entitled *Thalassa: A Theory of Genitality* (1924), created the idea that the return to the womb is the analysand's unconscious goal; the analysand wishes to reach this goal through "passive object love." When the analysand discovers that passivity toward the analyst does not bring about the desired fulfillment, a second "autoplastic masturbatory" phase sets in and the analysand attempts to turn away from any dependency on the analyst. Only at the end of the analysis can a capacity to find a new love object bring about the termination of the analysis.

A central point – the wish to return to the womb – characterized both books, and probably explains why Ferenczi and Rank, in spite of marked differences in thinking, could embark upon writing a joint book. Ferenczi's 1928 paper on termination, the first ever to address this stage, was written entirely within an emphasis on the absence of any conscious goals.

> The proper ending of an analysis is when neither the physician nor the patient puts an end to it, but when it dies of exhaustion, so to speak, though even when this occurs the physician must be the more suspicious of the two and must think of the possibility that behind the patient's wish to take his departure some neurotic factor may still be concealed. A truly cured patient frees himself from analysis slowly but surely; so long as he wishes to come to analysis, he should continue to do so.
>
> (Ferenczi 1928, p. 85)

Even in this paper, however, Ferenczi introduced many goals that an analyst should have in mind. Not satisfied with symptom analysis, he believed that no analysis can be ended without a complete character analysis (p. 80). He insisted that every male patient attain feelings of equality in relation to the analyst, and every female patient must get rid of her "masculine complex" without a trace of resentment (p. 84).

In 1935, Balint, Ferenczi's best-known disciple, published a paper entitled *The Final Goal of Psycho-Analytic Treatment*, in which the author maintained that an effective analyst should enable the analysand to gain the capacity for a "new beginning" (p. 192). In Balint's view, the libido was always object-seeking rather than pleasure-seeking. The self-erotic and narcissistic strivings from which so many men and women suffer are the results of disappointments in early object relationships – primarily the relationship to the mother. The goal of analysis is to work through these early disappointments, so that upon its completion a capacity to love without inner inhibitions has been newly acquired. A new emphasis on trauma is discernible in Balint's views. With one variation, the same idea is found in the writings of Loewald (1960) and Winnicott (1971). Winnicott emphasized particularly the renewal of the lost capacity to play, and Loewald the capacity to experience the analyst as a new object.

In Freud's view, and in the view of these psychoanalysts who followed his model, the analyst is a transference object upon whom unresolved psychic conflicts of the patient are projected. At the end of the analysis the nature of these projections is recognized and the transference is resolved. By contrast, in Loewald (1966), the emphasis of the analyst was never only a transference object but by her or his toleration of the patient whose aggression will always remain a new object to the patient and therefore is never eliminated. In every analysis both points of view are played out and upon termination they are experienced as distinct from each other.

I contributed to this discussion (Bergmann 1986) when it became clear to me that an analytic patient who develops a strong transference love toward the analyst is not necessarily capable of loving in real life. The fact that the analyst makes no demand to be loved by the patient, and accepts and tolerates aggression within the transference, can evoke love in the analysand that remains untransferable into real life.

In 1922, Karl Abraham and Max Eitingon created the first psychoanalytic institute according to a tripartite model which stipulated a personal analysis; a specified number of cases to be supervised by a training analyst; and systematic, psychoanalytic, course work.

It became mandatory for every analyst to undergo a training analysis, which removed some of these dangers. However, the analysis of the analyst could hardly be expected to eliminate all personal bias, and furthermore, every institute of necessity developed its own interpretation of Freud's work, fostering uniformity rather than creativity within that institute.

The third phase

After the Second World War, a new interest in the aims of psychoanalysis emerged in the United States. This attraction to the field did not arise out of intrinsic interest in the analytic process, but more as a result of new cultural forces that had to be dealt with. Before the Second World War, psychoanalysis had essentially been a private practice enterprise; but after the war, once the influence of analysis on several disciplines — psychiatry, psychology and social work — had led to remarkable progress, the American Psychoanalytic Association made every effort to continue to act as an influential force within these professions. It succeeded in dominating academic psychiatry, but this very success forced American psychoanalysts to consider the relationship between psychoanalysis and psychotherapy. Psychiatric residents could not be expected to become analysts, but they had to learn how to apply the principles of psychoanalysis in psychotherapy.

The hitherto prevalent opinion within psychoanalysis toward psychotherapy was expressed by Freud via a metaphor comparing psychoanalytic gold with psychotherapeutic copper. This metaphor gave psychotherapists who were influenced by analysis without becoming psychoanalysts themselves, a feeling of inferiority, and therefore did not adequately serve the needs of psychoanalytically oriented psychotherapists. The more successful the discipline of psychoanalysis became in its conquest, the more urgent it became to define the demarcation lines between the two modalities. The best-known paper dealing with this problem was Eissler's, entitled *The Effect of the Structure of the Ego on Psychoanalytic Technique* (1953): the so-called parameter paper. It included the following comment:

> If our knowledge of the structure of the ego were complete, then a variety of techniques – ideally adapted to the requirements of the individual disturbance – could be perfected; thus we could assure definite mastery of the

> ego over those areas in which it had suffered defeat, that is to say, assure complete recovery.
>
> (p. 104)

A corollary to this statement, however, is that such a full understanding of the ego is not possible; and, furthermore, every ego has its own structure. Therefore our success as therapists is also limited.

A year later, the *Journal of the American Psychoanalytic Association* published a number of papers on the relationship between psychoanalysis and psychotherapy. In these discussions, the issue of the goals of psychoanalysis played a major role. A new sense of victory was discernible in Alexander's (1954) paper:

> Psychiatrists came to recognize more and more the fundamental nature of Freud's discoveries, and psychiatric practice both officially and unofficially became highly influenced by psychoanalysis. Many psychoanalysts felt that through this change in the cultural climate our role and responsibility have changed. Now, when psychiatry is not only ready but eager to assimilate in an undiluted form the teachings of Freud and the work of his followers, we felt that it became our responsibility to guide and facilitate this process of incorporation.
>
> (p. 724)

Alexander singled out for attack what he called the "regressive-dependent component of the transference" (p. 732) – the very regression that Balint, Winnicott and other psychoanalysts considered a prerequisite for "a new beginning" (Balint 1935, p. 192). To prevent a regression from taking place, Alexander recommended that the frequency of analytic hours be changed when the analysand became too dependent. In fact, Alexander and his colleagues advocated the dissolution of analysis as a separate profession and favored its merging into psychiatry. The question of how much regression on the part of the patient the analyst should foster, or even allow, became a controversial topic with respect to the goals of analysis.

Rangell (1954) noted that dynamic psychiatrists view childhood in terms of interpersonal relationships, rather than in terms of psychosexual development. As a compromise, in opposition to Alexander's viewpoint, Rangell proposed the following definition of psychoanalysis:

> Psychoanalysis is a method of therapy whereby conditions are brought about favorable for the development of a transference neurosis, in which the past is restored in the present, in order that, through a systematic interpretative attack on the resistances which oppose it, there occurs a resolution of that neurosis (transference and infantile) to the end of bringing about structural changes in the mental apparatus of the patient to make the latter capable of optimum adaptation to life.
>
> (pp. 739–740)

Gill (1954) offered an almost identical definition:

> Psychoanalysis is that technique which, employed by a neutral analyst, results in the development of a regressive transference neurosis and the ultimate resolution of this neurosis by techniques of interpretation alone.
>
> (p. 775)

In the long run, the analysis of the transference neurosis as differentiating psychoanalysis from psychotherapy proved to be a concept that was impossible to maintain. Many analysands did not develop a transference neurosis and many patients in psychotherapy did.

Stone, in his by now famous paper *The Widening Scope of Indications for Psychoanalysis* (1954), raised the question of how much the classical analytic method can be modified and still be regarded as analysis (p. 575). He accepted Eissler's ideas of the need for parameters, but objected to the fact that all parameters must terminate and be interpreted before the end of analysis (p. 576). Stone's paper signaled permission to extend psychoanalysis beyond the limits of the neuroses.

In 1965, Wallerstein called for a distinction between "idealized goals" and "attainable goals." He noted that no person can be completely analyzed or attain perfect mental health. The psychoanalytic process may therefore be goalless, but its implicit goal is a radical change in character realignment.

Ernst Ticho (1972) called for a distinction between treatment goals and life goals, a distinction adopted in this paper. Life goals are those that an analysand would seek to obtain if he or she could put his or her potentialities to full use. Life goals were further divided into professional and personal ones, with personal goals involving the kind of person patients would like to become, as distinct from the professional goals they wish to address. The analysis itself should not be permitted to become a life goal. Treatment goals, on the other hand, aim to help the patient understand his or her neurosis, which in turn should enable the patient to differentiate between conscious and unconscious goals. The distinction between treatment goals and life goals, makes it possible for the analysand to achieve "unified treatment goals" (Ticho 1972, p. 315).

The distinction between life goals and treatment goals becomes crucial when a life goal of the analysand turns out to be beyond the reach of the treatment – for example, when a life partner cannot be found, when a phobia cannot be overcome, or even when the capacity to reach sexual orgasm cannot be obtained. Should the analyst continue to analyze with the hope that the life goal will become reachable? Or should we aim only at treatment goals, such as self-knowledge, giving the patient access to his or her unconscious through free associations and the interpretation of dreams?

When Ticho published his paper, the prestige of analysis within psychiatry was high, and it was also esteemed by the general public. But when analysis began to come under attack, the need to concentrate on life goals became urgent in order to show that analysis is cost effective in comparison with other treatment procedures (Bader 1994). For many years, Freud's decision to bring the treatment of the Wolf Man to an end had been regarded as a technical error; but in the new climate it was commended (Gunderson and Gabbard 1999, p. 692).

Weinshel (1990) described particularly well the changes that had taken place in the mainstream of American psychoanalysis. His main points (pp. 281–283) are:

1. We rarely speak any more of psychoanalytic "cures." We are much more likely to focus on changes, shifts, or compromise formations.
2. We do not, as a rule, talk about eliminating psychological conflict, but accept the presence of conflict as one of the givens of being alive. We no longer hope that the analysis will result in a more favorable resolution of the central conflicts that existed prior to treatment.
3. We do not think about analyses being complete but recognize that an analysis can be terminated successfully although more analytic work could be done.

4. We no longer insist that transferences be completely resolved.
5. We no longer think about "overcoming" resistances. We anticipate that analytic work will lead to greater access to the unconscious derivatives associated with resistances.
6. Insight is still a highly valued *desideratum*. We aim for the patient's achievement of it and we look for evidence of it in our analytic work, but it is no longer considered the *sine qua non* for a successful psychoanalysis.
7. The analysis of dreams is no longer considered "the royal road to a knowledge of the unconscious activities of the mind" (Freud 1900, p. 608).
8. We increasingly acknowledge the importance of the analyst's affective participation in the analytic work.

What is described represents a greater modesty and a more realistic assessment of what psychoanalysis can achieve. The trends enumerated above tend to obscure the demarcation between psychoanalysis and psychoanalytically oriented psychotherapy. At its very best, analysis can give the patient a new way of understanding him or herself, a kind of insight that enables the patient to understand what happened in his or her life that determined the unique nature of the patient's strivings.

There are a number of points in Weinshel's essay with which I do not concur. For one thing, the dream has retained for me a special position, and I continue to regard it as the most valuable communication from the unconscious of the analysand to the analyst (Bergmann 1966). I agree that Freud's archaeological metaphor no longer serves as a measure of progress in the analysis, but childhood memories – especially when they emerge in a dynamic context with current problems – are to me still of great significance. I also do not share Weinshel's belief that the concept of Kris's "good hours" has lost its pivotal position in psychoanalytic technique (Bergmann 1993a).

I will conclude my historical review by noting that, in 1995, Wallerstein published a book entitled *The Talking Cures*, which dealt at length with the evolving relationship between psychoanalysis and psychoanalytically oriented psychotherapy. Instead of regarding analysis as the best treatment anyone could hope for, as Freud did, the new approach offered the belief that

> treatment should be fitted to the clinical exigencies and needs of the patient, contrary to the stance of Freud's days, when psychoanalysis had been conceived as the only scientific and truly etiologic treatment approach to which the patient should be fitted if at all possible.
>
> (p. 88)

In 1996, Sandler and Dreher published a monograph subtitled "The Problem of Aims in Psychoanalytic Therapy." They concluded that mental health is specific to each patient and to his or her particular life situation, and the aims of psychoanalysis vary according to the value systems of both analyst and patient (p. 121). Analytic goals must take into account all the patient's personal limitations and particulars, as well as social or economic context (p. 122). In spirit, the book's philosophy is close to Weinshel's, emphasizing selectivity and modesty. Here, as well as in Weinshel's paper, analysts appear to be more realistically grounded.

As I see it, the issue of goals became important because of certain contradictions inherent in the very nature of Freud's creation of psychoanalysis. Insofar as the analyst is the guardian of the process of free association, efforts must be directed toward making it possible for the analysand to associate as freely as possible (A.

Kris 1982). If that approach is fully pursued, both analyst and analysand can become caught up in the thicket of the unconscious, years can pass, and the analysis may be in danger of succumbing to the primary processes. Therefore, the other function the analyst must keep in mind is support of the reality principle, which may at times become inimical to the process of free associations. Furthermore, in my own clinical approach, I have stressed my indebtedness to E. Kris; his 1956 paper was decisive in my development as an analytic clinician and analytic teacher, as I pointed out earlier.

Although psychoanalysts had long known that certain analytic hours were regarded by both patient and analyst as particularly productive, Kris was the first to examine such an hour systematically. He described such hours as generally beginning with the patient recounting a recent experience.

> One of the implications of Kris's concept of the good hour is that it is the analysand's property and cannot be willed either by analyst or analysand.
> (Bergmann 1993a, pp. 379–380)

I see the analyst not only as guardian of the patient's free associations, but also as midwife, facilitating the birth of the "good hour." The "good hour paper" had its roots in Hartmann's (1964) ego psychology; as long as neurosis prevails, the ego has to employ its energy in countercathexis, keeping unacceptable unconscious ideas and wishes in a state of repression. Analysis allows the ego to relax its grip, freeing the ego to employ its energy in integration and the undoing of isolation. Kris's good hour becomes more likely to occur once more energy is available to the ego for the work of integration. Analytic conceptualizing during the Hartmann era reached the high point of its contribution to technique with the concept of the good hour (Bergmann 2000).

I find it useful to divide the analytic process into three phases. In the initial phase the analyst is prepared to do everything in his or her power to ensure that the analytic process can get started. In practice, that means understanding the forces within the analysand that oppose the analytic process. If the unconscious mind's need to destroy the analysis is not made clear by the analyst, the analytic endeavor will be overcome by the repetition compulsion that is opposed to any change for the better in the intrapsychic equilibrium.

Once this temptation has been mastered and the analysand is no longer trying to destroy the analysis, the goal of the analyst shifts to preventing a compromise formation from taking place too early. In practice, it may be necessary to understand and overcome an unproductive stalemate that has set in during the middle phase of the analysis. Often, this requires the analysis of transference resistance, which may have achieved dominance over the analysand. The analyst can help by continuously emphasizing free association, and not deflecting the hour away from its inherent course. It is during this phase also that the analyst must work in such a way as to maximize the possibility of the number of good hours.

Finally, once this phase has accomplished its purpose, the analysis enters the termination phase. I pointed out (1997) the particular perils of this phase. Here, either leaving the termination process up to the analysand, as Ferenczi (1928) proposed, or its opposite – arbitrarily setting the date of the ending by the therapist, as Freud did with the Wolf Man – can be detrimental.

The distinction Ticho (1972) made between treatment goals and life goals needs emphasis: treatment goals vary and are dependent on particular stages in the analytic process; while life goals, which deal with such subjects as marriage, divorce, the wish to have children, single parenthood, and homosexuality, should be left strictly to the analysand to decide. Far too often, psychotherapists and psychoanalysts have found it difficult to leave all life goals to their patients themselves.

The maintenance of a sort of double stance – giving the analysand maximal free space to pursue his or her own life goals, and at the same time keeping control over the changing goals of the analytic process itself – lies at the very core of what it means to be a psychoanalyst. It constitutes our professional ego ideal.

As we enter the year 2001, we are well aware of very rapid changes taking place in our culture. Every present-day analytic case teaches us that the basic problems encountered by children in their formative years are not significantly different from those that Freud observed. Unloved children, children who suffer illnesses and other traumatic experiences, those subjected to social catastrophes, and those who encounter deviant parents and hostile siblings are with us now, just as they were in Freud's time. But as adults, these persons encounter a very different culture, one that offers different deprivations as well as different opportunities. In this new culture, the interaction between adult opportunities and early deprivations is very different. Thus, as analysts, we have the additional task of grasping the complexities of the changing culture encountered by both our patients and by us. This unique culture has imposed different life goals on our patients, and whether these life goals require a re-examination of our treatment goals remains to be seen.

Note

1 A German-language version of this paper was read at the annual convention of M.A.P. in Munich on November 12, 1999. First published as: Bergmann, M.S. (2001), "Life Goals and Psychoanalytic Goals from a Historical Perspective," *Psychoanalytic Quarterly*, 70: 15–34.

References

Alexander, F. (1954) Psychoanalysis and psychotherapy. *Journal of the American Psychoanalytic Association* 2: 722–733.

Bader, M.J. (1994) The Tendency to Neglect Therapeutic Aims in Psychoanalysis. *Psychoanalytic Quarterly* 63: 246–270.

Balint, M. (1935) The Final Goal of Psycho-Analytic Treatment. In *Primary Love and Psycho-Analytic Technique*. New York: Liveright, 1953, pp. 188–199.

Bergmann, M.S. (1966) The Intrapsychic and Communicative Aspects of the Dream – Their Role in Psycho-Analysis and Psychotherapy. *International Journal of Psychoanalysis* 47: 356–363.

Bergmann, M.S. (1987) *The Anatomy of Loving*. New York: Columbia University Press.

Bergmann, M.S. (1993a) Reality and Psychic Reality in Ernst Kris's Last Papers: An Attempt to Update his Findings. *Psychoanalytic Inquiry* 13 (4): 372–383.

Bergmann, M.S., ed. (2000) *The Hartmann Era*. New York: Other Press.

Bion, W. (1967) Notes on Memory and Desire. *Psychoanalytic Forum* 2 (3): 272–273.

Eissler, K. R. (1953) The Effect of the Structure of the Ego on Psychoanalytic Technique. *Journal of the American Psychoanalytic Association* 1: 104–143.

Fenichel, O. (1941) *Problems of Psychoanalytic Technique*, trans. D. Brunswick. New York: Psychoanalytic Quarterly.

Ferenczi, S. (1924) *Thalassa: A Theory of Genitality*. New York: Psychoanalytic Quarterly.

Ferenczi, S. (1928) The Problem of Termination of the Analysis. In *Final Contributions to Problems and Methods of Psychoanalysis*, Balint, M., ed. New York: Basic Books, 1955, 77–86.

Ferenczi, S. and Rank, O. (1925) *The Development of Psychoanalysis*, trans. C. Newton. New York: Nervous and Mental Disease Publishing.
Freud, S. (1900) The Interpretation of Dreams, Part I and Part II. S.E. 4–5: 1–625.
Freud, S. (1905c) On Psychotherapy. S.E. 7: 257–268.
Freud, S. (1912c) Recommendations to Physicians Practising Psycho-Analysis. S.E. 12: 111–120.
Freud, S. (1914a) Remembering, Repeating and Working Through. S.E. 12: 145–156.
Freud, S. (1914c) On the History of the Psycho-Analytic Movement. S.E. 14: 7–66.
Gill, M. (1954) Psychoanalysis and Exploratory Psychotherapy. *Journal of the American Psychoanalytic Association* 2: 771–797.
Green, A. (1999) On Discriminating and Not Discriminating Between Affect and Representation. *International Journal of Psychoanalysis* 80 (2): 277–316.
Gunderson, J.G. and Gabbard, G.O. (1999) Making the Case for Psychoanalytic Therapy in the Current Psychiatric Environment. *Journal of the American Psychoanalytic Association* 47: 679–703.
Hartmann, H. (1964) *Essays in Ego Psychology*. New York: International Universities Press.
Kris, A. (1982) *Free Association: Method and Process*. New Haven, CT: Yale University Press.
Kris, E. (1956) On Some Vicissitudes of Insight in Psychoanalysis. In *Selected Papers of Ernst Kris*. New Haven, CT: Yale University Press, 1975, 252–271.
Loewald, H. (1960) On the Therapeutic Action of Psychoanalysis. *International Journal of Psychoanalysis* 41: 16–33.
Loewald, H. (1966) Review of Arlow and Brenner. *Psychoanalytic Quarterly* 35: 430–436.
Rangell, L. (1954) Similarities and Differences Between Psychoanalysis and Dynamic Psychotherapy. *Journal of the American Psychoanalytic Association* 2: 734–744.
Rank, O. (1924) *The Trauma of Birth*. New York: Harcourt, Brace and Company.
Reik, T. (1935) *Der Überraschte Psychologe*. Leiden, Holland: A. W. Sijthoff's Uitgevers-maatschappij N. V.
Reik, T. (1948) *Listening with the Third Ear*. New York: Farrar, Straus & Co.
Reik, T. (1949) *Fragment of a Great Confession: A Psychoanalytic Autobiography*. New York: Farrar, Straus & Co.
Sandler, J. and Dreher, A. (1996) *What Do Psychoanalysts Want? The Problem of Aims in Psychoanalytic Therapy*. London: Routledge.
Stone, L. (1954) The Widening Scope of Indications for Psychoanalysis. *Journal of the American Psychoanalytic Association* 2: 567–594.
Ticho, E.A. (1972) Termination of Psychoanalysis: Treatment Goals, Life Goals. *Psychoanalytic Quarterly* 41: 315–333.
Wallerstein, R.S. (1995) *The Talking Cures*. New Haven, CT: Yale University Press.
Weinshel, E.M. (1990) How Wide is the Widening Scope of Psychoanalysis and How Solid is its Structural Model? *Journal of the American Psychoanalytic Association* 38: 275–296.
Winnicott, D.W. (1971) *Playing and Reality*. London: Tavistock.

CHAPTER 4

THE CHALLENGE OF EROTIZED TRANSFERENCE TO PSYCHOANALYTIC TECHNIQUE[1]

Classical analysis began as a treatment method for neuroses. Within the neuroses there is an expectable pattern for the development of the transference. In this expected pattern the transference will eventually bring up overt sexual wishes, but the process of sexualization of the transference is expected to be slow, hesitant and conflictual. The reason for this expected pattern is that neurotics have not resolved their Oedipus complex and feel guilty over their oedipal wishes, sexual as well as aggressive, as they appear in the transference. The development of the transference is expected to recapitulate the oedipal constellation, with the analyst in the role of the forbidden parent.

The women who have developed erotized transference early in the treatment and without the expected guilt have not followed the expected pattern. They have evoked countertransference reactions in the male analyst, as well as feelings of bewilderment and helplessness, and, eventually, hostility. Now that psychoanalytically oriented therapists have ventured to analyze patients within a wider scope than the neuroses, erotized transferences should be anticipated, and therapists should be ready to treat them.

The impact of Freud

Women developing erotized transference in treatment with male therapists have not fared well in psychoanalytic literature. The difficulty goes back to Freud himself, who in his 1915 paper *Observations on Transference-Love* said:

> There is, it is true, one class of women with whom this attempt to preserve the erotic transference for the purposes of analytic work without satisfying it will not succeed. These are women of elemental passionateness who tolerate no surrogate. They are children of nature who refuse to accept the psychical in place of the material, who, in the poet's words, are accessible only to "the logic of soup, with dumplings for arguments." With such people one has the choice between returning their love or else bringing down upon oneself the full enmity of a woman scorned. In neither case can one safeguard the interests of the treatment. One has to withdraw, unsuccessful; and all one can do is to turn the problem over in one's mind of how it is that the capacity for neurosis is joined with such an intractable need for love.
>
> (Freud 1915b, pp. 166–167)

It is evident from the tone of this paragraph that working with these women Freud lost his therapeutic neutrality as well as his empathy. The "logic of soup, with dumplings" and "elemental passionateness" are not psychoanalytic concepts. Freud goes on to suggest two further arguments the analyst can use in such a situation.

What we do above all, is to stress to the patient the unmistakable element of resistance in the "love." Genuine love we say would make her docile and intensify her readiness to resolve the problem of her case, simply because the man she was in love with expected it of her.

As a second argument against the genuineness of this love, we advance the fact that it exhibits not a single new feature arising from the present situation, but is entirely composed of repetitions and copies of earlier reactions, including infantile ones. We undertake to prove this by a detailed analysis of the patient's behavior in love (p. 167).

Neither argument has much validity. A mild positive transference may indeed create the desirable readiness; but transference love, like any other love, has an imperious quality all of its own. Nor is it true that transference love does not exhibit new features; the very fact that the analyst responds differently from the other significant persons in the history of the patient gives transference love a new quality. Freud felt that these two arguments would make women who are less violent in their love gradually readapt the analytic attitude. What makes one woman more violent in her love than another was beyond Freud's capacity to explore at that time. A page later Freud had misgivings about his whole line of argument.

> I think we have told the patient the truth, but not the whole truth regardless of the consequences. Of our two arguments, the first is the stronger. The part played by resistance in transference love is unquestionable and very considerable. Nevertheless, the resistance did not, after all, create this love; it finds it ready to hand, makes use of it and aggravates its manifestations. Nor is the genuineness of the phenomenon disproved by the resistance. The second argument is far weaker. It is true that the love consists of new additions of old traits and it repeats infantile reactions. But this is the essential character of every state of being in love.
>
> (p. 168)

It is rare for Freud to advance an argument and take it back a page later. To me it indicates that Freud felt helpless in this situation. Indeed, Blanton (1971) reported that Freud told him women in love are useless in analytic work. Freud did not even think it would help to refer the patient to another analyst; he was convinced that under the pressure of the repetition compulsion the patient would fall in love once again.

In 1910 and 1912 Freud had made the significant discovery that every person has his or her own "preconditions for loving." (In popular language, people often refer to these preconditions by saying that "he or she is not my type.") When object constancy has not been reached in childhood, and when the oedipal relationship has not been resolved, it is the situation rather than the individual that evokes the preconditions for loving. For example, some men find women attractive only when they belong to a rival. When the rivalry has been overcome, love subsides. Freud did not sharply separate preconditions for loving from preconditions for sexual attraction (Schafer 1977). Freud (1915b) himself inadvertently disclosed his own preconditions for loving: "When a woman sues for love to reject and refuse is a distressing part for a man to play; and in spite of neurosis and resistance, there is an incomparable fascination in a woman of high principles who confesses her passion" (p. 170).

There is a wonderful example of preconditions for loving in Shakespeare's *Measure for Measure*, when Angelo describes his falling in love with Isabella: "Never could the strumpet with all her double vigor, art and nature, once stir my temper; but this virtuous maid subdues me quite. Ever till now when men were fond I smiled and wondered how" (Act II, Scene II).

To return to Freud, there was something missing in this paper, which I did not see until I was invited to make these comments. What were these women threatening to do as a result of having fallen in love with their doctors? Presumably, they invited sexual relationships with their analyst, either of the more childlike pregenital type made familiar to us from Ferenczi's work (1933), or of a more adult genital type. This demand deserved special comment only if it evoked countertransferentially similar wishes in the analyst. It seems that Freud had primarily this danger in mind and therefore admonished the therapist not to experience transference love as a personal conquest. He was therefore fully aware that transference love was evoked by the analytic situation. I am not sure he knew fully that this love was evoked by the regressive nature of the psychoanalytic situation.

In my view the therapist confronted by erotized transference is facing two difficulties. The first is not to yield to the temptation; and the second is, after overcoming the temptation, not to feel aggressive toward the patient who has evoked the temptation. Both difficulties must be met if the work of analysis is to go on. The analysand may be so unhappy when her wishes are not gratified that she leaves the treatment. The possibility of the interruption of treatment is always present, but the danger is far greater when the love wishes are not allowed to become conscious.

Freud insisted on the basic rule that the patient tell him everything that occurred to her without censorship. Was not her falling in love the result of this demand? And if the demand to say everything leads to ever more explicit demands for love, should we not at this point ask ourselves whether the difficulty is not the result of a mismatch between the patient and the technique employed? To raise doubts about the basic rule when it ceased to be productive would have demanded a greater revision of psychoanalysis than Freud was willing to undertake.

It was many years later that Eissler (1958, p. 230) made the important observation that free associations work well only in a state of intrapsychic conflict.

Breuer and Freud (1895) regarded transference only as a false connection. Freud wished to investigate the origins of hysteria, not to get involved in amorous relationships. He first attempted to get rid of transference by calling it a false connection of the association process. In 1905, after the analysis of Dora, he accepted transference as a useful force in the therapeutic process. In 1914 he went a step further and suggested that the analyst use the transference to convert the infantile neurosis into a transference neurosis. It is evident from the earlier paragraph quoted from the 1915(b) paper that he did not regard erotized transference as a form of transference neurosis.

In my book *The Anatomy of Loving* (Bergmann 1987), in chapter 18 – "Transference love and love in real life" – I followed Freud's idea that transference love repeats infantile prototypes. I have added, however, that this love takes place in a state of regression brought about by the analytic situation. In real life, too, love is frequently evoked in regressive relationships. Patients who are hospitalized for organic conditions frequently fall in love with their nurses, as do pupils with teachers and secretaries with their employers. These figures recapitulate the parent-child relationship. I should add Bak's (1973) observation that love takes place after object loss – for example, after a parent's death. While I paid homage to the power of infantile prototypes, I added another motivating force that often opposes the wish for refinding in falling in love. When the original relationship to the parent left a residue of unhappiness and trauma, the wish will emerge that the lover cure the wounds the infantile objects have inflicted. In the unconscious, where contradiction does not exist, the two manifest themselves side by side, but once the attempt is made to translate these two contradictory wishes into a real relationship difficulties will ensue. The turbulence in many love relationships is explained by this contradiction. In the analytic situation, both wishes – the wish to refind, and the yearning for the healer – become powerful. There is still another set of contradictory wishes associated with falling in love. In falling in love, symbiotic wishes to merge become strong, but as Mahler (1971) has pointed out, the reawakened symbiotic wishes for oneness also reawaken the fear of the engulfing mother, creating conflict.

For centuries, men and women searched for mandrake roots and other love potions, and yet at the turn of century a Jewish Viennese physician uncovered love's secret. Love entered his consultation room, even though it was hardly welcome. What Freud discovered was that love can be evoked under a set of simple conditions: (1) Keep the environment as constant as possible. (2) Intrude as little as possible into evolving feelings and memories, particularly childhood memories. (3) Pay special attention to the recall of forgotten or repressed past loves. (4) Demonstrate to the person whose love you wish to evoke that after every disappointment, he or she developed defense mechanisms against future love.

It is a historical paradox that Freud, who found a way of cultivating a "hothouse" variety of love, became concerned when analysands insisted on sexual gratification.

A critical discussion of the literature after Freud

In *Transference and Reality* Nunberg (1951) described women who find fault with everything the analyst does: "Whatever I did or said was wrong. She found fault in everything. She corrected me constantly, trying to teach me what to do, how to behave, what to think and what to say" (p. 1).

At first glance these women are not the same as those Freud described in his paper. There is, however, a similarity. Here too the process of free association has come to a halt. These women use, or perhaps more accurately misuse, the basic rule of criticizing the analyst. Just as Freud felt helpless with his erotizing women, Nunberg was at loss when dealing with these fault-finding women.

Today we need not be as helpless as Nunberg was. I (Bergmann 1987) have shown that there are people who cannot fall in love with others but can love what they themselves have created. Ovid, the Roman poet, recounted the legend of the sculptor Pygmalion, beautifully illustrating this difficulty in loving. Pygmalion, horrified by the promiscuity of the women of his time, fashioned a statue of Aphrodite and beseeched the goddess to bring it to life. (George Bernard Shaw revived the same legend in *Pygmalion*, which was later again transformed into the musical *My Fair Lady*.) The women Nunberg described had as their precondition for loving the need to mold the therapist according to their own image. This wish is explainable if we take into account that many people, disappointed in their parents and wishing to remold them, as adults cannot relinquish this wish. Psychoanalysts who fall in love with their patients may belong to this type. The question is, do they love the analysand or what they themselves have accomplished?

Keiser (1953) discussed a case of a fifteen-year-old girl whose parents divorced when she was four. The father moved to a distant city, and the mother exposed the child to her own subsequent sexual relationships. Early in the analysis she had dreams in which incestuous relationships appeared in a manifest content. She quickly developed a transference neurosis in which sexual relationships with the analyst appeared disguised by the usual symbols. She also feared being irresistible and disrupting the analyst's life. Keiser's paper is historically important because it highlights the role of the superego in preventing the rapid emergence of erotized transference.

What is surprising in the history of the literature on erotized transference is that the soup and dumpling metaphor I quoted from Freud's paper of 1915 was never challenged. During the Hartmann period, erotization was seen as interfering with ego functioning. Rappaport (1956) exemplifies this period. Rappaport did not regard erotized transference as a form of transference neurosis. He saw but disapproved of the fact that these patients sought to refind a parent; if possible, a better parent than they had. He also deplored the fact that when these patients developed erotic feelings they were ego syntonic, insisting on close physical contact with the therapist. Greenson (1967) described women who came to analysis not to seek insight but to enjoy the physical proximity of the analyst (pp. 338–341). He noted that such patients react appropriately during the initial interview. They have a good history of achievement, an adequate social life, but an unsatisfactory love life. They develop an erotized transference in the first hour on the couch. Their sexuality, though very vocal, Greenson saw as "a last ditch defense against the abyss of homosexual love for the mother" (p. 340).

In my view Greenson oversimplified this situation. Of the three structures – ego, id and superego – only the ego can be induced to be interested in insight, for insight offers the ego weapons against id and superego. No analysand is ever interested only in insight. As to the second point, we will note later that the wish for physical contact is not as simple as Greenson assumed.

Swartz (1969) reported the case of a severely inhibited phobic young woman whose forbidding mother was incorporated into a harsh superego. When this harsh superego was analyzed, a flagrantly erotic attachment developed. Rappaport, who discussed this case, suggested that the patient "threw herself on the analyst's neck," demanding sexual relations to make him regret that he ever liberated her from her harsh superego. To Swartz the main problem of erotized transference was that it prevents the formation of an analyzable transference neurosis. One of the important warning signals that an erotized transference is about to develop is, in Rappaport's view, the loss of sexual interest by the analysands in their partners. Erotized transference can therefore be seen as an all-consuming transference neurosis rather than as the absence of it. Swartz, like Keiser, highlighted the importance of the superego as preventing the emergence of erotized transfer.

Blum (1973) represents a step forward. He noted that patients who develop an erotized transference have usually been seduced as children by adults. Unlike previous analysts, Blum recognized that erotized transference is a form of transference neurosis. Analysands trying to seduce the analyst are repeating actively what happened to them passively in childhood. Just to raise the possibility that they are reacting to a childhood seduction is often enough to dispel the erotized transference and get the analysis back on track. Blum's hypothesis, if tested and proven correct, would greatly enhance our power to deal with these patients.

Contemporary literature shows a deeper awareness of the forces behind erotized transference. Stern (1991) reports the case of a patient who told him she was convinced he would have sex with her once he trusted her enough not to tell anyone. The therapist sensed that this declaration was based on her feeling that, should the sexual liaison happen, she would be in control of the situation. He also sensed that the patient felt she could not get close to the therapist unless she granted him sexual favors. For his own sake, as well as hers, the therapist felt compelled to say, "In order to protect you and this treatment, you need to understand that I will not, now or ever, take sexual advantage of you in any way, recognizing as we do that this is both a terrifying and yet longed-for fantasy" (p. 475).

Although all therapists will empathize with Stern's position, it nevertheless remains true that analyzing the reasons behind the conviction would have been the therapeutically better approach. It is true, however, that to allow the process of free association to proceed, the therapist must always insist that he is the guardian of the therapeutic goal, as he is also the guardian of the free associations.

The important *Confusion of Tongues between Adult and Child* by Ferenczi (1933), is never mentioned in the literature on erotized transference. Ferenczi observed that when children behave seductively with adults, they are seductive in a childish way. It is the adult who misreads this seduction along adult lines and responds to the child as if the child were an adult sexual object. I would like to pursue Ferenczi's idea further. The interruption of the playful sexuality of the child by seduction has consequences on the whole capacity of these children to fantasize and symbolize. When later as adults they enter analysis, these patients develop an erotized transference. They are demanding, serious, and, above all, lacking in humor and gentleness. By their very form they betray their traumatic origin. If the analyst succeeds in reaching a deeper layer of the unconscious beyond the time when the seduction took place, a playful form of infantile sexuality will be uncovered. In such situations our patients become transformed into little girls who want to demonstrate to their father how pretty they are. If the analyst, in the role of the father, can reciprocate and be playful with the patient/daughter without arousing her sexually, a play space will open up. If we clarify this to our analysands they will sometimes be able to recapture in the transference the delightful seductiveness of the little girl that has little in common with the seductiveness of an adult woman.

There is no literature, to my knowledge, that deals with male homosexual erotized transference, but there is a substantial literature dealing with erotized transference between women. Greenacre (1954) found that male analysts overstepped the transference limits more frequently with women patients than women analysts did. Women analysts are more in danger of being drawn unconsciously into an overtly protective nursing attitude toward suffering patients. Women apparently showed greater courage than men in dealing with homosexual erotized transference. A particularly interesting example was presented by Lester (1985). In this case erotized transference emerged at the end of the second year of analysis in a dream that the patient was making love to a faceless but breasted woman. A few sessions later there came an erotized transference dream in which the analyst had a penis, and

> A persistent fantasy of putting her head on my lap developed around the same time. The patient learned to conjure up this fantasy in moments of stress and loneliness and claimed the fantasy was soothing. Often she would modify the fantasy to incorporate genital, sexual and aggressive impulses.
>
> (p. 287)

The erotized transference proper appeared in a dream. The fantasy was an attenuated version of what the dream conveyed. In reading this passage I wondered why the term "claim" was included. Was the analyst suspicious that the fantasy was not really a soothing one? It seems to me that we are not dealing here with erotized transference of the adult type, but rather with the love that Ferenczi discussed. Later in the analysis a split took place between the analyst cathected with negative transference feelings and the image of a lady cathected with libido. The fantasy of the lady had the character of a transitional object. It would be interesting to know whether the split took place for inner reasons or whether it was brought about by the analyst's disbelief in the soothing nature of the fantasy.

There is a deeper problem here for psychoanalytic technique: we wish our analysands to regress. In this case the patient regressed to the fusional symbiotic phase. The patient seemed to have rediscovered the soothing mother. Could this not have been taken as a sign that the good internalized object was about to be refound and would in time be projected onto a partner in real life? It would require further inquiry from the patient, that the fantasy was soothing because it represented regression to the fusional symbiotic phase. If so, it should have received more support from the analyst than the report indicates.

Apparently, a number of women analysts have found that their own analysis with male therapists did not sufficiently prepare them to deal with homosexual transference in their women patients. McDougall (1986) has pointed out that the homosexual strivings in the girl's preoedipal and negative oedipal phases consist of two complementary groups of wishes: the desire to possess the mother and all that the mother has, particularly her breasts; and the wish to be the opposite sex partner, to possess the genitalia of the father. In normal heterosexual development, this early stage with its contradictions is superseded by identification with the mother and rivalry with her for the father; that is, the oedipal phase proper. McDougall (1986) and Wrye and Welles (1989) show that the transition from the earlier to the later phase is not as simple as was assumed in the literature on feminine sexuality. Considerable repression is necessary if the homosexual layer is to be overtaken by the heterosexual one and for the ordinary oedipal phase to triumph. When in the course of analysis a woman patient regresses to this early phase, the woman analyst frequently encounters difficulties that have to be surmounted by an additional self-analysis. McDougall beautifully described a dream of her own that she had to analyze before she could proceed to work productively with her patient. Wrye and Welles likewise speak of complementary dreams countertransferentially evoked in the analyst dealing with such patients.

Person (1985) has pointed out that if this early homosexual level has not been reached in the analysis of women, the attitude toward men remains overidealized, dependent or worshipful; at the same time relationships with women remain problematic. Even more pertinently, she added, "The price may be the perpetuation of low-grade depression or a subjective sense of inauthenticity." These feelings in turn are based on an identification with the bad mother.

Clinical examples from my practice

I now give some examples that emerged in my teaching and control work. In one case, a woman in analysis with another woman developed a strong wish to suck at the analyst's breast. The analyst felt uncomfortable and interpreted the sucking wish as a defense against further free associations. I suggested that it was not possible to know so early whether the wish was based on a defense against free associations or on sexual wishes toward the breast, which in turn could be based on the repression of the symbiotic wish for union with the mother. In the next hour the analyst adopted a more tolerant approach, allowing the patient a greater opportunity to express the erotized wishes. It turned out that yearnings for the union with the mother predominated at that time.

In another case a woman developed an erotized transference to a male analyst. She told him that her father had been seductive in her adolescence, interested in her developing breasts. She also added that the father asked her to pose in the nude in photographs, and on her wedding day kissed her with kisses more becoming to the bridegroom. The analyst correctly connected her seductive behavior with him to these events, but did so in an authoritarian way, without giving the patient a chance to make this discovery on her own. Here too he acted prematurely, because he was himself afraid of the seductive nature of the transference.

In a third case, a woman analysand reported to her male analyst a masturbation fantasy in which she was sucking the penis of a man, but before ejaculation he withdrew and sprayed her face with semen. Here the analyst suggested that the man in the fantasy stood for himself, but did not analyze the fantasy itself. It would have been better to offer a reconstruction that behind the fantasy of the sprayed semen there lurked an unhappy memory, however dim, of a denied breast, which was transformed into a masturbation fantasy. Even if this reconstruction would have proven incorrect, it would have helped diffuse the erotized transference. To introduce into the transference fantasies that occur extratransferentially heightens the erotic component of the transference, and to do so without at the same time interpreting the unconscious meaning of the fantasy itself, leaves sexual arousal without a relieving insight.

One woman ended her analysis, and a few months later called the analyst. She made it clear, however, that she did not wish to pay for the hour. The analyst agreed to meet her for a drink. They met a few times like this; one thing led to another, and they ended by having an affair. During this relationship she realized that the analyst had no wish to divorce his wife and marry his ex-patient. It was only in her second analysis that she realized the fantasy of meeting the analyst after the analysis was completed had been there throughout the analysis, but had never been verbalized. The patient had been married when she entered analysis, but got divorced during the analysis. During the second analysis she realized that she had divorced her husband because she thought the analyst had been attracted to her and would eventually marry her. This fantasy, too, was not expressed. It was only after the analysis was over and she was exposed to the singles scene that she realized her divorce was a mistake. By that time, however, her husband was alienated.

What impressed me was not so much the affair, but the fact that the whole analysis was flawed because the analysand did not verbalize her conscious fantasies about the analyst. The behavior of the analyst after the analysis showed that her belief that the analyst was attracted to her was not pure fantasy; she had only miscalculated the depth of the attraction. The analyst failed the analysand probably because his own attraction prevented him from analyzing more vigorously why she wished to divorce her husband.

Erotized countertransference and countertransference love

I have suggested earlier that one of the varieties of love is falling in love with what one has created oneself. I called it "Pygmalion love." Narcissistic therapists who are incapable of falling in love with persons in the outside world are particularly open to the danger of falling in love with their own patients. By so doing they avoid the danger of rebuff that every lover in the real world must face. And second, they need not overcome their own narcissism, since the patient is, after all, at least in part, their own creation. The analyst who has helped a patient grow in his or her capacity to love beyond the analyst's own abilities will be prone to desire the patient, who has reached a stage he or she never reached. But the opposite is also true. Frustration can also lead to sexualization. Therapists can succumb to the illusion that they can cure by their sexuality what they could not achieve professionally.

Just as erotized transference is not identical to transference love, erotized countertransference is not identical to countertransference love. Erotized countertransference takes place frequently in inhibited therapists who are afraid of rebuffs in the outside world. Nevertheless, there is no denying that countertransference love is a genuine and often deep emotion. As one of my students put it: "The man of my dreams is lying on my couch." The ability of any therapist to treat someone with whom he or she is in love must in the best of circumstances remain limited, since love is not compatible with good reality testing. Conscientious therapists under the pressure of such a conflict often, for conscious or unconscious reasons, terminate the treatment prematurely.

In the last two decades, writings by McDougall (1980) and Chasseguet-Smirgel (1984) have revolutionized our understanding of perversion. (For similarities and differences of view of the two contributors see Whitebook 1991.) We know that a seductive attitude on the part of the parent, whether overt or covert, is conducive to the creation of the feeling that one is the "exception" in the sense in which Freud (1916) and Jacobson (1959) used this term. The exceptions do not recognize the validity of the oedipal taboo and feel compelled to transgress it. They also have failed to develop a superego that prohibits this transgression from within, and are held back only by the fear of punishment. Therapists who belong to this category will exploit their patients sexually and in other ways. Mental health professions must do all they can to eliminate such therapists from their ranks. But these therapists should not be confused with others, who have succumbed to countertransference love, even though the line of demarcation is not always easy to draw.

Since Euripides, the Greek tragedian, the Western world has known that incestuous love can be an overpowering emotion. Countertransference love is often of the incestuous variety. Celenza has described a case of a therapist offender that illuminates such an intrapsychic conflict. I recall that in a symposium on erotized acting out, I ventured to say that the acting-out therapist deserves our understanding as much as our condemnation. I was entirely alone in this point of view. The other speakers, as well as the audience, were only ready to condemn it. It seems that the profession needs a powerful collective defense against this temptation. I quote from Greenacre (1954):

> The (psychoanalytic) relationship is an artificial one, arranged and maintained for the definite purpose of drawing the neurotic reactions into a sharp focus and reflecting them upon the analyst and the analytic situation. It is, therefore, just as necessary to keep the field pure for the clear reflection of the memories emerging from the past, as it is not to contaminate the field of surgical operation, or to avoid getting extraneous dirt into a microscopic slide, which would blur or obscure the important findings, create artifacts and confuse interpretive understanding.
>
> (p. 680)

Although I agree with Greenacre's intention, it seems to me that a human relationship that mobilizes deep unconscious wishes and at times leads to temptation beyond control should not be compared to the clouding of the microscope or precautions taken in a surgical procedure.

Heterosexual women who are in treatment with heterosexual analysts and who develop a homosexually erotized transference belong to a different category. Here the problem is essentially a countertransference one, based on the fact that many women psychoanalysts did not in their own analysis get beyond the heterosexual oedipal level. They have built a reaction formation against their own homosexual yearnings, and therefore have difficulty in going deeper with their patients than their own analyst did with them. This is a general problem in psychoanalysis. Since psychoanalysis is reaching out to more difficult patients, many analysts have, in their own self-analysis, reached layers that were either insufficiently or not at all dealt with in their own analysis.

Discussion

Freud himself was a firm believer in the curative power of transference love. I (Bergmann 1987) have pointed out that in *Delusions and Dreams in Jensen's "Gradiva"* (1907) Freud stated his belief that "cure is accomplished in a relapse into love ... symptoms ... can be resolved and washed away by a fresh high tide of the same passion" (Freud 1907, p. 90). What is striking when we review this literature is that it is written mostly in the language of a one-person psychology: it is the woman who developed those erotized transferences. It is never indicated what the analyst did or did not do, either to provoke this love or to return it to workable channels.

Balint (1935) drew our attention to the fact that while psychoanalysis takes place between two people, the language it employs is that of a one-person psychology. I may add that the one-person psychology had two roots; first, that Freud analyzed himself and therefore used this language, and second, that psychoanalysis wished to emphasize the passive role of the psychoanalyst as being there but not affecting the flow of free associations. The literature on erotized transference has demonstrated, as many other studies have also done, that this is not the case. Bibring (1936) showed that many analyses proceed differently depending on whether the analyst is a man or a woman. In fact, analysts affect the flow of free associations in at least two different ways: first by whether they are male or female and young or old, by the manner of their speech, by the metaphors they use, and by the style of their office and attire; second, by what they select to interpret and what they ignore.

Erotization serves many purposes, one of them being a defense against other instinctual wishes; for example, a heterosexual erotized transference may be a defense against homosexual wishes, or aggressive wishes.

Erotized transference may be a last-ditch defense against the danger of melancholia or against an impending breakdown of the self (Bak 1973). It is of considerable importance for the therapist to discover what is behind the erotized transference. I would add that the need to defend against one affect with another is a sign that the ego is not defending itself by ordinary defense mechanisms, but has reached a more vulnerable stage (Jacobson 1957). The breakdown may already have begun before the analysand entered the analysis. In this case erotized transference represents a desperate attempt to forestall the breakdown by the mobilization of all the libidinal resources at the command of the patient. Such a case is analogous to erotomania that is mobilized to avoid paranoia.

In my experience, the seduction takes place by two very different parents. The first suffer from a lacuna in the superego, and the second are so depressed that seduction is a way of establishing contact with the child. The depressed mothers can relate to the child only briefly by awakening sexual excitement in the child and in themselves (Coen 1981).

In patients developing erotized transference, other problems should also be expected. Because these patients were seduced, they did not have a chance to develop the incest taboo; therefore, their superego does not object to the sexualization of the transference. Reality testing was either insufficiently developed before treatment began or weakened as a result of the treatment. These patients are not aware of the reality consequences of what would happen to them should the seduction be successful. The capacity of the ego of these patients to delay gratification and to sublimate is not sufficiently developed. When the ego's capacity to test reality is weakened, it leads to a loss of the "as if quality" of the analytical relationship. Instead of the analyst being seen as if he or she were the parent, the analyst is experienced in erotized transference as the parent. This is in essence the process that also takes place when transference neurosis becomes a transference psychosis.

Even though transference love is, strictly speaking, evoked by the transference situation, it is still a form of love. The only difference is that therapists and analysands have entered into a contract that whatever feelings are evoked in either one of them – be it love or aggression – will be examined and put in the service of the analysand's therapy. Positive transference may sometimes have a curative effect in that the analysand may, to curry favor, give up some symptomatic behavior. But a cure so obtained turns out to be a broken reed, and the symptoms reappear when transference turns negative. Transference love is only useful if the ego of the analysand has succeeded in sublimating this love for purposes of treatment. If the process of sublimation does not take place or remains very weak, the analysis is in danger of remaining intellectual, in which case it will not become a personal experience and will have little impact. I was often surprised to discover that whenever the real nature of transference love was not denied by the therapist, but clearly identified, the erotized transference subsided markedly. When we make such a statement we approach the analysand from the side of the ego, whereas if we suggest that the sexual wish is a violation of the oedipal taboo, we only increase the guilt feelings of the analysand. All that an analyst need do is insist that the analysand continue analyzing this love. In due time it will become evident whether it is a defense against homosexuality; a re-enactment of the infantile seduction; or from another, unexpected source.

Erotized transference is likely to take place when countertransference feelings have been evoked in the analyst and the analysand has perceived correctly that the attempt to seduce the analyst has some chance of succeeding. In this case the analysand may be carrying out the unconscious wishes of the analyst (Person 1985).

Regarding the handling of the erotized transference, diagnosis is essential, since erotized transference in a psychotic patient can turn so quickly into a paranoia based on the projection of the sexual wishes onto the analyst. In borderline patients with a more intact ego, the analyst must show sufficient concern to convey to the patient that the patient matters, provided this care is not experienced as a seduction. The analyst should also examine whether there was something in what he or she said or did that rightly or wrongly evoked the erotized transference. The analyst should examine the erotized transference from the point of view of a two-person psychology. If the analyst finds that it was something that he or she did, the analyst should help the analysand to discover the point where the erotized transference was evoked. The question itself reduces guilt and directs the attention of the analysand back to the analytic situation. (For a very interesting discussion of the controversy around "conveying love" see Miller and Post 1990.)

If the analyst feels reasonably sure that an erotized transference is not a prelude to a breakdown, I suggest that the analyst allow considerable expression to the erotized transference in order to ascertain whether it is defensive in nature or whether it is in the service of the establishment of symbiotic wishes. Following the idea expressed by Ferenczi in 1929, we may hope that many patients with erotized fantasies will eventually come to see them as fusional symbiotic urges in which the sought-after "good mother" was refound. Even if the role of defense is prominent, we should try to help the analysand uncover the symbiotic core behind the defense. Under favorable conditions, erotized transference can be transformed into symbiotic longings.

Note

1 Originally printed as Bergmann, M.S. (1994) "The Challenge of Erotized Transference to Psychoanalytic Technique," *Psychoanalytic Inquiry*, 14: 499–518. Reprinted by permission of Taylor & Francis, LLC.

References

Bak, R. (1973) Being in Love and Object Loss. *International Journal of Psychoanalysis* 54: 1–8.

Bergmann, M.S. (1987) *The Anatomy of Loving: The Story of Man's Quest to Know What Love Is*. New York: Columbia University Press.

Bibring, G. (1936) A Contribution to the Subject of Transference Resistance. *International Journal of Psychoanalysis* 17: 181–189.

Blanton, S. (1971) *Diary of My Analysis with Sigmund Freud*. New York: Hawthorn Books.

Blum, H. (1973) The Concept of Erotized Transference. *Journal of the American Psychoanalytic Association* 29: 61–76.

Breuer, J. and Freud, S. (1895) Studies on Hysteria. S.E. 2: 1–335.

Chasseguet-Smirgel, J. (1984) *The Ego Ideal: A Psychoanalytic Essay on the Malady of the Ideal*. Trans. P. Barrows. New York: W.W. Norton.

Coen, S.J. (1981) Sexualization as a Predominant Mode of Defense. *Journal of the American Psychoanalytic Association* 29: 395–411.

Eissler, K.R. (1958) Notes on Problems of Technique in the Psychoanalytic Treatment of Adolescents. *Psychoanalytic Study of the Child* 13: 223–254.

Ferenczi, S. (1933) Confusion of Tongues Between Adult and Child. In *Final Contributions to Problems and Methods of Psychoanalysis*, Balint, M., ed. New York: Basic Books, 1955, 156–167.

Freud, S. (1907) Delusions and Dreams in Jensen's "Gradiva." S.E. 9: 7–95.

Freud, S. (1915b) Observations on Transference-Love: Technique of Psycho-Analysis. S.E. 12: 159–171.

Freud, S. (1916) Some Character Types Met with in Psychoanalytic Work. S.E. 14: 309–333.

Greenacre, P. (1954) The Role of Transference: Practical Considerations in Relation to Psychoanalytic Therapy. *Journal of the American Psychoanalytic Association* 21: 671–684.

Greenson, R. (1967) *The Technique and Practice of Psychoanalysis*. New York: International University Press.

Jacobson, E. (1957) Denial and Repression. *Journal of the American Psychoanalytic Association* 5 (no. 1): 61–92.

Jacobson, E. (1959) The Exceptions: An Elaboration of Freud's Character Study. *Psychoanalytic Study of the Child* 14: 135–154.

Keiser, S. (1953), A Manifest Oedipus Complex in an Adolescent Girl. *Psychoanalytic Study of the Child* 8: 99–107.
Lester, E. (1985) The Female Analyst and the Erotized Transference. *Journal of the American Psychoanalytic Association* 66: 283–293.
Mahler, M.S. (1971) A Study of the Separation-Individuation Process and Its Possible Application to Borderline Phenomena in the Psychoanalytic Situation. *Psychoanalytic Study of the Child* 26: 403–424.
McDougall, J. (1980) *A Plea for a Measure of Abnormality*. New York: International Universities Press.
McDougall, J. (1986) Eve's Reflection: On the Homosexual Components of Female Sexuality. In *Between Analyst and Patient*, ed. H. C. Meyers. Hillsdale, NJ: The Analytic Press.
Miller, J.P. and Post, S.L., eds (1990) How Theory Shapes Technique: Perspectives on a Self-Psychological Clinical Presentation. *Psychoanalytic Inquiry* 10: 457–624.
Nunberg, H. (1951) Transference and Reality. *International Journal of Psychoanalysis* 32: 1–9.
Person, E.S. (1985) The Erotic Transference in Women and in Men: Differences and Consequences. *Journal of the American Academy of Psychoanalysis* 13: 159–180.
Rappaport, E. (1956) The Management of an Erotized Transference. *Psychoanalytic Quarterly* 25: 515–527.
Schafer, R. (1977) The Interpretation of Transference and the Condition of Loving. *Journal of the American Psychoanalytic Association* 25: 335–362.
Stern, D.A. (1991) Technical Implications for Certain Types of Erotized Treatment Relationships. *Psychoanalytic Psychology* 8: 463–476.
Swartz, J. (1969) The Erotized Transference and Other Transference Problems. *Psychoanalytic Forum*, 3: 307–318.
Whitebook, J. (1991) Perversion, Destruction, and Reparation: On the Contributions of Janine Chasseguet-Smirgel and Joyce McDougall. *American Imago* 48: 329–350.
Wrye, H.K. and Welles, J.K. (1989) The Maternal Erotic Transference. *International Journal of Psychoanalysis* 70 (4): 673–84.

CHAPTER 5

TERMINATION

The Achilles heel of analysis[1]

The psychoanalytic literature dealing with termination is reviewed in support of the central idea of the author that psychoanalysis, and particularly the literature on technique, has so far failed to offer a paradigm for termination. As a result, psychoanalytic practitioners are left without guidelines as to how to bring the psychoanalytic process to an end. In the second part, the reasons and conditions that are responsible for the clinical fact that many analyses are not self-terminating are discussed. Two main reasons are given: most wishes to terminate are reaction-formation against deeper dependency needs. In the course of a psychoanalysis, these are eliminated as resistance, allowing repressed dependency needs to surface. Genuine wishes for independence are difficult to foster. For many analysands, transference love is the best love relationship that life has offered. Understandably, they are reluctant to give it up. In other analyses, the psychoanalyst has inadvertedly entered into an equilibrium in the analysand's life. This too makes termination difficult. In real life, only death and hostility bring a libidinal relationship to an end. The kind of termination psychoanalysis demands is without precedent.

A historical survey and statement of the problem

In retrospect, we should have been more surprised than we were that Freud's papers on technique never included one on termination. Had we idealized Freud less, we would have realized earlier that psychoanalytic technique lacks anything like a "royal road" toward termination. In the early days of psychoanalysis, there were only two kinds of terminations. Either the analysand interrupted the course of the analysis on his own – an act usually attributed to the analysand's resistance – or the analyst at some unspecified date informed the analysand that the analysis was finished or coming to an end. How many analysands never finish their analysis, we do not know, but we do know that Dorothy Burlingham's (1989) analysis with Sigmund Freud continued for many years, daily, until close to Freud's death.

Hurn (1971) and Blum (1989) concluded that psychoanalysis lacks a paradigm for termination. Blum (1989) found:

> During Freud's lifetime there was an opening and middle phase of clinical analysis. There was no description of a concluding or terminating phase in an otherwise open-ended, timeless analytic process.
>
> (p. 275)

> Termination had not been taught or supervised in analytic training. Prior to 1950 it had been assumed that anyone who could conduct analysis properly could terminate it correctly. A terminated case was not required for institute graduation, nor for certification in the American Psychoanalytic Association. (p. 283)

The first psychoanalysts to address difficulties in termination were Ferenczi and Rank (1924). In keeping with Freud's (1914a) idea that during psychoanalysis the infantile neurosis is transformed into a transference neurosis, they advocated that the analyst should set the termination date the moment this transformation occurs. They believed that only then could a repetition of clinging to the early object be avoided. The termination date must be set this early if fixation on the mother is not to give way to transference fixation. They advocated that analysis must end before it can become a vehicle for the repetition compulsion.

Ferenczi (1928) published the first psychoanalytic article devoted to the process of termination:

> The proper ending of an analysis is when neither the physician nor the patient put an end to it, but when it dies of exhaustion ... A truly cured patient frees himself from analysis slowly but surely; so long as he wishes to come to analysis he should continue to do so ... The patient finally becomes convinced that he is continuing analysis only because he is treating it as a new but still a fantasy source of gratification, which in terms of reality yields him nothing. (Ferenczi 1928, p. 85)

He emphasized that neurotics will relapse into illness after termination as long as reality and fantasy are not rigidly separated.

In subsequent psychoanalytic literature, it was Ferenczi rather than Rank who was always quoted when the desire to return to the womb was considered an important unconscious wish, as one can see today in the writings of Bela Grunberger (1971) and Janine Chasseguet-Smirgel (1986). The type of ending that Ferenczi advocated was revived by Goldberg and Marcus (1985) and called "natural termination."

After the publication of Ferenczi's diary (1988), it is easy to see that Ferenczi's view of termination was already influenced by his feeling of disappointment in his analysis with Freud.

Arlow (1991) believes that Freud's (1937a) "Analysis, Terminable and Interminable" is a contribution to technique. I myself do not see this paper as a guideline towards termination. Rather, it is an argument against Ferenczi's reproach that Freud failed to bring his analysis to a satisfactory conclusion, and a philosophical statement expressing Freud's belief in the death instinct and other forces that limit analyzability. Freud regarded penis envy in women and passivity in men as a "rock bottom" that is immune to psychoanalytic change. In discussing the Wolf Man, Freud noted, "It was a case of treatment inhibiting itself. It was in danger of failing as a result of its partial success" (Freud 1937a, p. 217). Premature terminations happen because the good is the enemy of the better.

In 1937, ego psychology had only recently begun. It is striking to see how much weight Freud assigned to the abnormal ego that treats recovery itself as a danger. He maintained that psychoanalysis achieved its best results when the ego of the patient has not been significantly deformed by the neurotic illness. Mistakenly he thought that this is the case in traumatic neurosis (1937a, p. 220).

In the optimistic phase prior to "Analysis Terminable and Interminable," psychoanalysts were preoccupied with what psychoanalysis should achieve rather than what it can achieve. Nunberg (1930) devoted the last page of his book to the changes that should be brought about through analysis. Termination results when (1) what was hitherto unconscious becomes conscious, (2) the representations of the instinct enter consciousness more easily and consequently the id is under less tension, (3) the ego that does not have to spend energy on defenses becomes stronger, (4) fantastic thinking subject to primary process is replaced by realistic thinking subject to secondary process, (5) the ego is enriched through assimilation of repressed material, and (6) the severity of the superego is mitigated tolerating the repressed. It is not difficult to see that these were idealized statements rather than empirical observations.

In his paper *On the Synthetic Functions of the Ego* (1930), Nunberg stressed that the ego brings the striving of the id into accord with the demands of the superego. In this view, the strengthening of the ego brings peace where intrapsychic conflict had reigned.

Glover (1955) devoted two chapters to the terminal phase. He observed that "the opportunities of watching a classical analysis coming to a classical termination are much less frequent than is generally supposed" (p. 140). The reason such terminations are rare is that many analytic cases never go beyond transference manifestations, and unless a transference neurosis takes hold, a classical termination Glover thought to be impossible. The great majority of analyses end for external reasons, when a symptomatic improvement occurs, or when the patient defeats the analyst in an oedipal struggle expressed in a premature termination.

A somber attitude is found in Waelder's (1960) elementary book on psychoanalysis. He stated:

> If the scientific goal of psychoanalysis is the complete understanding of a person's psychic life, normal and pathological and a complete reconstruction of the development of the personality, no analysis is ever complete. From a therapeutic point of view, when the pathological structures have been understood both dynamically and genetically, if all has been worked through and the psychopathology has disappeared or become controllable, therapeutic termination has been achieved. In actual practice this is not always possible. Psychoanalysis should therefore be terminated when one has reached the point of diminishing returns.
>
> (pp. 242–243)

This echoes Freud's statement (1937a, p. 219) that analysis should terminate when it reaches a stage where no further change could be expected.

In his monograph, *The Theory of Psychoanalytic Technique*, Karl Menninger (1958) devoted the end of a chapter to "the termination of the contract, the separation of the two parties," where he expressed surprise at the vast difference of opinion about the average length of an analysis. He designates as tragic, or even farcical, analyses that last over ten years. In Menninger's view, termination begins when a change of direction has taken place from regression to progression. The love the analysand sought from the analyst he is now ready to seek elsewhere. He recognizes that the analysis did not fulfill his wishes, but did what was needed for him to reach a better understanding of himself.

> I have gotten what I paid for; I can do for myself ... I can endure foregoing what must be foregone and accept and enjoy without guilt such pleasures as are accessible to me.
>
> (Menninger 1958, p. 159)

Most papers on termination discuss what analysis should achieve rather than what it does achieve. Warnings to psychoanalysts abound in this literature. We should beware of "symptomatic cure," "flight into health," and "transference cure."

In the first international congress after the Second World War, an important symposium on termination took place. I have observed that most psychoanalytic schools are initially far more certain of the result they can obtain than they are later in their development. The symposium showed that by that time, ideas of termination were cast in terms of the different schools that had come into existence. Melanie Klein (1950) had emphasized that the analyst is introjected into the analysand as a persecutory as well as an idealized object. The split between the two must diminish if a reliable termination is to be reached. Only then can good objects – as distinguished from idealized objects – be securely established. This view advocates a permanent resolution of the conflict that can withstand the test of time.

Although psychoanalytic ego psychology stressed the significance of attaining secondary ego autonomy and the enlargement of the conflict-free sphere of the ego, Hartmann (1939) lowered the sights by noting that "a healthy person must have the capacity to suffer anxiety and to be depressed" (p. 6). Aarons (1965), following in Hartmann's footsteps, suggested that "the analysand's ego functions must attain a position of maximum secondary autonomy." Similarly, Zetzel (1965) stated that "the analyst as an object for continued object ego identification must be retained within the area of autonomous ego functions" (p. 50).

Under the influence of Arlow and Brenner (1964), the entire vocabulary of the Hartmann era, with its emphasis on secondary autonomy and conflict-free spheres, was pushed aside. The aim of analysis shifted to bring about a change from pathological compromise formation to a relatively healthy one.

Brenner (1976) asked when an analysis should be terminated, or how much one should expect to alter a patient's psychic conflict for the better (p. 173). He answered that it is a question of balancing pros and cons, for symptoms often disappear as do characterological problems, "but psychic conflict that results from instinctual wishes never disappears" (p. 176).

I interpret Brenner's remark to mean that the beneficial results of psychoanalysis cannot be looked upon as a permanent achievement. What has in fact been achieved is a balance of forces that hold true for certain conditions but can be overturned in less favorable ones. Brenner's view mirrors the circumstances of our outer world, for we now believe less in the permanence of any social order.

Within the Brennerian orbit, termination is arbitrary, but the statement that psychic conflict never disappears, although true, must be modified in practical terms. The conflict ceases to be significant when (1) it is no longer expressed in symptoms or character traits, (2) misuse of reality as an arena for the expression of intrapsychic conflict has come to an end, (3) anxiety and depressive affects no longer dominate the intrapsychic picture. This can happen only when the ego, in Nunberg's (1930) earlier formulation, is strong enough to dominate the other intrapsychic agencies. Under Brenner's (1976) influence, we have to recognize that health is not the peaceful state of *Pax Romana*, but the result of a new ego dictatorship over other components of the personality. The power of basic fantasies over a person has been broken, but they still exist and may at some future date rebel against the ego.

Arlow's (1969) growing emphasis on the significance of unconscious fantasy function, and the view that unconscious fantasies are hierarchically organized like different editions of a book around a small number of infantile wishes, also influenced thinking on termination. Abend (1988) urged a greater emphasis on specific fantasies that arise when the termination phase is considered. He suggested that as long as the wish to terminate is fueled by unconscious fantasies, the termination is bound to be premature. He noted, however, that these termination fantasies do not always emerge with sufficient clarity, leaving a residue of primary process fantasies associated with termination.

How can termination best be achieved? Fleming and Benedek (1966), in keeping with the ethos prevalent in the 1960s, emphasized mutual agreement rather than the psychoanalyst setting an arbitrary date. They felt setting a date in advance activated the mourning process, which is the very essence of the termination work. Their views were influential and echoed in subsequent literature.

Most analyses terminate at the end of the analytic year or when the analysand embarks upon a new life goal such as a new job, marriage, or the birth of a child. However, such termination has been criticized as being based on an outer rather than an inner state. Loewald (1962), like Fleming and Benedek, stressed that the replacement of the real analyst by an internalized one can only be achieved through a process of mourning. What needs emphasis is that, without the support and presence of the analyst, mourning may turn into depression or hostility toward the analyst after termination.

A decisive new step in the real world tends to eliminate the mourning process. Because so many analysands cannot terminate, Kubie (1968) suggested that the work of termination be undertaken by a new analyst. To bring psychoanalysis closer to life, many analysts have resorted to a termination based on weaning. Stone (1961) suggested that, in certain cases, the process of weaning be emulated by the gradual reduction of hours.

In an article written in 1969, I suggest that impending termination is often communicated by a dream. In such situations, dreams are reported because the patient can communicate only in code due to inner conflict (p. 363). Following the primary process, a dream can express both a wish to leave and a fear of loss. This was emphasized in a recent book by Bond, Franco and Richards (1992). They devoted a chapter to "indicators of pretermination as revealed in dreams" and another to "the good termination dream."

In summary, there are several reasons the termination date should be set in advance. The first is to wait out the elation often associated with termination and allow the mourning process to be worked through. The second is a growing belief that there are specific primary process fantasies associated with termination that require time to emerge. These fantasies have a tendency to remain repressed until the analysand is convinced he really is terminating. A third function of the termination process is to assist the ego in accepting the reality principle and relinquishing hopes for a glorious termination that is beyond the capacity of the ego (Orens 1955).

I am fully aware that no historical survey can be free from the bias of the summarizer. My aim in citing the literature was to confirm that psychoanalysis never developed the technique of termination to the same level as transference analysis or analysis of defenses. If my argument is convincing, then my title "The Achilles heel" is justified.

Why psychoanalysis need not be a self-terminating process

Psychoanalysis is the only significant human relationship that terminates abruptly. In real life, we encounter three types of termination of human relationships: geographical separation, transformation of a friendly or love relationship into a hostile one, and death. The analysand, however, is supposed to bring about separation under conditions of love and gratitude. All life experience runs against such a termination. To be sure, the child separates from the parent, but this separation occurs in stages and is never complete. Psychoanalysis makes demands of internalization that are not asked for in any other human relationship.

By analyzing defenses, the analytic process eliminates the neurotic wishes to terminate; the analysis exposes fear of reliance on the analyst, a host of paranoid fears, and finally works through the fear of many analysands that they will be forsaken. When this stage of security and trust is reached, a passive regression within the analysis becomes possible. We can then hope for a new beginning with a genuine nondefensive separation process. In practical terms, it is easier to terminate an analysis if the possibility of a newer love relationship or a reordering of an older love relationship is realistically possible. When this is not the case, termination is more difficult.

There are analysands for whom transference love, in spite of its lack of physical intimacy, is the best love relationship they ever had because of the potentialities for fantasy and idealization. When at some point the analyst feels no new insights are forthcoming and pressures the analysand to terminate, the analysis may terminate but the analysand quickly seeks a new analyst so the state of transference love can continue.

I have indicated (Bergmann 1987) that the selection of a love object depends on two different capacities: the capacity to combine the refinding of an old love object with the capacity to hope that the new love object will heal the wounds the old one has inflicted, as well as the ego's capacity to tolerate a compromise formation where the selected object is good enough, even though it falls short of all one's wishes. When neither the first nor the second condition is attainable, transference love will be preferred to love in real life.

Under such conditions, there is great pressure on the analysand to start a new analysis. Given that analysts today are divided into warring schools, the analysand is likely to find a sympathetic analyst of a different school who will agree that the limitations of his previous analysis were due to the previous analyst's school. New hope is kindled, and a new beginning will be made that may or may not result in a better termination.

In a previous publication (Bergmann 1988), I observed that Annie Reich (1958) was the first to recognize that transference may not always be resolvable. This is true when the analyst represents "the first really reliable object relationship in the patient's life" (p. 236). In many cases, the state of transference love may not successfully translate into a capacity to love in real life. Because the analyst makes fewer demands on the analysand than persons in real life, and asks for less reciprocity, many people can develop transference love but are incapable of translating it into real life. I (Bergmann, 1988) further noted:

> Every analysand enters analysis with some combination of primary process fantasies of what the analysis will accomplish and realistic secondary process realizable hopes. As the transference deepens and transference neurosis gains

> in strength, the primary processes become increasingly important. However, the decision to terminate is by its very nature a secondary process decision. (p. 149)

We have learned from Freud (1905d, p. 222) that all findings are refindings. To the extent to which the analyst has become "a primary love object," the analysand, upon termination, may look to refind a love object modeled after the analyst. Such a transfer may or may not be appropriate from the point of view of the ego; for example, when an analyzed woman finds a much older person because the analyst was old. Dewald (1982) stressed that successful termination requires the process of mourning on the part of the analysand as well as the analyst. A too-early refinding of a new object often results if the analysand is trying to avoid the mourning process. Novick (1982) deepened our understanding of the termination process when he stated: "It is not the analyst as a real or transference object who is relinquished and mourned, but a part of the self, often the infantile self which is guiltily discarded." Loewald (1988) also stressed mourning as the key to termination. But he added the observation that in some cases the transference neurosis comes into full bloom under the pressure of the vacillation to terminate or not to terminate. For at that moment the past becomes acutely alive. It is during this period of threatening termination that passive homosexual wishes may emerge for the first time. Thus, the prolonged analysis that never reaches the termination phase shields the analysand from many painful feelings and deepening insights.

If we move from a one-person psychology to a two-person psychology, as Balint (1969) suggested, we will note that both analysts and analysands must contend with two opposing forces. The first is the struggle against a utopian solution – the high expectation that both have about what psychoanalysis ought to achieve rather than what it realistically can achieve. The other and opposite danger is a premature loss of faith, as succumbing to a depression or a sense of defeat before the repetition compulsion. Both patient and analyst may be in danger of bowing prematurely before the power of the repetition compulsion; or of the superego of the analysand that does not permit progression beyond a certain point. Often, this point is reached when the analysand senses that his capacity for enjoying life or success has gone past what the analyst has achieved. An analysand may terminate the analysis out of fear of an oedipal victory. Cases of such clinical stalemates are frequently discussed in supervision and clinical seminars. New insights into a case gained by the therapist often bring about a new hope of curability.

We should differentiate between preconditions for psychoanalysis and preconditions for termination of analysis. Many analysands develop the capacity for free association, are capable of expressing and utilizing transference interpretations, and do well in analyzing their dreams. Yet they are unable to terminate because the preconditions for termination are very different from those for analyzability. Unfortunately, we cannot judge ahead of time whether a given analysand will develop the capacity to replace the analyst by self-analysis and continue his inner development after termination. Our theory assumes that the analyst is a fantasy object, and when the power of fantasy recedes, real objects offering mutuality and real gratification will be sought, but this is not always true in all situations.

I wish to emphasize one further aspect of the problem that has not, to my knowledge, been discussed in the literature on termination. Most patients seek psychotherapy or psychoanalysis when a pre-existing equilibrium in their lives has ended for outer or inner reasons. The disequilibrium has evoked feelings of anxiety or depression, and analytic help is sought because the patient alone cannot find a new balance. It happens quite frequently that the analysis itself helps establish an equilibrium.

For example, an analysand enters analysis because of unbearable marital conflict or because of conflict between the marriage and extramarital relationships. The analysis establishes a new equilibrium, and instead of extramarital relationships, the analysand now finds that he or she can tolerate the marriage, provided the complaints about the marital partner and some of the love feelings frustrated in the marriage can be directed toward the analyst. The analyst as the other love object is more acceptable and safer than an extramarital love object. When this situation is not understood, or even if it is understood and subject to psychoanalysis, it may still happen that the restoration of a new equilibrium without the analyst's participation is beyond the capacity of analyst and patient to achieve. This can result in a prolonged analysis or, if the analysis is terminated, the pre-existing analytic equilibrium demands refinding. Because human perfection is never obtained, the analysand will seek the lost equilibrium by a new analysis.

In the hopeful cases, it is the new ego, as Nunberg (1930) has foreseen, that brings about termination in its quest for a richer life after termination. But we may not always be able to effect this. The ego's capacity to bring about termination is a new and highly complex ego function that must be implanted, nurtured and supported by the analyst throughout the duration of the analysis. Freud (1937a) recognized many of the forces that limited the power of psychoanalysis. To these we must add another: the inability of many to acquire the necessary ego strength for termination. If we do not succeed in fostering this capacity, we face the danger of the sorcerer's apprentice, who can cast the spell but does not know how to bring the magic he has evoked to an end.

Particularly difficult, but also deeply moving, are the former analysands who return to us when they are confronted with terminal illness. Now the aim is no longer cure, but to die in close relationship with a person who did not disappoint the analysand. Such returns, which incidentally occur more frequently when the analyst himself grows older, represent the final battle between libido and aggression. As the life force itself begins to ebb, these returning analysands have convinced me with particular force that the analyst remains the libidinal object often of last resort.

In spite of the large literature on termination, no paradigm of termination has been made part of the professional equipment of the psychoanalytic practitioner. In this absence, the psychoanalyst is under the pressure of his superego to terminate treatment, often prematurely, to escape the inner accusation that he exploits the analysand for libidinal or financial purposes. At the same time, he is under the opposite pressure, based on the idealization of psychoanalysis, that more would have been achieved had he or she been more experienced or knowledgable. Though there are general signs that the analysand has entered the termination phase, the termination moment is still a matter of art rather than science. Some analysts and analysands are better at guessing when the optimal point has been reached than others. Premature terminations and unproductively prolonged analyses cannot, at the present time at least, be avoided.

Acknowledgments

For the ideas expressed in this article, I alone am responsible. But I owe a debt of gratitude to my participation in the seminar on prolonged analysis conducted under the sponsorship of the Psychoanalytic Research and Development Fund. I express my gratitude to its chairman, Dr. Sidney Furst, and the participating doctors, Joseph Coltrera, Eleanor Galenson, Alexander Grinstein, Philip Herschenfeld, Deanna Holtzman, Daniel Jacobs, Peter Neubauer, Henry Nunberg, Mortimer Ostow, Bernard Pacella, Leo Stone, Arthur Valenstein, and the late Annamarie Weil.

Note

1 Originally published in Bergmann, M.S. (1997) "Termination: The Achilles Heel of Psychoanalytic Technique," *Psychoanalytic Psychology*, 14 (2): 163–174. http://dx.doi.org/10.1037/h0079713. Copyright © 1997 American Psychological Association. Reproduced with permission.

References

Aarons, Z. (1965) On Analytic Goals and Criteria for Termination. *Bulletin of the Philadelphia Association for Psychoanalysis* 15: 97–109.

Abend, S.M. (1988) Unconscious Fantasies and Issues of Termination. In H. Blum *et al.*, eds. *Unconscious Fantasy, Myth and Reality*. Madison, CT: International Universities Press.

Arlow, J.A. (1969) Unconscious Fantasy and Disturbances of Conscious Experience. *Psychoanalytic Quarterly* 38: 1–27.

Arlow, J.A. (1991) Perspective on Freud's "Analysis Terminable and Interminable" after 50 Years. In *On Freud's "Analysis terminable and interminable,"* J. Sandler, ed. New Haven, CT: Yale University Press, pp. 73–88.

Arlow, J. and C. Brenner (1964) *Psychoanalytic Concepts and the Structural Theory*. New York: International Universities Press, Inc.

Balint, M. (1969) Trauma and Object Relationship. *International Journal of Psychoanalysis* 50: 429–437.

Bergmann, M.S. (1987) *The Anatomy of Loving: The Story of Man's Quest to Know What Love Is*. New York: Columbia University Press.

Bergmann, M.S. (1988) On the Fate of the Intrapsychic Image of the Psychoanalyst After Termination of the Analysis. *Psychoanalytic Study of the Child* 43: 137–153.

Blum, H.P. (1989) The Concept of Termination and the Evolution of Psychoanalytic Thought. *Journal of the American Psychoanalytic Association* 37: 275–295.

Bond, A., Franco, D. and Richards, A. (1992) *Dream Portrait: A Study of Nineteen Sequential Dreams as Indicators of Pretermination*. Madison, CT: International Universities Press.

Brenner, C. (1976) *Psychoanalytic Technique and Psychic Conflict*. New York: International Universities Press.

Burlingham, M.J. (1989) *The Last Tiffany: A biography of Dorothy Tiffany Burlingham*. New York: Atheneum.

Chasseguet-Smirgel, J. (1986). *Sexuality and Mind: The Role of the Father and the Mother in the Psyche*. New York: New York University Press.

Dewald, P.A. (1982) The Clinical Importance of the Termination Phase. *Psychoanalytic Inquiry* 2: 441–461.

Ferenczi, S. (1928) The Problem of Termination of the Analysis. In *Final Contributions to Problems and Methods of Psychoanalysis*, Balint, M., ed. New York: Basic Books, 1955, 77–86.

Ferenczi, S. (1988) *The Clinical Diary of Sándor Ferenczi*, ed. J. Dupont. Cambridge, MA: Harvard University Press.

Ferenczi, S. and Rank, O. (1924) *Entwicklungsziele der Psychoanalyse: Zur Wechselbeziehung von Theorie und Praxis*. Leipzig: Internationaler Psychoanalytischer Verlag.

Fleming, J. and Benedek, T. (1966) *Psychoanalytic Supervision*. New York: Grune & Stratton.

Freud, S. (1905d) Jokes and Their Relation to the Unconscious. S.E. 8: 9–236.

Freud, S. (1914a) Remembering, Repeating and Working Through. S.E. 12: 145–156.

Freud, S. (1937a) Analysis, Terminable and Interminable. S.E. 23: 211–253.
Glover, E. (1955) *The Technique of Psychoanalysis*. New York: International Universities Press.
Goldberg, A. and Marcus, D. (1985) "Natural Termination": Some Comments on Ending Analysis without Setting a Date. *Psychoanalytic Quarterly* 54:46–65.
Grunberger, B. (1971) *Narcissism*. New York: International Universities Press.
Hartmann, H. (1939) Psychoanalysis and the Concept of Health. In *Essays on Ego Psychology*. New York: International Universities Press, 3–18.
Hurn, H.T. (1971) Toward a Paradigm of the Terminal Phase: The Current Status of the Terminal Phase. *Journal of the American Psychoanalytic Association* 19: 332–348.
Klein, M. (1950) On the Criteria for Termination of a Psychoanalysis. In *Envy and Gratitude and Other Works*. New York: Delacorte, 43–47.
Kubie, L.S. (1968) Unsolved Problems in the Resolution of the Transference. *Psychoanaytic Quarterly* 37: 331–352.
Loewald, H. (1962) Internalization, Separation, Mourning, and the Superego. *Psychoanalytic Quarterly* 31: 483–504.
Loewald, H. (1988) Termination Analyzable and Unanalyzable. *Psychoanalytic Study of the Child* 43: 155–166.
Menninger, K.A. (1958) *Theory of Psychoanalytic Technique*. New York: Basic Books.
Novick, J. (1982) Termination: Themes and Issues. *Psychoanalytic Inquiry* 2: 329–365.
Nunberg, H. (1930) The Synthetic Functions of the Ego. In *Practice and Theory of Psychoanalysis*. New York: International Universities Press, 120–136.
Orens, M. (1955) Setting a Termination Date: An Impetus to Analysis. *Journal of the American Psychoanalytic Association* 3: 661–665.
Reich, A. (1958) A Special Variation on Technique. In *Psychoanalytic Contributions*. New York: International Universities Press, 236–249.
Stone, L. (1961) *The Psychoanalytic Situation: An Examination of its Development and Essential Nature*. New York: International Universities Press.
Waelder, R. (1960) *Basic Theory of Psychoanalysis*. New York: International Universities Press.
Zetzel, E.R. (1965) The Theory of Therapy in Relation to a Developmental Model of the Psychic Apparatus. *International Journal of Psychoanalysis* 46: 39–52.

CHAPTER 6

PSYCHOANALYSIS IN OLD AGE

The patient and the analyst[1]

My admission

Before I begin, I have to tell you that this chapter has a special significance for me. It is an admission paper to a very exclusive club called "Gerontocracy" – those who have remained creative in old age. So far, its members are Sophocles, Goethe, Verdi, Bertrand Russell and George Bernard Shaw. Since I am one hundred years old, I am entitled to membership, but only if this chapter is good enough.

The current economic meltdown has made it clear that we live in a society that cannot plan. The marriage between capitalism and democracy is in trouble. The current problem of old age has a sociological aspect. Progress in medicine has prolonged life beyond expectation, but our social capacity to make these last years productive – or at least tolerable – has lagged significantly behind the capacity of medicine to keep old people alive.

Old age is often associated with illness, loneliness and bereavement. As a result, many middle-aged men and even more women spend a great deal of their life's energy taking care of those aging parents. "Honor thy father and thy mother" has become a burdensome commandment. After decades of separation, parent and child are now once more in very close contact. Wounds of infancy that have not completely healed are often reopened and oedipal conflicts reawakened. A large literature within psychoanalysis and in popular culture has emerged describing the horror of old age. I do not wish to contribute to this literature. The aged and aging population offers a professional challenge to psychoanalytic therapy, and I want to examine this challenge. This vast caretaking population often requires what we are accustomed to call supportive psychotherapy to help alleviate their burden, but this therapy will not be the subject of this chapter.

The older patient population falls into two groups: those so burdened by what old age brought that they need support, and those who need and can achieve new insight and some change. Fortunately, there are therapists willing to give patients in the first group support, but we do not ask these patients to be capable of intra-psychic change. It is important that we do not confuse the two populations and the two tasks.

The older patient in analysis

Freud, it is well known, did not believe that older people should be analyzed. In *Sexuality in the Aetiology of the Neuroses*, published in 1898 (before *The Interpretation of Dreams*), he says:

> Psycho-analytic therapy is not at present applicable to all cases. It has, to my knowledge, the following limitations. It demands a certain degree of maturity and understanding in the patient and is therefore not suited for the young or for adults who are feeble-minded or uneducated. It also fails with people who are very advanced in years, because, owing to the accumulation of material in them, it would take up so much time that by the end of the treatment they would have reached a period of life in which value is no longer attached to nervous health. (p. 282)

Freud feared that their analysis would only lead to the recognition of past mistaken and lost opportunities, without the capacity to use this new knowledge gained by psychoanalysis for new and more productive ends. He feared that under such conditions, the analysis would not "pay for itself." I find this attitude of Freud's too commercial, as if psychoanalysis has to be financially profitable to be worth the effort and expense. Instead, I have adopted the slogan of the shipping industry when they were competing with transatlantic airlines: "Getting there is half the fun." Psychoanalysis should return benefits from the first hour when the patient meets the analyst who knows how to listen, not condemn, and who knows that he or she must know a great deal about a patient before venturing an opinion or an interruption. Or, to put it in the language of the structural phase, we know now that insights obtained in the course of an analysis can be appropriated by the superego to punish the patient for opportunities lost; they can also be grabbed by the id and lead to acting out, or be used by the ego to master past traumatic events. Which one of the three possibilities takes place will not depend on age but on the patient's psychic structure and the analyst's skill. As therapists, we are responsible for delivering our understanding in such a way that the patient's ego can make use of them and not for the superego to attack the patient or for the id to endanger the patient by acting upon the revelations. We must make sure our interpretations are of use to the ego and not subject to the commands of the id or the superego.

Having said all that against Freud, he is not so easily dismissed. As we get older, we become more dependent on the very environment we have created. A couple may be unhappy together, but they have a house they are attached to, they have children and pets in common, and a circle of friends they fear losing. They fear the empty house, the loss of the caretaker in illness, and that they do not have enough libido for a new relationship. So let us assume that after due deliberation the analysand decides that no change is possible. Does that mean the whole endeavor had been for naught? The American ethos would be inclined to say yes. I would argue that there is a difference between having examined the situation constructively, and having reached a decision that no change is possible and having been afraid to attempt this examination. The issue is whether the examined life is richer than living in fear of such an examination. Psychoanalysis has its roots in the conviction that the examined life, regardless of whether it was fulfilling or not, is richer than a life in which such an examination was not undertaken out of the fear that such an endeavor would result in depression.

The termination of analysis has always been an interest of mine and I have written two papers on this subject, but lately I have terminated some cases where the patients, after analysis, decided not to break up a long and difficult marriage. Such endings are difficult for both patients and analysts. Such terminations are not associated with a sense of joy and achievement, but even under such conditions the examination of one's life and facing reality without the need to repress or deny is, in my experience, worthwhile.

One of the main characteristics of old age is the disappearance of the future as a dimension. We are not always aware of it, but our lives consist of remembering or reanimating the past, a sense of the present, and hopes for the future. In old age the future as a dimension disappears, and there is nothing to hope for. The loss of the future tends to accentuate the past, popularly known as "memory lane." This compulsory re-examination, this looking back, can often become needlessly painful. There is much to be said in favor of not undertaking this re-examination alone, but rather with a benign and objective therapist. The therapist's main function in the examination of the life lived is to not allow it to fall under the domination of the superego and result in a depression.

I have noticed that as I have gotten older, my patients have also gotten older. What are the problems of the patients who seek our help in their upper sixties and beyond? If my practice is any guide, and if we exclude those who have been hit by cruel old age and largely need supportive therapy (that is, ordinary aging men and women), the most prevalent problem is the relationship to their adult children. Often, their children are clinging and unable to move away from home into a world that appears too strange, too hostile, or too rejecting. In other words, neither they nor their parents have mastered the final step of separation. Many of these children have become accusatory or hostile, without the capacity to move away. One benefit of analyzing older patients is that their relationship to their adult children may undergo a change for the better. I have observed that an analysis of an older patient results in a different strategy in dealing with them than that used for children or younger patients.

The next problem of this population is in the sphere of love. In a long marriage, the formerly romantic partner often becomes either parent or child, but is no longer the sexual partner: For the woman, the husband has increasingly become a father figure; for the man, the wife becomes a mother figure. In these cases, the incest taboo has caught up with the couple. Freud visualized the Oedipus complex as the kernel of the infantile neurosis: if it is not overcome in childhood, it threatens adult sexuality by transferring the oedipal taboo to the adult relationship. The oedipal taboo will manifest itself in impotence, premature ejaculation or frigidity, or in a cessation of sexual intercourse. In long relationships, therefore, the partners are in danger of being transformed from sexual lovers into each other's parents. Thus, after many years, the oedipal taboo that may have been successfully overcome returns. Husbands slip and call their wives by their mother's name, and women refer to their husbands by their children's name. Psychoanalytic help may be necessary to prevent such a return of the Oedipus complex and the incest taboo. When this help is not available or fully successful, a new love relationship may be sought, which often creates new guilt. I remember one of these patients realizing, "My trouble is I have a woman I love and the other woman I cannot live without.." Psychoanalytic work revealed that the wife became the early mother, without whom the patient could not exist, while the other woman could be loved because she represented the mother after separation. Both were mother figures who stood in for the mother at different periods of the man's life. Once this dichotomy was understood, the choice could be made. It is characteristic of the primary processes that the same wishes for two different aspects of the mother type can be activated at the same time.

Existential patients

I come now to another category of older patients, whom, for lack of a better term, I will designate as "existential patients." Their basic complaint is that they have not lived their lives fully, and do not want to die without having fully lived.

Here we often see a degree of depersonalization, as if somebody else has been living their lives. Often, sexual inhibitions are involved, or there is an excessive need to please others. Psychoanalytically speaking, we can see in these patients an excessive use of ego defense mechanisms, which have become too expensive and strong and have exacted so much energy from the person that the feeling of aliveness was jeopardized. Our society, with its emphasis on success, may have contributed to this problem. As life comes to its end and there is nothing left to conquer, this feeling that life was partly or largely wasted can become overwhelming. Such patients need our help to mourn, for they have not allowed themselves this experience. In summary, the older patient often needs our help and we can make the difference between a deepening intrapsychic conflict in old age and one that can be mastered.

The prospect of retirement is often the reason why elderly people need therapy. Work offers all of us certain gratifications. A workplace is often an outlet for needs to love or be loved, and for many people it is also an outlet for aggression. To be suddenly deprived of this outlet will disturb the inner equilibrium and require therapeutic help. I am familiar with a case in which a woman looked forward to retirement as a chance to explore foreign countries, but upon retirement discovered that her husband was afraid of flying. In another instance, a manufacturer was very successful financially, having worked very hard since he was in his teens; his work was synonymous with his life. Now it is time for retirement. Should he sell his factory or give it to his workers as a cooperative? Or should he give it to some relatives for whom he never cared? And what will he do if he does not get up every morning to go to work? To the wife, being together with an ever-anxious, repetitive husband is boring and being together twenty-four hours a day is unbearable. She needs analysis to find new ways of sublimation.

In a third example, a man who held an important political position ten years ago, but has since experienced painful political defeats is now reaching eighty years old. He fears a depression is coming, based on a reliving of his defeats in reality and in his dreams. A few years ago, when newly discovered drugs were hailed as the solution to depression, many thousands of people were put on a combination of medications – but the limitation of this solution has now been experienced and the need for therapy in old age is more urgent.

The fear of death

Psychoanalytic patients, and even patients undergoing psychotherapy that is modeled on psychoanalysis, become acquainted with Freud's "basic rule." They know they are supposed to say everything that comes to mind, censoring nothing that occurs to them. When the analyst is aging, what occurs to them all too often is the fear of the analyst's death. If my own experience is any guide, this need not be detrimental to the therapist. Dealing with one's own death from the point of view of a number of patients tends to objectify it and make it less personal.

Freud differentiated between primary processes and secondary processes. Secondary processes obey Aristotelian logic and accept the reality principle, while primary processes follow the pleasure principle and disregard the reality principle. Nowhere is the difference between the two processes more prominent than in the attitude towards death. The secondary processes tell us that everything that is alive is destined to die; only the inanimate does not die. To be alive means to be born, to develop and grow old, and eventually to die. The primary processes do not accept this inevitability, however. One of my patients has special difficulty in accepted that at one moment one is alive, but at the next moment one is not. When analysts are old a certain fear of their death has to be regarded as normal. Only if it goes beyond a certain degree, or when it serves as a defense against either the transference or as a defense against the treatment process as such, should we call it into question.

A different problem is presented by those patients who fear, and cannot come to terms with, their own deaths. Here the primary processes have gained dominance. When patients suffer from insomnia we usually say that we sleep well when we are unconsciously in contact with our internalized good objects, and cannot sleep well when we are under the sway of our internalized bad objects. Something similar goes on when the fear of one's own death is powerful: one fears being overwhelmed by these internalized bad objects. Narcissism also plays a role; one cannot tolerate that the party (life) can go on undisturbed even when one can participate no longer.

As to my own philosophy of life and death, I no longer remember when I first realized that the two belong together. Only what is alive can and must die; the inanimate alone knows no death. Some butterflies live only a few hours, while the redwoods in California live hundreds of years; but everything that lives is subject to death. We are the only species that knows death is inevitable, and yet history shows that we have done so very much to deny this knowledge, beginning with the Egyptian pyramids and up to the belief in an afterlife and heaven and hell. All are denials of the simple fact that life is final. Why is it, then, that we encounter patients who are afraid of death, or that we ourselves are afraid? Think of Hamlet's famous soliloquy, "To be, or not to be":

> To sleep: perchance to dream: ay, there's the rub;
> For in that sleep of death what dreams may come
> When we have shuffled off this mortal coil,
> Must give us pause.
>
> (Act III, Scene I: 65–68)

What happened to Hamlet happens to some of our patients: the denial of death has backfired and become transformed into a fear of the afterlife.

Why is it that some people can accept death as inevitable and life as final, while others cannot? Why is it that some people do not mind donating their corpse to a hospital for residents to learn how to operate, while others cannot? If my clinical experience is any guide, it is our capacity to have good internal objects that enables us to accept death, and here it is helpful if as children we were wanted by our parents, particularly the mother.

It is very much to the credit of psychoanalysis that it had something new to say on this subject. We sleep well and are rested in the morning when we sleep with our good objects, which love us and wish us well. We are restless, have nightmares, and are tired in the morning when we have slept with our bad objects. Hamlet's fear of death turns out to be the fear of the power of bad objects. In contrast to Hamlet, I cite *Because I Could Not Stop for Death* (1890), one of the poems I cherish by Emily Dickinson; here are the first eight lines from the first published version:

> Because I could not stop for Death,
> He kindly stopped for me;
> The carriage held but just ourselves
> And Immortality.

We slowly drove, he knew no haste,
And I had put away
My labor, and my leisure too,
For his civility.

We thank the poet for her capacity to transform her fear of death into these wonderful lines. What Emily Dickinson did in this poem has a psychoanalytic term: she libidinized death. Note the line, "The carriage held but just ourselves." To the poet, death has become a monogamous lover. This is not an outright denial of death, but by transforming death into a romantic companion, it is a form of denial. Freud did something similar in his 1913 paper, *The Theme of the Three Caskets*:

> We might argue that what is represented here are the three inevitable relations that a man has with a woman – the woman who bears him, the woman who is his mate and the woman who destroys him; or that they are the three forms taken by the figure of the mother in the course of a man's life – the mother herself, the beloved one who is chosen after her pattern, and lastly the Mother Earth who receives him once more. But it is in vain that an old man yearns for the love of woman as he had it first from his mother; the third of the Fates alone, the silent Goddess of Death, will take him into her arms.
>
> (Freud 1913a, p. 301)

Freud personified death as a mother figure, but in Western art death is usually represented as a jealous man who separates the happy lovers. In The Bible, when a man dies, he is "assembled unto his fathers," not his mothers.

There is no goddess of death who takes us into her arms. I admit that it is not likely that I will ever persuade my unconscious to accept what I just told you, that life and death are intertwined and cannot be separated. My dreams tell me that in my unconscious I have not even accepted the death of my parents.

In an often-quoted passage in *Beyond the Pleasure Principle* (1920), Freud felt "compelled" to say, "The aim of life is death and looking backward, that inanimate things existed before living ones" (p. 38). The hidden difficulty here is in understanding what Freud means by the word *aim,* which might be closer to what we would call *direction.* I aimed (intended) to get this paper published, but it is not in the same sense that the aim (direction) of my life is death. I do not believe that the organic living world has a wish to return to the inorganic, as Freud thought. The Darwinian view of the survival of the fittest speaks against it, but older folks can also develop a desire for it, perhaps because it is an aim of life. However, psychoanalysis considers those who wish to die as depressed and suicidal, and regards these wishes as pathological. If the aim of life is death, then depression should be a normal, expectable state. It is surprising that after the concept of the death instinct was formulated, the question of depression was not re-examined. Once more Shakespeare extends his hand:

Falstaff: I would it were bed-time, Hal, and all well.
Prince: Why, thou owest God a death.
Falstaff: 'Tis not due yet: I would be loath to pay him before his day.
What need I be so forward with him that calls not on me?

(*Henry IV, Part I,* Act V, Scene I: 125–128)

In this matter, I side with Falstaff rather than Freud. We need not be forward with death; death is not the aim of our lives. But regardless of what our primary processes whisper to us, our secondary processes tell us that life and death are intertwined; neither one exists without the other. Freud (1900), citing this quote by Shakespeare, made the famous slip, "*Du bist der Natur einen Tod schulding*" ("you owe nature a death") (p. 205). Two pages later, "since life is short and death inevitable" (p. 207) leads Freud to the Latin "*carpe diem*" ("seize the day").

Practicing as an elderly analyst

We owe to Ferenczi's article *The Unwanted Child and the Death Instinct* (1929) the insight that human babies do not enter life with a strong instinct to survive. We have to be persuaded by the mother's love that life is worthwhile, and for the rest of our life we remain dependent on love to successfully combat the death instinct in us, hence the permanent fear of succumbing to depression. In old age, death is always near, something like a neighbor. It falls to the ego both to resist the fear of death and the attraction of it.

In a symposium not so very long ago, I thanked the profession of psychoanalysis for protecting me from "the swimming pools of Florida" when my co-speaker told the audience, "I just bought an apartment in Florida." Only half jokingly, I said, "We analysts can never retire; it takes us so very long to become any good."

The other change is that the anonymity of the analyst has changed. New patients look us up on the internet, and some even look for who my father was. The waiting room is no longer just a waiting room but now a cell phone zone. In the past my patients came because they wanted to be analyzed; now it is more common for them to come to me for a more personal relationship rather than to be "merely" analyzed.

With these preliminaries out of the way, I believe I can point to two major differences that are due to old age. Eroticized transference, which caused so much trouble for Freud (1915b), does not appear except in the latent content of dreams. However, the most important difference is the frequency with which the fear of my death appears. Sometimes this is the main theme, hour after hour. It is difficult for patients to bring this topic up, but the demand to free associate – to say everything that occurs to them – leaves them no choice. Many times, I find this preoccupation helpful in making my death more objective, but at times it can be difficult to hear, particularly when the theme repeats itself in many sessions on the same day.

It is important to help patients recognize that in our unconscious, death is not a biological necessity but a desertion, to say, "If I die I am not leaving you, I just cease to exist. Death is not a desertion." Both my patients and I myself need to hear this.

I once more call upon Shakespeare; King Lear expresses his wish to retire from responsibilities thus:

> To shake all cares and business from our age,
> Conferring them on younger strengths while we
> Unburdened crawl toward death.
>
> (Act I, Scene I: 37–39)

Lear, like many old men, experiences life as a burden, and the phrase "crawl toward death" implies that he equates future retirement with a return to infancy. Shakespeare does not give this abdication wish a happy ending, and for a very interesting reason. As the fool tells him, "thou madest thy daughters / thy mothers" (Act I, Scene IV: 156–157). In psychoanalytic language, Lear's abdication wish has activated his oedipal wishes, with his daughters replacing his mother. In my experience, this wish to regress is stronger in men than in women. Some men see retirement as equivalent to carefree childhood and the days when there was yet no obligation to work, and as a result they were free from superego pressure.

The idea of retirement seems to be a combination of two very different trends of thought. The first is that old age makes effective work more difficult. We retire because we cannot perform as well as we used to. Tasks that were easy when we were young become difficult in old age. However, there is also another idea: that work itself is a burden. We get paid for work because it is opposed to the pleasure principle. Here we encounter some important differences. Artists are supposed to love their work; that is why it is so hard to unionize musicians: they love to play even if they are not being paid. In psychoanalytic terms, when work itself yields pleasure we can call it sublimation. Our language also acknowledges a third group, workaholics, people who work not because they enjoy it but because not working evokes in them anxiety or depression. Where do we, therapists, stand? With artists or with those who consider work a burden? The contribution I can make to this discussion is that our work becomes more pleasurable as we get older. The work of therapy is difficult if we do not know what to do; our work becomes more enjoyable as we increasingly master our trade. We also develop our personal style only over time, and this brings us closer to being artists.

Note

1 This chapter was originally published as M.S. Bergmann, "Psychoanalysis in Old Age: The Patient and the Analyst," *Clinical Implications of the Psychoanalyst's Life Experience: When the Personal Becomes Professional* (2013), ed. Steven Kuchuck, New York: Routledge. Reprinted by permission of Taylor & Francis Group, LLC.

References

Ferenczi, S. (1929) The Unwelcome Child and His Death Instinct. In *Final Contributions to the Problems and Methods of Psychoanalysis*, ed. Balint, M. New York: Basic Books, 1955, 102–107.

Freud, S. (1898) Sexuality in the Aetiology of the Neuroses. S.E. 3: 261–285.

Freud, S. (1900) The Interpretation of Dreams, Part I and Part II. S.E. 4–5: 1–625.

Freud, S. (1913a) The Theme of the Three Caskets. S.E. 12: 291–301.

Freud, S. (1915b) Observations on Transference-Love: Technique of Psycho-Analysis. S.E. 12: 159–171.

Freud, S. (1920) Beyond the Pleasure Principle. S.E. 18: 7–64.

PART III

HISTORY OF ANALYSIS

CHAPTER 7

REFLECTIONS ON THE HISTORY OF PSYCHOANALYSIS[1]

I have chosen the history of psychoanalysis as my topic in order to address a point of urgency in current psychoanalysis: the danger of becoming a latter-day Tower of Babel. That famous tower was intended to reach Heaven, but the project was abandoned when God confounded its builders' languages as a punishment for their pride. In my view the fact that different schools of psychoanalytic thought and practice compete, calls for a re-evaluation of the history of psychoanalysis.

Historical survey

The question I am posing is: what was there in the structure and history of psychoanalysis that led to the establishment of different schools within it? I will not in this presentation take a stand on the relative merits of the various psychoanalytic schools, but will examine psychoanalysis as a study in the history of ideas.

In studying the psychoanalytic past, I found it useful to differentiate three types of contributors: heretics, modifiers and extenders. The heretics, rare in recent years but prevalent in Freud's lifetime, were typically close to Freud for some time, made important contributions, and then bolted to start their own schools. They include Adler, Stekel, Jung, Rank and Wilhelm Reich. During Freud's lifetime there were only heretics and extenders. Modifiers appeared after Freud's death when no one, not even Anna Freud, could lay claim to being the only heir to Freud's legacy.

Modifiers recast psychoanalytic theory or modified psychoanalytic practice, but did not leave the psychoanalytic field. A typical strategy for a modifier is to claim that his or her modification is implicit in Freud's writings or flows directly out of Freud's ideas. While modifiers create controversy in psychoanalysis, they also keep it alive and protect it from stagnation. Early modifiers were Ferenczi and Federn; later ones were Hartmann, Melanie Klein, Winnicott, Lacan and Kohut. Many modifiers are influenced by movements that take place outside psychoanalysis and attempt a synthesis between psychoanalysis and another discipline. Bowlby (1960) attempted to coordinate psychoanalysis with ethology; Lacan's modifications can be seen as an attempt to recast psychoanalysis in the language of structural linguistics.

Extenders, the third group, usually extend psychoanalysis into areas as yet unexplored, but their findings do not demand modification. Unlike modifiers, they evoke no enmity and their contributions are appreciated. Some of the important extenders are Karl Abraham, Hermann Nunberg, Robert Waelder and Otto Fenichel.

My first task in this survey is the examination of the way psychoanalysis was discovered. In his *Introductory Lectures on Psychoanalysis*, Freud (1916-17a, p. 2) enumerated three major blows that science inflicted on man's self-esteem. Copernicus showed that Earth was not the center of the universe. Darwin proved that man descended from the animal kingdom. Freud assigned the third blow to himself: he showed that man is not master in his own house because he does not know his unconscious. It was in the company of Copernicus and Darwin that Freud wished to be remembered. History has not yet rendered its verdict; possibly Freud will be remembered in a different context, in a line extending from Plato to Schopenhauer and Nietzsche (Bergmann 1987, p. 155; Makari 1991).

Was psychoanalysis, like the New World, waiting to be discovered? Greek and Chinese science endured a long time without a Copernicus, a Darwin, and certainly without a Freud. Great as a man may be, he is the creature of his culture and a child of his time. However, within each given culture it is legitimate to ask how much time would have passed before another man would have made the same discovery, or even if the particular discovery would have been made at all. A good example is Darwin's relation to Malthus. Darwin acknowledged his survival of the fittest theory to be only the doctrine of Malthus applied to the entire animal and vegetable kingdom. Did Darwin need Malthus's dictum of 1795 – that population increases at an exponential rate while food supplies can at best be augmented at a linear rate – as an impetus to discover natural selection and the survival of the fittest?

In 1837, the year Queen Victoria ascended the throne, Darwin returned from a six-year, forty-thousand-mile voyage around the world. The idea of survival of the fittest occurred to him in 1839, but was not published until twenty years later. Alfred Russell Wallace made the same discovery independently of Darwin and mailed him the results. Wallace too had read, and was influenced by, Malthus. If we take Darwin as a prototype of a scientific discoverer we see immediately how different the situation was with Freud. No one came close to his deciphering dreams, with the possible exception of Popper-Linkeus. And even Popper-Linkeus was not interested in the therapeutic use of dreams; he wanted to use them only in the service of social reform (Freud 1932).

There were other psychiatrists – Jean-Martin Charcot, Pierre Janet, Eugen Bleuler and Adolf Meyer – who treated hysterics. But it is safe to say that none of them would have exerted the kind of influence on the Western world that Freud did. As a step in the development of psychiatry, Freud's discoveries were entirely unexpected. Freud was treating a relatively insignificant part of the world's population. His patients were middle-class, well-educated, articulate, and by-and-large secular Jews. They were more articulate and introspective than the hysterics Charcot treated. They helped Freud make observations and discoveries, and formulate theories that changed the way Western man understands himself.

The building blocks from which psychoanalysis was structured – the meaning of dreams, the significance of infancy for adult functioning, and the ubiquitous presence of transference reactions – could all have been discovered by others at other times. It was Freud's combining them into one discipline that went beyond the realm of discovery. It is this very complexity of psychoanalysis that makes it vulnerable to modification.

Possibly something like the Oedipus complex would have been discovered by a later observer, but I doubt it would have been named after a Greek hero. As I have demonstrated (Bergmann 1992), Freud read *Oedipus Rex* during his adolescence, when he first fell in love with Gisela Fluss. What he discovered in his self-analysis were attenuated derivatives of the Oedipus complex: love for the mother and jealousy of the father. The impact of Sophocles' masterpiece made it possible for Freud to reach the radical conclusion of a wish for sexual union with the mother and murder of the father, a remarkable transmission of insight across two thousand years of human history. Looking back at the past, I see no royal road leading from hysteria to psychoanalysis. A path is discernible, but it could have been traversed by one man only. If the discovery of psychoanalysis was less determined, it follows that its future will also be less predictable.

A different picture emerges if we change our focus from psychiatry to the broader ferment that characterized the nineteenth-century world of art and letters. When the art historian Erwin Panofsky tried to explain the rise of neo-Platonism as a dominant philosophy during the Renaissance, he found only one other movement that exerted a similar influence: psychoanalysis in our time. Whether we begin with philosophers like Schopenhauer, Nietzsche and Feuerbach, the plays of Ibsen or Strindberg, the novels of Dostoyevsky, Schnitzler, Proust, or even the music of Wagner, immersing ourselves in this world makes clear that the appearance of Freud is a possibility. The optimism of the Enlightenment has turned to introspection and a new interest in the morbid. It is at the point where Enlightenment and German Romanticism meet that Freud's antecedents are to be found. As Fenichel (1941) said, the subject matter of psychoanalysis is the irrational. Its methodology, however, is rational. Psychoanalysis offered a synthesis between Enlightenment and Romanticism; this synthesis constituted its main appeal.

How close psychoanalysis came to being engulfed by the irrational is illustrated by an exchange of letters between Jung and Freud in 1910. On February 11, 1910, Jung urged Freud "to revive among the intellectuals the feeling for symbol and myth and ever so gently to transform Christ back into the soothsaying God of the vine ... What infinite rapture and wantonness lie dormant in our religion waiting to be led back to their true destination!" Two days later Freud replies, "You must not regard me as the founder of a religion. My intentions are not so far-reaching .... I am not thinking of a substitute for religion; this need must be sublimated" (McGuire 1974, pp. 294–295). The correspondence illustrates the danger of a remerger between psychoanalysis and the irrational. Freud resisted Jung in the name of the spirit of rational enlightenment. The exchange also throws light on the psychology of one future heretic. Freud refused Jung's need for idealization. With this refusal Jung's libido, we may assume, had to turn back upon himself. If Freud would not assume the task of converting psychoanalysis into a new religion, Jung would. The Jungian heresy represents an attempt to merge psychoanalysis with the irrational. There will be further attempts along the same lines.

Let us turn back to September 21, 1897, when Freud informed Wilhelm Fliess that he had lost faith in his "neurotica." He has realized "that there are no indications of reality in the unconscious so that one cannot distinguish between truth and fiction that has been cathected with affect" (Masson 1985, p. 264). This day may well be the birthday of psychoanalysis. It is one of the glorious moments in the history of psychoanalysis, yet something happened that we need to re-examine. Schimek (1975) has shown that the majority of Freud's women patients did not report to him conscious memories of seduction. It was Freud who made this construction out of their associations. Schimek comes close to saying that the seduction theory was an iatrogenic illness, for Freud's female patients experienced his unrelenting and penetrating pressure to reveal to him their hidden memories of a seduction. Even earlier, Sadow *et al.* (1968) showed that the seduction theory, which they charitably called "the seduction hypothesis," was a construction. Psychoanalysis proper, therefore, owes its origins to a construction that failed. Historically it is incorrect to speak of the seduction hypothesis; it was not a hypothesis but a belief. Ferenczi in his diary (1988) remarked that when Freud discovered that hysterics lie he stopped loving his patients (p. 93). It was not the clinical material that persuaded Freud to change his mind, but his self-analysis. An event intrapsychic to Freud – his self-analysis – colored the way he interpreted events in the outer reality, the associations of his patients. The subsequent demand that the analyst be analyzed was intended to protect future patients from the dangers of similar distortions. The lesson not learned that still haunts us today is that there is no royal road leading from the raw data of psychoanalysis – the memories told, the fantasies confessed, the dreams reported – to the constructions made or ignored by the analyst. Different models lead to different constructions.

At this historical juncture the concept of unconscious psychic reality as determining much of human behavior became central to psychoanalysis (Freud 1900, pp. 613, 620; 1913b, p. 159). As to technique, Anna Freud commented in 1943:

> The two main foundation stones of psychoanalytic technique were the substitution of free association for hypnosis, and the reduction to a minimum of the real relationship between analyst and patient.
>
> (p. 630)

The question of the role of reality, and particularly traumatic reality versus wish-fulfillment fantasy, has remained with us ever since. Eventually psychoanalysts became accustomed to a mixed theory of neurosis consisting of the instinctual structure and the influence of reality in early childhood. Nevertheless a measure of vagueness remained as to how much responsibility is to be assigned to each factor. Psychoanalysts can concentrate, as Arlow (1969) has taught, on the analysis of hierarchically arranged unconscious fantasies as the central unit of the psychoanalytic endeavor; or one can emphasize the infant's adaptation to the peculiaritics of the adults in his life as the interpersonalists or the object relations theorists urge us to do. It will be argued that one should do both, and see the persistence of the unconscious fantasy as a response to parental deprivation or indulgence, but, as a matter of fact, if we emphasize one we will tend to de-emphasize the other. At this point controversy emerges.

My second stop deals with Freud's case histories. Freud interpreted Dora's dreams brilliantly, but who besides Freud could have done so? The encounter was tragic, as Erikson (1962) pointed out. Freud understood her dreams, but not her actuality. Kris (1951) noted that the Rat Man was subjected to massive indoctrination. The Wolf Man relapsed into psychosis while in analysis with Brunswick (1928). Ironically we also count Schreber, a man Freud never met in person, as a case history. It has become painfully evident that Freud's case histories are of historical importance, but no longer examples to be emulated. Today only modifiers write case histories.

As the third moment in the history of psychoanalysis I select the paper Freud delivered at the Second Psychoanalytic Congress in Nuremberg in 1910.

> You know of course that the psychoneuroses are substitutive satisfactions of some instinct the presence of which one is obliged to deny to oneself and others. Their capacity to exist depends on this distortion and lack of recognition. When the riddle they present is solved and the solution is accepted by the patients these diseases cease to be able to exist ... In place of a single sick person, let us put society – suffering as a whole from neuroses ... The

> success which the treatment can have with the individual must occur equally with the community. Sick people will not be able to let their various neuroses become known.
>
> (Freud 1910c, p. 148)

Early psychoanalysis, as this passage indicates, had a Utopian core, and this core will reappear in many modifiers. Freud, the "godless Jew," the secular prophet, speaks these lines. Strange as it may seem to us today, Freud thought enlightenment and shame would be the curative factors for the whole of society. At this point psychoanalysis revealed itself most clearly as the daughter of enlightenment. It is at this moment in its history that it became allied with other powerful Utopian movements that captured the imagination of the young on the eve of the First World War – surrealism, socialism, progressive education, and the belief in an early sexual enlightenment of children. It was this Utopian aspect that won psychoanalysis many of its adherents. Eventually these attitudes would coalesce around the popular books written by Wilhelm Reich.

Karen Horney's (1937) *Neurotic Personality of Our Time* also belongs to this category. The touchstone for all Utopian books within psychoanalysis is the role they assign to the Oedipus complex. In all these books it is assumed that if the child is given proper parental care, the Oedipus complex will cause no particular stress. Kohut (1977) shared this view. He spoke of the oedipal phase as a joyful experience despite its anxieties, provided the parents react with pride to the child's developmental achievement (pp. 229–230). Behind this debate we find the same juxtaposition of intrapsychic conflict characteristic of our humanness, against the concept of pathology created by environmental forces.

The next decisive moment I would single out is the year 1914, important in history as the year in which the First World War broke out, and, according to Peter Gay, the year in which the twentieth century proper began. In this year, when the guns of August destroyed the world of the nineteenth century, Freud made two important contributions. The first was the paper *On Narcissism: An Introduction* (1914d). Now psychoses were renamed narcissistic neuroses not open to psychoanalytic influence. Psychoanalytic endeavors were limited to the transference neuroses. In time this dichotomy became a focal point for controversy. Both Kernberg (1980) and Kohut (1971) argue that narcissistic neuroses are not identical to psychoses, and the Kleinians will show that psychoanalysis can treat more severe disturbances beyond the transference neurosis.

In the other significant paper of that year, *Remembering, Repeating and Working Through*, Freud (1914a) maintained a delicate balance, recognizing acting as a form of remembering, but therapeutically less desirable than recollection. Psychoanalysis became a technique that deliberately aimed to intensify transference manifestations into a transference neurosis that would actualize the infantile neurosis around the figure of the analyst. The possibilities and desirabilities of this transformation gave rise to another group of controversies. The introduction of the term "working through" was significant because it implied that merely making conscious what was unconscious does not in itself suffice for cure.

Freud was less optimistic in 1914 than he was in 1910. Nevertheless he was convinced that the infantile neurosis can yield to the transference neurosis, and once this change has come about the transference neurosis will be worked through and result in psychoanalytic cure. For a long time the ability to form a transference neurosis was the hallmark of the good analysand, and the development of the transference neurosis the dividing line between psychotherapy and psychoanalysis proper. Eventually this point too will become a focus of controversy, this time in the realm of technique. Are only transference interpretations mutative (Strachey 1934), or should one, for optimal results, balance transference interpretations with extratransference ones? By now it has become evident that one obtains a completely different kind of analysis depending on the path pursued.

Beyond the Pleasure Principle (Freud 1920) represents a turning point in the history of psychoanalysis. Freud became pessimistic. The repetition compulsion recognized in 1914 as the active force behind the transference neurosis was re-evaluated. What in 1914 was a positive force aiding the psychoanalyst in his endeavor to make the analysand experience the analysis emotionally, was now seen as operating in the service of the death instinct and therefore antagonistic to the psychoanalyst's efforts. In the transference neurosis, the analysands repeated their painful experiences that never led to pleasure. The analytic repetition no longer guarantees that the ego will obtain mastery over the traumatic experience. For the first time we hear from Freud a pessimistic note: reconstructions without memories do not solve the therapeutic problem (Freud 1920, p. 18). Furthermore, all too often the most essential memories can never be remembered and have to be re-enacted. Overcoming the repetition compulsion became the major task of the analyst.

The Ego and the Id (Freud 1923b) marked not only the establishment of the structural hypothesis and the beginning of ego psychology, but also the beginning of object relations. Using the language of metapsychology, Freud found that "object cathexis can be replaced by identification" or "objects can be set up inside the ego," bringing about character change. The ego assumed features of the love object and demanded love from the id (pp. 28–30). The relationship between the self and the internalized object representations is at the core of the psychoanalytic object relations theory. In 1923 Freud emphasized the weakness of the ego, but in 1926 he laid the foundations for psychoanalytic ego psychology. Nevertheless the therapeutic pessimism expressed in 1920 reappeared in Freud's *Analysis, Terminable and Interminable* (1937a).

Up to 1920 the relation between technique and theory was nearly perfect. The theory stated that repression – more precisely the return of the repressed – was responsible for the formation of the symptom. As Freud put it (1932, p. 221), if what is repressed contrives to force its way into consciousness or action, we are no longer normal. It was an act of genius for Freud to see that the same road that leads to abnormality also leads to cure, provided it takes place under the guidance of the analyst and in the safety of the analytic situation. The analogy to inoculation, never verbalized, is evident. And like an excessive dosage, a premature interpretation can bring out the disease rather than the cure. This simple harmony does not prevail in the structural formulation. The division of the psychic apparatus into superego, ego and id opened the way to two different approaches in technique. Franz Alexander and James Strachey advocated modifying the superego by encouraging the analysand to project his superego onto the analyst, who would then give back to the patient his own and more benign superego. In the other camp were the ego analysts who believed that all progress must be made through modifications of the ego. In 1934 the two contrasting points of view were presented side by side in papers written by Strachey and Sterba. At that historical juncture psychoanalysis lost its unity of approach and the controversy between ego and superego psychoanalysts came to a head in the Marienbad Symposium of 1936 (Glover *et al.*, 1937).

Hitherto psychoanalysis was regarded as superior to all therapies since it alone was causal, a technique in which investigation and cure go hand in hand. Psychoanalysis alone cured, while other therapies were merely ameliorative. All this source of pride was called into question in Freud's last contribution to technique (1937a). It is not surprising that younger generations of ego psychoanalysts, as well as the followers of Melanie Klein, could not accept this pessimistic appraisal.

I thus arrived at an unexpected conclusion. Freud's about-face in 1920 came as a shock to the psychoanalytic movement, causing disarray. Until now only certain leading disciples occasionally bolted to create their own schools. But now the full implications of Freud's thinking could not easily be fathomed. It was inevitable that different schools would emerge.

During the same period, psychoanalytic technique came under the influence of Wilhelm Reich's character analysis (1927, 1928). Reich evoked powerful reactions in his patients by showing them, and even caricaturing for them, the rigidities in their speech and movement. Kris (1951) called Reich's approach prestructural. Anna Freud in 1936 designated it as "permanent modes of defense." With the advent of ego psychology this technique of confrontation was rejected. Fenichel's (1941) book on technique stabilized the controversy between Wilhelm Reich and Anna Freud. The Kleinians, however, continued to interpret what ego psychologists call "dormant conflicts."

One of the important tasks facing psychoanalytic historians is the re-evaluation of Ferenczi's role based on his diary and the Ferenczi-Freud correspondence. The controversy between the two goes far beyond the question of "abstinence" versus indulgence. Ferenczi demanded that the analyst "take seriously" the infantile need for help (Ferenczi 1988, p. 260). He accused Freud and his followers of working to establish the transference: when the "patient is going through agonies, he sits calmly in the armchair, smoking a cigar and making conventional remarks in a bored tone; occasionally he falls asleep" (p. 178). The most radical and least acceptable of Ferenczi's modifications was the idea of mutual analysis. It emerged, in my opinion, out of the incomplete analysis he had with Freud. It was the state of mutual analysis he wished to establish with Freud, and when this wish was thwarted he attempted to carry it out with his own patients. Ferenczi attempted to restore the childhood trauma to the position it lost after Freud gave up the seduction theory.

In *Thalassa: A Theory of Geniality* Ferenczi (1924) speculates that both sleep and sexual intercourse represent a regression to the period of birth and the prenatal existence. It also recapitulates ontogenetically the philogenetic adaptation to terrestrial existence. Ferenczi's idea of genitality is different from Freud's, but close to Freud's thinking in *Beyond the Pleasure Principle* (1920). In their 1924 booklet Ferenczi and Rank present (their protestation to the contrary notwithstanding) a major deviation from the standard technique. Instead of insight, they elevate the emotional experience of the analysand as central to treatment. Ultimately Ferenczi reached the conclusion that the primal scene is traumatic not because it is overstimulating or because the child feels deserted, but because the child experiences the inadequacy of his own sexual organs to gratify the adult. Ferenczi here meets Adler halfway. From the diary, Ferenczi emerges as the ancestor of many future psychoanalytic modifiers. Two of his late papers *The Unwelcome Child and His Death Instinct* (1929) and *Confusion of Tongues Between Adult and Child* (1933) mark the beginning of object relations theory. Had the climate been propitious, he could have been more influential. Through his disciple, Michael Balint, he exercised an influence in the subsequent history of psychoanalysis. The idea that the psychoanalyst should allow the regression to go as far back as necessary until new beginnings emerge spontaneously, we traditionally associate with Balint and Winnicott – but it goes back to Ferenczi.

Central to Balint's thought was the reformulation of the libido theory. Instead of conceptualizing libido as pleasure-seeking, Balint saw it as object-seeking. With this reformulation in the 1930s, the object relation theory came into its own. Through this conceptualization the role that parents play, hitherto excluded when Freud gave up the seduction theory, returned to the psychoanalytic fold.

Freud worked with two often contradictory metaphors and models. His favorite metaphor was the archaeological one. In a more pessimistic vein he spoke of the archaeological metaphor, implying that all that was repressed is still alive in the unconscious and pressing upward to consciousness through various derivatives. This metaphor dominates *Civilization and its Discontents* (1930) and *Constructions in Psycho-Analysis* (1937b).

In a more optimistic vein, Freud used the transformational model. Here he stressed the flexibility of instincts and the possibilities of sublimation. This model dominates Freud's papers on masochism, female sexuality, and *The Dissolution of the Oedipus Complex* (1924b). In *Transformations of Instinct as Exemplified in Anal Erotism* (1917b) he told women that their penis envy could be transformed into the wish for a child, making them maternal; or into a love for a man, making them feminine.

A psychoanalytic developmental theory should be able to explain why some themes persist in the unconscious while others are capable of transformation. We have not gone very far beyond Freud, and I would suggest that this is an important task facing the younger generation of psychoanalysts (Bergmann 1989).

The history of psychoanalysis after Freud's discoveries shows how dominant ideas capture the imagination of generations of psychoanalysts and are usually carried to an extreme until a disappointment takes place, only to give room to new ideas. To give examples: Wilhelm Reich's ideas that resistance interpretations should always precede content interpretation, and his insistence that the character armor be pierced before content interpretations are made, is no longer part of psychoanalytic technique. The belief dear to psychoanalytic pioneers that child analysis, like an inoculation, is a prophylactic against adult neurosis is no longer a shared belief. The idea that psychoanalysis should be defined as the therapeutic technique that aims to maximize the role of the transference neurosis no longer holds the dominant position. The idea that psychoanalysis will become a general psychology through the study of the conflict-free sphere that so excited Rapaport and led to the entrance of clinical psychologists into psychoanalysis, is no longer an active vision. The frustratingly silent psychoanalyst advocated by Karl Menninger's (1958) book on technique has lost favor. Throughout psychoanalytic history every excess taught us something new and in that sense was beneficial. The study of the history of psychoanalysis is still in its infancy and the process of change within psychoanalysis has not been carefully scrutinized.

Psychoanalysis prospered because after the Second World War a generation of Americans believed they were entitled to the pursuit of happiness and a better life than that of their parents. Now that the wheel has turned, and we are no longer sure every generation will have it better than the previous one, the climate of opinion is distinctly less favorable to the psychoanalytic enterprise.

As long as the psychoanalytic focus was on the oedipal fixation, it was relatively easy to see that every person represents his or her individual variation on that theme. When this specific variation was understood and accepted by the analysand, the analysis came to an end. When later on the interest shifted first to the mechanisms of defense of the ego, and from there to preoedipal pathology, developmental deficits, and eventually also to the psychotic core which most if not all of our patients have, the analysis became increasingly long and the termination point murky.

The painful discovery was made that many were analyzable in terms of developing the capacity for free association of verbalization of their transference reactions, but nevertheless incapable of internalizing the process so that a good termination could be achieved. These considerations affect psychoanalysis in the marketplace in terms of cost effectiveness. The process of intrapsychic change and the resolution of the transference (Bergmann 1988) proved more difficult than the psychoanalytic pioneers assumed. Disappointed in the results of an analysis, and yet unable to give up the hope aroused by psychoanalysis, many analysands looked to another school for another chance. Earlier generations of psychoanalysts were typically attracted to psychoanalysis after reading a book by Freud – mostly *The Interpretation of Dreams* (1900) – but in the last decade younger colleagues have emerged to whom Freud's writings no longer spoke. These younger psychoanalysts were drawn by the concepts and language of one of the modifiers: Melanie Klein, Kohut, Balint, Winnicott or Lacan.

After the Second World War the sense of professional identity of the practicing psychoanalyst changed. The psychoanalytic pioneers were inspired by a sense of identification with Freud and felt co-engaged in one of the great discoveries of the century. Their successors were practitioners rather than discoverers, members of a profession whose services were available to the rich and the not-too-severely-disturbed of the general population. The poor and the unanalyzable were cared for by psychiatrists, social workers and psychologists.

The modifiers

The prolonged controversy between Melanie Klein and her followers on one side, and Anna Freud and the ego analysts on the other, is of particular interest because both claimed Freud – but different parts of Freud – as their point of origin. We are in a better position to study the controversy now that it has been published (King and Steiner 1991). We owe Waelder's paper of 1936 a special debt of gratitude because, so early in the history of this controversy, he demonstrated the vast scope of this debate. What was at stake were (1) the psychological significance of the first year of life, (2) the role of fantasy (psychic reality) and reality in the life of the infant, (3) the role of projection and introjection during early infancy, (4) the nature of evidence in psychoanalysis, (5) the nature and structure of memory, (6) the connection between the psychosexual phases and the development of the ego, (7) the relevance of direct observation of children in the development of psychoanalytic theory, and (8) the evolution of the superego.

It is noteworthy that Melanie Klein appears in the Freud-Jones correspondence as early as 1925 (Steiner 1985). That is two years after the publication of *The Ego and the Id* (Freud 1923b). Melanie Klein therefore emerged during the period of uncertainty created by Freud's reformulations. The problem merits deeper study than I can give it here, but there can be little doubt that Melanie Klein's followers felt that she answered questions about the more disturbed patients who were agitating psychoanalysts. Klein as well as her followers saw themselves as extenders. As Riviere (1936) put it,

> I can claim that my hypothesis makes use of all Freud's findings and does not convert any of the principles he has laid down; but they extend the application

> of these principles in some directions where he himself has so far preferred not to pursue them.
>
> (p. 396)

To Anna Freud and many of her colleagues, however, the Kleinians appeared as heretics about to overthrow or at least hopelessly muddle Freud's heritage. In his reply to Riviere, Waelder (1936) stated:

> To all this it may be replied that the theories in question abandon none of the views with which we have long been familiar but merely add to them. I do not think, however, that it is possible simply to add to the body of our knowledge without altering it in any respect.
>
> (p. 124)

Melanie Klein's system was derived from Freud's dual instinct theory and his emphasis on the death instinct. She modified Freud to state that at birth the death instinct is more powerful than libido. The libido is transmitted to the child by the love of the mother. The fusion of aggression and libido creates the depressive position. Strange as it may seem, the best confirmation of Klein's belief about the power of the death instinct in early childhood came from Hartmann's camp. Spitz (1945, 1946) showed by direct observation that human infants develop marasmus and die if they do not receive maternal love.

Anna Freud (1943, p. 631) summarized her disagreement with Klein succinctly. For Melanie Klein the importance of preverbal fantasies is overwhelming compared with happenings after the acquisition of speech, and since these very early fantasies can emerge only in transference most if not all analytic work takes place through transference interpretations. Transference along Freudian lines assumes that the first contacts between analyst and patient are governed by normal relational attitudes. It is the deepening of the transference that evokes emotions from deeper layers. For Klein the transference is there at the moment of encounter. It is at its height when the analyst is a pure fantasy object. Experience diminishes rather than enhances the power of transference. Finally, Freudian technique aims to undo repression; Kleinian technique aims to undo projection and introjection.

Heinz Hartmann and Melanie Klein are modifiers who see themselves as Freud's heirs. Modifiers and their followers tend to engage in the irrational battle as to who is Freud's true heir. At times the argument resembles more a theological debate than a scientific discussion. They developed psychoanalysis in two opposite directions. The third modifier of note after the Second World War was Franz Alexander, best known for the term "corrective emotional experience" (Alexander and French 1946). In its crude form it did not survive, but historically Kohut's self-psychology can be seen as a mutation of Alexander's point of view. Freudian analysts believe that cure depends on the reliving of the traumatic past in the transference. Self-psychologists see the analyst as a new self-object who, through empathy, can avoid or at least postpone the appearance of the traumatic repetition compulsion in the analysis. This is one of the great dividing lines in the history of psychoanalytic technique. In the subsequent literature, regardless of interpretations, all analysts increasingly grant some curative role to the fact that the analyst is a kind of person the patient had never encountered before.

Freud (1914d) postulated that secondary narcissism is augmented by the withdrawal of libido from the external world and, conversely, in states of being in love narcissistic libido is converted into object libido. Kohut questioned this convertibility and postulated that narcissism had its own developmental line. It is of historic interest to note that a generation earlier, Thomas Mann, in the novel *Joseph and His Brothers*, described the evolution of such a narcissist into a man who saves Egypt from hunger. It seems likely that Kohut was influenced by Mann.

Hartmann and his co-workers are today at the center of a controversy. There are those who believe that Hartmann's ego psychology is at the very core of the identity of American psychoanalysis. It has given American psychoanalysis an inestimable edge over psychoanalysis on the Continent and in South America (Young 1989).

There are also those who believe that Hartmann and his followers have turned away from the unconscious, the most valuable part of psychoanalysis, to advocate conformity and adaptation. It is argued that they misread and misunderstood Freud and buttressed their misunderstanding by the English *Standard Edition* of Freud's works, a translation that does not mirror Freud's thinking faithfully. Finally, they defined analyzability so narrowly that only a few can pass through the eye of that needle. Even more sharply, Hartmann was accused by Edelson (1986) of neglecting the empiricism of the psychoanalytical situation as a source of data, in favor of abstract theorizing – thus setting psychoanalysis back for a whole generation.

Hartmann (1939, pp. 3–21) saw psychoanalysis as developing along a straight line. He divided its history into three periods. During the first, attention was directed toward the drives and their development (psychosexual phases). This was primarily an analysis of the id. From 1926 on, the emphasis shifted to the ego from the point of view of its defenses against the id. The third period was reached in his own book. In this third era the ego and its autonomous development are the center of psychoanalytic interest. I want to draw your attention to the fact that this is a typical statement for a modifier: to see himself as standing at the apex of psychoanalytic development.

What makes a cohesive group of those who follow Hartmann is not only shared concepts and ideas, but also the set of passionately held beliefs they have in common:

1. The truly great discoveries of psychoanalysis are behind us; what is needed now is systematization.
2. The area of promise for new psychoanalytic ideas will come primarily from infant and child observations (Hartmann 1950). Waelder (1936) went so far as to state that the final proof of psychoanalytic interpretations will come from direct observation of children. This emphasis on observation was designed to counteract the Kleinian influence. (In 1977 Kohut reacted sharply against this point of view, emphasizing that only the psychoanalytic interview yields the data that psychoanalysis needs.) The new emphasis on developmental psychology yielded a number of important new concepts, such as the development of the infant from need satisfaction to object constancy, and the gradual separation between self and object representation. Most of the work of Spitz, Margaret S. Mahler and Edith Jacobson was derived from these differentiations.
3. Hartmann's concept of neutralization of both the sexual and aggressive drives, and his concept of the autonomous ego and its conflict-free sphere, are the main bridges that lead from psychoanalysis as a theory of neurosis to psychoanalysis as a general psychology. Drive neutralization was conceptualized as essential for the building-up of object relations and the reaching of object constancy. Rapaport (1951, pp. 364–365) made neutralization the main explanation for the difference between primary and secondary processes.

Contrary to assumptions, the Hartmann era, if not Hartmann himself, was interested in technique. The ego analyst interprets only what is already or almost preconscious; therefore the interpretation is parsimonious. The Kleinians interpret what is unconscious; therefore their interpretations are lengthy and cover a much larger territory. Psychoanalytic ego psychologists became interested not only in the pathology of the patient, but also the way he solved the problems he faced in childhood and adulthood; that is, an interest also in the healthy, functioning part of the ego (A. Reich 1958a).

Kris (1956a, 1956b) re-evaluated the role of memories. All memory undergoes modification in the process of development. The function of memory itself can become libidinized with the important implication that recall of childhood memories by themselves need not be curative. The concept of neutralization enabled Kris to throw new light on the "good" psychoanalytic hour. This resulted in an important change of technique; namely helping the analysand to develop the integrative functions of his own ego. These functions in turn make the analysand increasingly independent of the analyst and foster the termination process: an analysis ending in the capacity for self-analysis.

There were creative analysts working in the US who did not follow Hartmann, Kernberg, Waelder, L.S. Kubie, M. Kanzer and others – H.W. Loewald, Serge, G.S. Klein and Schaffer – who were in opposition. In my view Arlow and Brenner's re-emphasis on the centrality of compromise formation already belongs to the retrenchment of a post-Hartmann era.

In *The Evolution of Psychoanalytic Technique* (Bergmann and Hartman 1976) I maintain that all discussions of theory are translatable into differences of technique. Anna Freud (1976) was the most vehement opponent of the so-called "widening scope." She opposed Stone (1954) and Green (1975). The debate with Melanie Klein and her followers crystallized around the timing of interpretations. But within my perspective it appears that another dimension is relevant. Could it be that Anna Freud's frame of reference supports the confinement of psychoanalysis to the neuroses, while the Kleinian frame is more suitable for the treatment of borderline conditions?

Winnicott can be seen as a modifier of Melanie Klein. Like the Kleinians, he interpreted dormant conflicts; but unlike them, he was more careful not to evoke the patient's hostility by massive interpretations. His classic of 1953 on the transitional object was still the work of an extender, but when in 1955 he spoke of the true and false self he introduced new moral categories into psychoanalysis that were alien to the traditional value-free language of Freud. He became one of the most important modifiers, pointing out that only patients who receive "good-enough" infant care can undergo psychoanalysis.

Wrestling with the complex heritage

What conclusions are we entitled to draw from this historical survey? If my idea that there was nothing inevitable about the discovery of psychoanalysis is accepted, it should follow that there is also no way to predict the direction in which psychoanalysis will evolve.

In the history of psychoanalysis heretics appeared before modifiers. It is likely that the concept of modifier became a reality in organized psychoanalysis after the controversies between Kleinians and ego psychologists did not result in a split. The outcome demonstrated that after Freud's death no one, not even his daughter, could claim to be his only legitimate heir. While self-psychology has the status of a modification, the interpersonalists and Lacanians have the status of heretics. But this could change if we find productive ways of communication among dissident modifiers. So far, however, organized psychoanalysis survived a number of modifications but has not yet developed a productive technique of communication among different modifiers. The next generation of psychoanalysts will have to find ways to subject the modification to rational procedure so that their contributions can be tested against each other.

Case conferences demonstrate that we have reached such a degree of sophistication that any clinical material can be interpreted in a variety of ways. At this point in psychoanalytic history we cannot rely on case material to settle theoretical questions. One of the important tasks facing the younger generation of psychoanalysts is to find ways to give back to the case history its pivotal significance. This will require more candid and explicit reporting of clinical data.

If the historical point of view presented here is accepted, it follows that the different schools were not the result of mere chance. But inherent in the complex structure of psychoanalysis it should be possible to study them in an objective manner. There is a paradox here that must be faced: psychoanalysis, a rational method of approaching the irrational, has nevertheless not saved us from an irrational attachment to cherished psychoanalytic ideology. I have found it useful to test different theories by asking the following questions:

1. In the view of the theory, how does psychopathology originate?
2. Does the theory lead to the conclusion that some forms of mental illness are not treatable by this method?
3. What does the theory regard as the ideal therapeutic process?
4. What is the theory's model of the mind (Gedo and Goldberg 1973), including its view of human nature and developments during the first years of life?
5. What steps are used by the adherents of the theory to convert the pathology of the patient into the model of mental health held by the theory?

On the whole I find it less productive to search for the common denominator or even compare the theories of the various schools, but useful to study what analysts of various schools say to their patients – particularly in moments of therapeutic crisis. I do not see the existence of different schools of analysis as the curse of the Tower of Babel, but as a unique opportunity to compare the clinical usefulness of different approaches to divergent clinical groups.

The long historical battle between the wider or narrower scope, regardless of personal predilection, has, in my opinion, *de facto* been settled. Patients with borderline diagnoses are increasingly seeking psychoanalytic help. Psychoanalysis cannot maintain its future position as the leading healing profession unless it finds better ways of applying its findings beyond the neuroses. Otherwise we may well remain confined to a double aristocracy of patients suffering only from psychoneuroses and able to afford seeing the analyst four or five times a week. Important beginnings in the treatment of borderline patients have been made by Kernberg. Not accidentally, he has shown how different thinkers' work can be synthesized. There have been others (Pine 1990) who also contributed to this field. Working with more disturbed patients may show how the insights of different schools can be productively used.

If we can admit that the unknown still outweighs the known, we may succeed in reorganizing psychoanalysis from a body of practitioners into a body of workers aware that even though psychoanalysis is soon to celebrate its centennial, our divisions indicate there is still much to be learned about the alleviation of intrapsychic distress. Graduation from a psychoanalytic institute should indicate not only professional competence, but also a capacity to work with colleagues and a sense of obligation to study the many as yet unanswered problems in the field. As individuals our experience is bound to be limited, but collectively we can test hypotheses provided we create a climate in which failures can be reported as freely as successes.

Also, we must overcome the inertia of leaving basic issues unresolved over many decades. If we cannot arrive at clarification, we should at the very least know where the uncertainty begins. The survival of psychoanalysis will also depend on our ability to educate a new generation who are less partisan and more willing to look at the evolution of psychoanalysis from a historical viewpoint. I have tried to contribute to this aim. Thus an inquisitive and rational approach to current diversities, if accepted as a challenge, can become a source of new hope. And hope is essential for our survival.

Note

1 Plenary address presented at the Fall Meeting of the American Psychoanalytic Association, New York, December 20, 1991. First published as Bergmann, M.S. (1993), "Reflections on the History of Psychoanalysis," *Journal of the American Psychoanalytical Association*, 41: 929–955.

References

Alexander, F. and T.M. French (1946) *Psychoanalytic Therapy*. New York: Ronald Press.

Arlow, J.A. (1969) Unconscious Fantasy and Disturbances of Conscious Experience. *Psychoanalytic Quarterly* 38: 1–27.

Bergmann, M.S. (1987) *The Anatomy of Loving: The Story of Man's Quest to Know What Love Is*. New York: Columbia University Press.

Bergmann, M.S. (1988) On the Fate of the Intrapsychic Image of the Psychoanalyst After Termination of the Analysis. *Psychoanalytic Study of the Child* 43: 137–153.

Bergmann, M.S. (1989) Science and Art in Freud's Life and Work. In *Sigmund Freud and Art: His Personal Collection of Antiquities*, ed. L. Gamwell and R. Wells. New York: Harry M. Abrams, pp. 173–183.

Bergmann, M.S. (1992) *In the Shadow of Moloch: The Sacrifice of Children and its Impact on Western Religions*. New York: Columbia University Press.

Bergmann, M.S. and Hartman, F., eds (1976) *The Evolution of Psychoanalytic Technique*. New York: Basic Books.

Bowlby, J. (1960) Grief and Mourning in Infancy and Early Childhood. *Psychoanalytic Study of the Child* 15: 9–52.

Brunswick, R.M. (1928) A Supplement to Freud's "History of an Infantile Neurosis." *International Journal of Psychoanalysis* 9: 439–476.

Edelson, M. (1986) Heinz Hartmann's Influence on Psychoanalysis as a Science. *Psychoanalytic Inquiry* 6: 575–600.

Erikson, E.H. (1962) Reality and Actuality. *Journal of the American Psychoanalytic Association* 10: 454–461.

Fenichel, O. (1941) *Problems of Psychoanalytic Technique*, trans. D. Brunswick. New York: Psychoanalytic Quarterly.

Ferenczi, S. (1924) *Thalassa: A Theory of Genitality*. New York: Psychoanalytic Quarterly.

Ferenczi, S. (1929) The Unwelcome Child and His Death Instinct. In *Final Contributions to the Problems and Methods of Psychoanalysis*, ed. Balint, M. New York: Basic Books, 1955, 102–107.

Ferenczi, S. (1933) Confusion of Tongues Between Adult and Child. In *Final Contributions to Problems and Methods of Psychoanalysis*, ed. Balint, M.. New York: Basic Books, 1955, 156–167.

Ferenczi, S. (1988) *The Clinical Diary of Sándor Ferenczi*, ed. J. Dupont. Cambridge, MA: Harvard University Press.

Freud, A. (1943) Memorandum. In *The Freud-Klein Controversies 1941–1945*, eds P. King and R. Steiner. London: Routledge, 1991, pp. 629–634.

Freud, A. (1976) Changes in Psychoanalytic Practice and Experience. In *The Writings of Anna Freud, Vol. VIII: Psychoanalytic Psychology of Normal Development*: 176–185. New York: International Universities Press.

Freud, S. (1900) The Interpretation of Dreams, Part I and Part II. S.E. 4–5: 1–625.

Freud, S. (1910c) The Future Prospects of Psychoanalytic Therapy. S.E. 11: 141–151.

Freud, S. (1913b) Totem and Taboo. S.E. 13: 1–161.

Freud, S. (1914a) Remembering, Repeating and Working Through. S.E. 12: 145–156.

Freud, S. (1914d) On Narcissism: An Introduction. S.E. 14: 73–102.

Freud, S. (1916–17a) Introductory Lectures on Psychoanalysis, Parts I and II. S.E. 15: 9–239.

Freud, S. (1916–17b) Introductory Lectures on Psychoanalysis, Part III. S.E. 16: 243–463.

Freud, S. (1917b) Transformations of Instinct as Exemplified by Anal Erotism S.E. 17: 127–33.

Freud, S. (1920) Beyond the Pleasure Principle. S.E. 18: 7–64.

Freud, S. (1923b) The Ego and the Id. S.E. 19: 3–66.

Freud, S. (1924b) The Dissolution of the Oedipus Complex. S.E. 19: 173–179.

Freud, S. (1930) Civilization and its Discontents. S.E. 21: 57–145.

Freud, S. (1932) My Contact with Josef Popper-Linkeus. S.E. 22: 218–224.

Freud, S. (1937a) Analysis, Terminable and Interminable. S.E. 23: 211–253.

Freud, S. (1937b) Constructions in Psycho-Analysis S.E. 23: 257–269.

Gedo, J.E. and Goldberg, A. (1973) *Models of the Mind*. Chicago: University of Chicago Press.

Glover, E., Fenichel, O., Strachey, J., Bergler, E., Nunberg, H. and Bibring, E. (1937) Marienbad Symposium on the Theory of the Therapeutic Results of Psychoanalysis. *International Journal of Psychoanalysis* 18: 125–189.

Green, A. (1975) The Analyst, Symbolization and Absence in the Analytic Setting (On Changes in Analytic Practice and Analytic Experience). *International Journal of Psychoanalysis* 56: 1–22.

Hartmann, H. (1939) Psychoanalysis and the Concept of Health. In *Essays on Ego Psychology*. New York: International Universities Press, 3–18.

Hartmann, H. (1950) Comments on the Psychoanalytic Theory of the Ego. In *Essays on Ego Psychology*. New York: International Universities Press, 1964, 113–141.

Horney, K. (1937) *Neurotic Personality of Our Time*. New York: Norton.

Kernberg, O.F. (1980) *Internal World and External Reality: Object Relations Theory Applied*. New York: Aronson.

King, P. and Steiner, R. (1991) *The Freud-Klein Controversies 1941–45*. New York: Tavistock/Routledge.

Kohut, H. (1971) The Analysis of the Self: A Systematic Approach to the Psychoanalytic Treatment of Narcissistic Personality Disorders. *Psychoanalytic Study of the Child*, Monograph No. 4. New York: International Universities Press.

Kohut, H. (1977) *The Restoration of the Self*. New York: International Universities Press.

Kris, E. (1951) Ego Psychology and Interpretation in Psychoanalytic Therapy. In *Selected Papers of Ernst Kris*. New Haven, CT: Yale University Press, 1975, 237–251.

Kris, E. (1956a) On Some Vicissitudes of Insight in Psychoanalysis. In *Selected Papers of Ernst Kris*. New Haven, CT: Yale University Press, 1975, 252–271.

Kris, E. (1956b) The Personal Myth: A Problem in Psychoanalytic Technique. In *Selected Papers of Ernst Kris*. New Haven, CT: Yale University Press, 1975, 272–300.

Makari, G.J. (1991) German Philosophy, Freud, and the Riddle of the Woman. *Journal of the American Psychoanalytic Association* 39: 183–213.

Masson, J.M., ed. (1985) *The Complete Letters of Sigmund Freud to Wilhelm Fliess 1887–1904*. Cambridge, MA: The Belknap Press of Harvard University Press.

McGuire, W., ed. (1974) *The Freud/Jung Letters. The Correspondence Between Sigmund Freud and C. G. Jung*, trans. R. Manheim and R.F.C. Hall. Princeton: Princeton University Press.
Menninger, K.A. (1958) *Theory of Psychoanalytic Technique*. New York: Basic Books.
Pine, F. (1990) *Drive, Ego, Object, and Self: A Synthesis for Clinical Work*. New York: Basic Books.
Rapaport, D. (1951) The Autonomy of the Ego. In *Collected Papers*, ed. Gill, M.M. New York: Basic Books, 1967, 357–367.
Reich, A. (1958a) A Character Formation Representing the Integration of Unusual Conflict Solutions into the Ego Structure. In *Annie Reich: Psychoanalytic Contributions*. New York: International Universities Press, 1973, 250–270.
Reich, W. (1927, 1928) Report on the Seminar for Psychoanalytic Therapy. *Int. Ztschr. fr Arztliche Psychoanal.* 13: 241–244; 40: 438–440.
Riviere, J. (1936) On the Genesis of Psychical Conflict in Earliest Infancy. *International Journal of Psychoanalysis* 17: 395–422.
Sadow, L., Gedo, J.E., Miller, J., Pollock, G.H., Sabshin, M. and Schlessinger, N. (1968) The Process of Hypothesis Change in Three Early Psychoanalytic Concepts. *Journal of the American Psychoanalytic Association* 16: 245–273.
Schimek, J.G. (1975) The Interpretations of the Past: Childhood Trauma, Psychical Reality, and Historical Truth. *Journal of the American Psychoanalytic Association* 23: 845–865.
Spitz, R.A. (1945) Hospitalism – An Inquiry into Genesis of Psychiatric Conditions in Early Childhood. *Psychoanalytic Study of the Child* 1: 53–74.
Spitz, R.A. (1946) Hospitalism: A Follow-up Request. *Psychoanalytic Study of the Child* 2: 113–17.
Steiner, R. (1985) Some Thoughts about Tradition and Change Arising from the Examination of the British Psychoanalytical Society's Controversial Discussions 1943–1944. *International Journal of Psychoanalysis* 12: 27–71.
Stone, L. (1954) The Widening Scope of Indications for Psychoanalysis. *Journal of the American Psychoanalytic Association* 2: 567–594.
Strachey, J. (1934) The Nature of the Therapeutic Action in Psychoanalysis. *International Journal of Psychoanalysis* 15: 127–159.
Waelder, R. (1936) The Problem of the Genesis of Psychical Conflict in Earliest Infancy. In *Psychoanalysis: Observation, Theory, Application: Selected Papers of Robert Waelder*, ed. S.A.G. Guttman. New York: International Universities Press, 1976, 121–188.
Young, M. (1989) Heinz Hartmann, M.D.: An Introduction and Appreciation. *Psychoanalytic Quarterly* 58: 521–525.

CHAPTER 8

THE CONFLICT BETWEEN ENLIGHTENMENT AND ROMANTIC PHILOSOPHIES AS REFLECTED IN THE HISTORY OF PSYCHOANALYSIS[1]

One of the questions the study of history poses is whether subsequent ages understand an age better than the age understood itself. Since this question cannot be satisfactorily answered, we may suggest that we understand an earlier epoch differently than the epoch understood itself. We understand Freud's age differently than the way Freud and Abraham understood it. I invite you to look at familiar facts from a perspective that the two philosophies, Enlightenment and Romanticism, shaped the history of psychoanalysis. To study Freud's work within a larger context is not to diminish his contribution. In Freud the past was reborn in a new form. To deny Freud his full intellectual ancestry was one of the mistakes of the early Freudian hagiography.

Enlightenment and Romanticism

The literature on the Enlightenment is immense. For me, Ernst Cassirer's book *The Philosophy of the Enlightenment* (*Die Philosophie der Aufklärung*, 1932) is particularly valuable. According to Cassirer:

> The age venerated reason and science as man's highest faculty. This slogan, *Sapere Aude* (dare to know) ... Kant called the motto of the Enlightenment.
> (p. XI)

> It encounters the world with fresh joy and the courage of discovery, daily expecting new revelations. Yet its thirst for knowledge and intellectual curiosity are directed not only toward the external world. The thought of this age is even more passionately impelled by other questions of the nature and potentiality of thought itself.
> (pp. 4–5)

> The 18th century is imbued with a belief in the unity and immutability of reason. Reason is the same for all thinking subjects, all nations, all epochs and all cultures.
> (p. 6)

> Enlightenment is man's exodus from his self-incurred tutelage. Tutelage is the inability to use one's understanding without the guidance of another person.
> (p. 163)

Kant emphasized that a man must strive to become an autonomous individual; when he achieves such an autonomy, he will be governed by reason. By contrast to reason, our emotions are egoistic and antisocial. It is the task of reason to impose restraint on emotions. The Enlightenment had a favorable view of the potentialities of human nature. Any residual tendency to take account of the evil in men was met with the conviction that it will be eventually eliminated as men become guided by reason. The Enlightenment was opposed to the more pessimistic view of Christianity that Original Sin and its continuation in sexual lust makes men forever subject to sin and dependent on God's mercy. The Enlightenment refused to accept the biblical conviction that "the imagination of men's heart is evil from his youth," or the view of Aristotle, expressed in his politics, that the depravity of man is inexhaustible. As the Enlightenment put a high premium on reason, reason itself became emotionally charged. It was the ideology of the founders of the American Revolution.

The young Freud – that is, the Freud before the First World War – shared the optimism of the Enlightenment.

> The psychoneuroses are substitutive satisfactions of some instinct, the presence of which one is obliged to deny to one's self and others. Their capacity to exist depends on this distortion and lack of recognition. When the riddle they present is solved and the solution is accepted by the patients these diseases ceased to be able to exist.
>
> (Freud 1910c, pp. 148–149)

If the Enlightenment claimed France as its country of birth, and the English philosophers as its citadel, then Romanticism claimed Germany as its homeland, even though the impact of Romanticism on English and French art was great (Clark 1973). The same can also be said of English and French poetry (Bowra 1950). In Winckelman's famous words, "Art should aim at noble simplicity and calm grandeur." For the Romantics, art should excite the emotions, particularly the emotion of fear because fear was regarded by them as the source of the sublime. Shelley in the poem *The Beauty of the Medusa*, spoke of "the tempestuous loneliness of terror," and Goethe made the statement that "*Das Beste im Menschen liegt im Schaudern*" (the best in man is found in his shudder). To Poe, the death of a beautiful woman is unquestionably the most poetic topic in the world (Praz 1970). The iconography of Romantic art emphasized witches, torturers, shipwrecks and assassinations.

The Romantic philosophers put much less faith in the rationality of man and were not convinced that humanity is continuously progressing. They valued the irrational, the unconscious, bisexuality and human intuition. Man, to them, was part of nature. They were interested in mystical ecstasy, poetic and artistic inspiration, somnambulism and dreams. Truth was another name for reality, and was to be discovered by exercising the faculty of imagination. Creative imagination, in turn, was closely connected to insight into an unseen reality behind visible things. Man's spirit must be released from the bonds of habit. Romantic to its very core is Keats ending of his *Ode to A Grecian Urn*:

> Beauty is truth, truth beauty,--that is all
> You know on Earth and you need to know

The Romantics discovered the splendor of childhood, a period regarded as insignificant by the thinkers of the Enlightenment. Wordsworth's famous quote is apt: "The child is father to the man." The Romantics tended to think in polarities, a way of thinking that characterized Freud. The Romantics emphasized local communities, national feelings and folklore. Romanticism held a strong appeal to poets and artists, such as William Blake, Edgar Allen Poe and Fyodor Dostoyevsky; and composers including Wagner and Chopin. In Germany it included the writers Johann Gottfried von Herder and the Grimm Brothers, and the philosophers Schopenhauer and Nietzsche. Like impressionist art, Romanticism emphasized nature at a time when industrialization began to threaten it. The Romantics valued empathy (*Einfühlung*), experience (*Erlebnis*) and parapsychology. Romantic is Goethe's famous declaration: "*Das grösste Gluck der Menscheit ist doch die Personlichkeit*" (Humanity's greatest bliss is the personality). Ellenberger (1970) has described what he called "romantic medicine," views that psychiatrists working in mental hospitals developed during the nineteenth century.

With the publication of *The Interpretation of Dreams*, Freud, without being aware of it, stepped into a major philosophical controversy between the natural sciences and the Enlightenment on one side, and the Romantic philosophers arrayed on the other. Under the banner of the natural sciences, psychoanalysis entered the domain that the nineteenth century had acceded to Romanticism – the world of dreams, fairytales, myth and religion. Fenichel (1945) put it thus: "The subject matter of psychoanalysis is the irrational, but its methods are rational." Before Freud, the victories of the natural sciences were confined to the external world of physics, chemistry and astronomy. It was also applied to the investigation of the human body by the rational approach of physiology and medicine. The human psyche was to be studied by the rational methods of natural science. The territory was to be wrested from the realm of Romanticism and religion. This promise created enthusiasm among Western intellectuals, as well as strong opposition. Freud's father Jacob belonged to the Hebrew Enlightenment, *Haskala* (Bergmann 1976). Freud's education in the *Gymnasium*, with its emphasis on Latin, Greek and the German classics, was imbued by the ideas of the Enlightenment. Freud had a further reason to be attached to it: the Enlightenment opened the walls of the ghetto, and promised the emancipated Jews equality as citizens, along with the end of anti-Semitism.

Siegfried Bernfeld (1944), in his paper *Freud's Earliest Theories and the School of Helmholtz*, deserves gratitude for one of the earliest endeavors to place psychoanalysis within the context of scientific thought. Bernfeld noted that the history of psychoanalysis usually begins with the meeting of Freud and Charcot, when Freud won the scholarship to Paris (1885–86). It was in Paris that Freud encountered both hypnosis and hysterical patients. Freud was almost thirty years old when he met Charcot. Bernfeld suggested that in order to understand the world of Breuer and Freud we must know more about the atmosphere that prevailed in Ernst Brücke's laboratory, where Freud was employed as an assistant for seven years before his encounter with Charcot. Freud's teacher, Ernst Brücke (1818–92) – who Freud once said influenced him more than any other person – was strict as a man and as a scientist. Bernfeld discovered a memoir written in 1842 by Dubois, another prominent physiologist:

> Brücke and I pledged a solemn oath to put into power this truth: no other forces than the common physical and chemical ones are active within the organism. In those cases which cannot at the time be explained by these forces one has either to find the specific way or form of their action by means of the physical

> mathematical method, or to assume new forces equal in dignity to the physical-chemical forces inherent in matter, reducible to the force of attraction and repulsion.
>
> (p. 348)

Freud's work was an attempt to live up to the Brücke oath. Freud tried to the best of his capacities, as he developed psychoanalytic metapsychology, to understand the human psyche the same way as scientists try to understand nature. The "Project" upon which Freud had embarked in 1895, just after the publications of the *Studies on Hysteria*, bears the proud title *A Project for a Scientific Psychology*. The opening sentence reads, "The intention is to furnish a psychology that shall be a natural science." (Freud 1985, p. 295) Freud is speaking as Brücke's disciple.

On the other hand, when, as a student, Freud decided to become a physician, he was under the impact of *Naturphilosophie*, a movement that Bernfeld described as "pantheist monism, close to mysticism."

Nietzsche's idea of the eternal return hovers over Goethe's essay on nature. In his ideology, Freud was a strict natural scientist, but not without being attracted to the irrational, the part of life that was at the core of Romantic philosophy.

It was *The Interpretation of Dreams* (1900) that forced Freud to confront the philosophy of Romanticism head-on. He acknowledged that "Dreams received a warmer recognition when the human mind was dominated by philosophy and not by the exact natural sciences." (p. 63) Freud equates all philosophy with Romantic philosophy. There we see the battle between Enlightenment and Romanticism beginning within Freud himself. For a time, Enlightenment emerged victorious. For here, in tenets of the Enlightenment, was the belief that there is only one overarching truth that can be arrived at by rational methods. This belief appears in *The Interpretation of Dreams* in Freud's conviction that every manifest content of a dream is translatable into only one latent meaning by the technique of free associations. The possibility that there are many latent meanings dependent on the undertaking of the analyst would have been anathema within the orbit of Freud's thinking at the time.

The great monument of the Enlightenment is chapter 7 of *The Interpretation of Dreams*, which is more abstract and in which Freud developed the metapsychology of the dreaming process. The papers on metapsychology continue as a scientific tradition.

Thomas Mann (1922) may well have been the first to comment on the unique position of psychoanalysis between Romanticism and Enlightenment:

> Freud's interest as a scientist in the affective does not degenerate into a glorification of its object at the expense of the intellectual sphere. His anti-rationalism consists in seeing the actual superiority of the impulse over the mind, power for power; not at all in lying down and groveling before that superiority, or in contempt for mind. It gives no occasion for confusion, nor is itself prey to any. Its interest in impulse is unmistakably and unchangeably not a subserviency which denies mind and clings to "nature"; on the contrary, it works in the interest of the triumph it envisages in the future for mind and reason; it serves – I use the poor proscribed word in its largest sense, independent of the wave-play of the time – it serves "enlightenment."
>
> (pp. 193–194)

Mann characterized psychoanalysis as Romanticism that has become scientific, and characterized Freud as a "*Selbstdenker*," a man who thinks his won thoughts.

When Freud, after substituting free associations for hypnosis, recognized the enormous role that resistance plays against psychoanalytic cure, he was confronted with the irrational side of man in a way the philosophers of the Enlightenment were never forced to consider.

There is no evidence that Freud ever thought that what he discovered in his analytic work was in any way incompatible with the philosophy of the Enlightenment. In *An Outline of Psycho-Analysis* (Freud 1940), his commitment to natural science and his belief in the death instinct are discussed without any sign of discomfort between the two. Where Freud saw no contradiction, I see a major incompatibility. It was not long after the International was founded that "wild analysis" (Freud 1910e) presented a danger. To avoid countertransference in psychoanalysts toward their patients it was decided that each one of them must themselves be psychoanalyzed. The implicit assumption behind this move was that both analyst and anlysand are in danger of succumbing to the power of the irrational. The psychoanalysis of the analyst was thought to be the guarantee that this would not happen. Our history did not entirely live up to these expectations. Psychoanalyzed psychoanalysts may be less subject to the temptations of the analytic situation, but they are not immune to them.

Freud recognized the full power of the aggressive drive and the death instinct, and saw this instinct in a perpetual battle with the life drive without any assurance that libido – equated with the life drive – will emerge victorious; in fact, he moved psychoanalysis away from Enlightenment.

Madeleine and Henry Vermorel (1986), in a paper entitled *Was Freud a Romantic?* warned of a danger of "an amputation of the romantic dimensions of psychoanalysis." They cited Freud's 1919 paper, *The Uncanny* as the most Romantic of Freud's writings. They consider the dual instinct as derived from Schelling. The word "*trieb*" (drive) as used by Freud, they believed, derived from Novalis. And such terms as "*Urfater*" (primal father) and "*Urphantasie*" (primal fantasy) were derived from Goethe's "*Urphenomena*" (primal phenomena). They also consider bisexuality as a Romantic idea transmitted to Freud through Fliess, whom they consider a Romantic physician. Freud's adherence to Lamarck they describe as an example of the Romantic influence upon him. As an example, they cite Freud's *Thoughts for the Times of War and Death* (1915c, p. 296): "The man of prehistoric times survives unchanged in our unconscious." Romantic is also the statement in the same essay:

> This attitude of ours towards death has a powerful effect on our lives. Life is impoverished, it loses in interest when the highest stake in the game of living, life itself, may not be risked.

The Uncanny (1919b) is perhaps Freud's most Romantic work, as well as the paper *The Theme of the Three Caskets* (1913a):

> The three forms taken by the figure of the mother in the course of a man's life – the mother herself, the beloved one who is chosen after her pattern, and lastly the mother earth, who receives him once more. But it is in vain that an old man yearns for the love of woman as he had it first from his mother; the third of the fates alone, the silent goddess of death, will take him into her arms.

That we are received by "mother earth" upon death is a truly Romantic statement.

Strenger (1989) covered the same territory with a different emphasis. To Strenger, Freud embodies the Classical attitude; and Ferenczi, and later Kohut, the Romantic vision. He counseled the avoidance of the extremes of both the Classical and the Romantic vision.

> It is our tasks as analytic therapists, no less than as human beings, to bear the tension between the perspectives on ourselves from within and without, and hence between the classic and the romantic attitude.
>
> (p. 608)

Schopenhauer, Nietzsche and Jung, and the ancestry of psychoanalysis

Freud's loyalty to the "scientific method" made it impossible for him to acknowledge how much psychoanalysis owes to Schopenhauer and Nietzsche. Wagner, who for the first time in Western literature glorified a brother and sister incest, paved the way for the acceptance of psychoanalytic ideas. In *Die Walküre*, when Brünnhilde acts contrary to the wishes of her father Wotan, she claims obedience to his "secret will." The term "secret will" is what Freud will call an unconscious wish. Brünnhilde is punished to fall into a deep slumber surrounded by fire, and become the wife of a man who will find and waken her. Here too we are dealing with a Freudian insight, but before Freud. As long as Brünnhilde was identified with her father, carrying her own spear and shield, she could not become anybody's wife. She must separate herself from her father and be awakened by her future husband to become a woman. Tristan's wish to join his mother in his *Liebestod* should also be considered a Freudian insight before Freud. Traditional psychoanalytic wisdom would have claimed that Wagner anticipated Freud. However, a historical understanding of the epoch should result in our understanding that like Nietzsche, Wagner too prepared Freud for his discovery.

On April 1, 1908, the Vienna Psychoanalytic Society devoted a meeting to the relationship between Nietzsche and psychoanalysis. There Freud disclaimed any knowledge of Nietzsche's work. "Occasional intents at reading it were smothered by an excess of interest." (Nunberg and Federn 1962, p. 359). On October 28, 1908, a second meeting was devoted to Nietzsche. There Freud praised Nietzsche: "The degree of introspection achieved by Nietzsche had never been achieved by anyone, nor is it likely ever to be reached again" (Nunberg and Federn 1967, pp. 31–32). However Freud demarcated the difference between Nietzsche and psychoanalysis:

> What disturbs us is that Nietzsche transforms "is" into "ought," which is alien to science. In this he has remained after all, the moralist; he could not free himself of the theologian.

There too Freud reiterated (speaking in the third person):

> That he has never been able to study Nietzsche, partly because of the resemblance of Nietzsche's intuitive insights to our laborious investigations, and partly because of the wealth of ideas which has always prevented Freud from getting beyond the first half page whenever he tries to read him.
>
> (Nunberg and Federn 1967, p. 32)

Freud has often been condemned for failing to face directly this indebtedness to Nietzsche. But to admit that intuition played an important role in psychoanalysis as it did in Nietzsche's work would have threatened the whole scientific basis of the psychoanalytic edifice.

In 1912, Lou Andreas Salome joined Freud's circle of pupils and became a psychoanalyst. As a young woman, she was very close to Nietzsche; she was one of the very first non-medically trained people to be trained as a psychoanalyst.

Ellenberger (1970) lists examples of Nietzsche's influence. Nietzsche was passionate in his efforts to unmask conventions and get at the truth. In the *Genealogy of Morals,* Nietzsche described men as "wild beasts, magnificent blond beasts, craving booty and victory." With the founding of society, the instincts could no longer be discharged outwardly and this was the origin of guilt feelings. Even the thirst for knowledge Nietzsche saw as the self-destructive instinct in man. He saw science as inimical to life. The passage where Nietzsche wrote about the repression of instincts could have been written by Freud, but the idea that the epistemological wish, the wish to know, is inimical to life, Freud would have rejected. Psychoanalysis is based on the idea that knowledge of the unconscious or that making the unconscious conscious contributes to human freedom. Robert Waelder (1929) saw Freud as a successor to Dostoyevsky and Nietzsche as the discoverers and explorers of the unconscious. However, he also saw Freud as different from them because he "converted intuitive surmise into knowledge, experience into insight, and artistic hunches into science" (p. 377).

Much has been written about the relationship between Nietzsche's idea of "the eternal return" and Freud's repetition compulsion. Just how close Freud came to Nietzsche ultimately hinges on whether we accept the idea of Nietzsche about the "eternal return" or the "eternal recurrence" (Kaufmann 1950) as identical with Freud's repetition compulsion. Chapelle (1993) has written a small book to demonstrate that the two are almost identical. These issues are complex and require clarification. The idea behind Nietzsche's "eternal recurrence" goes back to Greek philosophy, particularly to Pythagoras and Heraclites. The pagan religions that dominated the Middle East were all cyclical in nature and based on the seasons of the year; they exemplify eternal recurrences. Buddhism, with its belief in reincarnation, is another example. By contrast, Jewish monotheism was not cyclical but historical. It implied progression from the creation of the world, to revelation on Mount Sinai and the establishment of law, to the final coming of the Messiah. All monotheistic religions are historical.

For Nietzsche, the idea of the "eternal return" was a powerful conviction; it was an insight that he was convinced redeemed his life. He left us a record of this experience, the record of his resistance to it:

In political terms, Nietzsche's eternal recurrence was a great discovery. In his time, Nietzsche's idea of the eternal return held great appeal. Thomas Mann converted it into a long prologue to his two-volume book *Joseph in Egypt.*

I come now to Freud's repetition compulsion:

> The manifestation of a compulsion to repeat (which we have described as occurring in the early activities of infantile mental life as well as among the events of psychoanalytic treatment) exhibit to a high degree an instinctual character and, when they act in opposition to the pleasure principle, give the appearance of a "daemonic" force at work.
>
> (Freud 1920, p. 35)

Freud's repetition compulsion is associated with trauma and is experienced "beyond the pleasure principle." The question arises whether the death instinct and the repetition compulsion, as described by Freud, are still compatible with the outlook of the Enlightenment, or whether at this point Freud made a major concession to Romanticism.

Because this issue is of some importance, I made a study of Freud's use of the word "daemonic." With the aid of the concordance to the *Standard Edition*, I found that he used the term eighteen times. The earliest appearance of the word occurs when Freud discusses some forms of hysteria, such as the violent blasphemies of nuns during the Middle Ages (Freud 1892–93, p. 126). In *The Interpretation of Dreams* Freud used the term when he quoted Aristotle's view that dreams are not divine but daemonic, since nature itself is daemonic, not divine. In his book on Leonardo da Vinci (1910b), Freud described the Mona Lisa's smile as "daemonic." (p. 108). The connection between the repetition compulsion and the word "daemonic" appears for the first time in 1919, in the paper *The Uncanny*, where Freud says, "a compulsion powerful enough to overrule the pleasure principle, lending to certain aspects of the mind their daemonic character." (Freud 1919b, p. 238). It seems that Freud used the term "daemonic" only as a metaphor.

In 1910, Jung, still a disciple of Freud, became intoxicated with Nietzsche's *Birth of Tragedy Out of the Spirit of Music*. He wished to transform psychoanalysis into a Dionysian fraternity. On February 11, 1910, he wrote to Freud:

> The ethical problem of sexual freedom really is enormous, and worth the sweat of all noble souls. But 2,000 years of Christianity can only be replaced by something equivalent. An ethical fraternity, with its mythical nothing, not infused by any archaic-infantile driving force, is a pure vacuum and can never evoke in man the slightest trace of that age-old animal power which drives the migrating bird across the sea and without which no irresistible mass movement can come into being.
>
> (Jung 1910)

Jung's letter can be seen as the invasion of Romanticism into psychoanalysis. Freud answered soberly two days later:

> My intentions are not so far reaching ... I am not thinking of a substitute for religion: this need must be sublimated. I did not expect the fraternity to become a religious organization any more than I would expect a volunteer fire department to do so.
>
> (McGuire 1974, pp. 294–295)

After Jung left psychoanalysis, the Romantic streak in his work became more pronounced and eventually led to his anti-Semitism.

In *The Role of the Unconscious*, written shortly after breaking with Freud, Jung wrote:

> these specifically Jewish doctrines are thoroughly unsatisfying to the German mentality; we still have a genuine barbarian in us who is not to be trifled with: and whose manifestation is no comfort to us and not a pleasant way of passing the time. Would that people could learn the lesson of this war.
>
> (Jung 1918, p. 14)

Jung took Freud's idea of repression and transformed into Romantic concepts "upper and lower parts," and "darker" and "brighter" sides. The secular mixture of psychoanalysis is discarded and the religious concept of "redemption" is introduced. Jung differentiates between the need of German bloodlust from the overcivilized Jew – the two becoming incompatible, a view that easily becomes anti-Semitic.

Jung became something equivalent to Hitler's court psychologist, and his utterances became more overtly anti-Semitic. Just the belief that there is a gulf that cannot be bridged between Germans and Jews demonstrates the return to Romanticism. In Jung's analytical psychology Romanticism re-entered the field of psychotherapy with a vengeance. For understandable reasons, Jung could embrace Nietzsche and proclaim his indebtedness to him.

Scientific method and psychoanalytic technique

When Freud wrote his papers on technique (1912c) he made a number of statements that later proved to be a stumbling block, and psychoanalysis paid a heavy price for them. They had the purpose of maintaining the scientific status of psychoanalysis as a natural science and were intended to prevent it from sliding back into the dangers of Romanticism.

> I cannot advise my colleagues too urgently to model themselves during psychoanalytic treatment on the surgeon who puts aside all feelings, even his human sympathy and concentrates his mental forces on the single aim of performing the operation as skillfully as possible.
>
> (p. 115)

The mirror and the surgeon metaphors have often been cited against Freud as proof of his detachment and the lack of personal involvement in his work. They were designed to uphold the scientific status of psychoanalysis. The resistances of the patient had to be overcome, and transference worked through, in such an aseptic atmosphere in order that psychoanalysis be recognized as a science. In a chapter of his book on technique, significantly entitled "The termination of the contract," Karl Menninger (1958) described the kind of termination that Freud's metaphors aimed to achieve.

> He has reacted to the analyst as if he were his mother, his father, his brother, his teacher, his sister, his wife. Gradually these illusions have tended to fade in intensity. The analyst becomes more and more just the analyst. The doctor who has patiently listened to me.
>
> (p. 172)

In the history of psychoanalysis Menninger's view can be described as carrying the transference view of psychoanalysis to an extreme. This view should be contrasted with Loewald's 1960 point of view of the analyst as a new object who leaves a permanent impact on the patient precisely because no pervious person in their life behaved like the analyst did. I found that Loewald was more correct than Menninger, but Menninger's patient does not return to analysis while Loewald's is more likely to come back for further analysis.

In his seminal paper of 1960, Loewald expressed what amounted to a fundamentally new point of view:

> If "structural changes in the patient's personality" means anything, it must mean that we assume that ego development is resumed in the therapeutic process in psychoanalysis. And this resumption of ego development is contingent on the relationship with a new object, the analyst.
>
> (p. 221)

In these few lines, Loewald expressed two revolutionary ideas. The first was that psychoanalysis aims at the resumption of ego growth. This was not part of Freud's vocabulary. As Freud saw it, all that psychoanalysis could do was to remove the extra burden that the neurosis adds, so that the neurotic can face the ordinary miseries that life offers without an extra burden. To use an analogy, Freud saw psychoanalysis as removing an extra tax that neurosis imposes, but expected the analyzed person to share all the difficulties of real life. Erikson first introduced the ideas that we keep on developing throughout our lives if we are not handicapped by a neurosis. In Erikson's view, human development did not stop with the repression of the Oedipus complex, but continued through the life cycle, including marriage and old age (Erikson 1959).

Loewald's second idea, no less revolutionary, was that psychoanalytic cure is contingent on the relationship with the analyst as a new object. The analyst as a new object was not subject to the same kind of termination and resolution of the transference that Freud envisioned. Loewald (1960) became critical of the classical approach:

> While the fact of an object relationship between patient and analyst is taken for granted, classical formulations concerning therapeutic actions, and concerning the role of the analyst in the analytic relationship, do not reflect our present understanding of the dynamic organization of psychic apparatus.
>
> (p. 222)

With these formulations, object relations theory was introduced into the mainstream of psychoanalysis in the United States. In Great Britain Michael Balint (1968, p. 156) suggested that the model of psychoanalysis as a one-person psychology with the analyst acting as an observer, be changed into a two-person psychology with analyst and analysand in a perpetual interaction with each other. Thus a new paradigm no longer rooted in natural science with new problems took hold.

Within the context of the Enlightenment, the neutral psychoanalyst may well have his origins in the ideal of the historian. Cassirer (1932) quotes Pierre Bayle's (1647–1706) credo for historians writing in the spirit of Enlightenment.

> All those who know the laws of history, will agree that a historian who wishes to fulfill his tasks faithfully must free himself of the spirit of flattery and slander. He must, as far as possible, adopt the state of mind of the Stoic who is moved by no passion. Impervious to all else, he must heed solely the interests of truth.
>
> (pp. 208–209)

In 1919 Freud added another admonition: "Analytic treatment should be carried through as far as possible under privation – in a state of abstinence" (Freud

1919a, p. 162). He maintained that every improvement diminishes the wish of the analysand to go deeper.

> Cruel that it may sound, we must see to it that the patient's suffering ... does not come to an end prematurely ... we must reinstate appreciable privation; otherwise we run the danger of never achieving any improvement except quite insignificant and transitory ones.
>
> (p. 163)

The view of mankind that emerges from the 1919 paper is no longer that of the Enlightenment. It was the crucial role that resistance plays that convinced Freud that the irrational is a major force to be reckoned with.

The incursion of Romanticism into psychoanalytic technique can also be traced back to the debate between Freud and Ferenczi as to the relative significance of insight (*Einsicht* in German) as opposed to genuine experience (*Erlebnis* in German). Insight can become a weapon in the hands of the ego to free itself from the shackles of the repetition compulsion; while experience is a subjective way of feeling relief from psychic tensions. Although experience may be feared as dangerous, it is usually welcome. By contrast, insight is usually resisted, even by the ego itself. For Freud, insight was crucial, while for Ferenczi, experience mattered most. Insight represents the victory of the rational realm over the irrational, while experience is a value of Romanticism (Hynal 1988).

After 1920, the study of culture became increasingly important to Freud. In *An Autobiographical Study* (1925c), Freud observed:

> My interest after making a lifelong detour through the natural sciences, medicine and psychology, returned to the cultural problems which had fascinated me long before when I was a youth scarcely old enough for thinking.
>
> (p. 72)

In 1920, Freud announced his dual instinct theory with his emphasis on the eternal struggle between the life and the death instinct, and when, in 1923, he developed the structural point of view – with its emphasis on the intrapsychic conflict between superego, ego and id – without intending to do so Freud broke his links to the optimistic tenets of the Enlightenment. But the inference of the Enlightenment remains strong, particularly in his book *The Future of an Illusion* (1927a) in which his abiding loyalty to the Enlightenment comes out more strongly than elsewhere:

> Religion is comparable to a childhood neurosis, and he [Freud] is optimistic enough to suppose that mankind will surmount this neurotic phase, just as so many children grow out of their similar neurosis. The voice of the intellect is a soft one, but it does not rest till it has gained a hearing. Finally, after countless succession of rebuffs, it succeeds. This is one of the few points on which one may be optimistic about the future of mankind.
>
> (p. 53)

A strange, and I could almost say no longer appropriate, optimism pervades the 1927 book.

Freud continued to fear that psychoanalysis might become a philosophy and lose its status as a science. A chapter in *The New Introductory Lectures on Psycho-Analysis* (1933) is entitled "The question of a *Weltanschauung*."

> Weltanschauung is an intellectual construction which solves all the problems of our existence uniformly on the basis of one overriding hypothesis which accordingly, leaves no question unanswered, and in which everything that interests us finds its fixed place ... psychoanalysis as a specialist science, a branch of psychology – a depth psychology, or psychology of the unconscious – it is quite unfit to construct a Weltanschauung of its own. It must accept the scientific one
>
> [...]
>
> psychoanalysis has a special right to speak for the scientific Weltanschauung at this point, since it cannot be reproached with having neglected what is mental in the picture of the universe. Its contribution to science lies precisely in having extended research to the mental field.
>
> (pp. 158–159)

According to Freud's definition of *Weltanschauung*, science – with its awareness of how much is still unknown – cannot become a *Weltanschauung* since it cannot answer all questions. Freud himself had a philosophy of life that he developed with increasing vigor after 1920. It was the *Weltanschauung* that contributed to making the twentieth century the century of Freud (Nelson 1957).

In 1924 Freud attempted a major reinterpretation of the place of masochism in human life. He wrote:

> Masochism comes under our observation in three forms: as a condition imposed on sexual excitation, as an expression of feminine nature, and as a norm of behaviour.
>
> (Freud 1924a, p. 161)

The phrase "comes under our observation" is the language of science, as if Freud were using a particularly powerful microscope; but in fact Freud is here combining three different phenomena under one roof. It is a creative act of synthesis that no one before him had attempted. The language remains the language of science and observation, while the integrating power of the observer goes beyond the data of observation.

After Freud

After the Second World War the center of gravity of psychoanalysis shifted to North America, and the debate between Enlightenment and Romanticism lost much of its relevance.

When Freud died on September 23, 1939, two roads were potentially open to psychoanalysis. It could have continued to live off Freud's heritage, making small additions to what he and his co-workers had already discovered; or it could develop significantly beyond Freud, but at the cost of sacrificing its own inner unity.

In his Freud lecture, Leo Stone (1961) took issue with Freud's metaphor of the surgeon:

> I do not believe that any patient, except in a morbid sense, can ever accept even the possibility (not to speak of the fact) that the analyst is not at all interested in the course of her or his personal life and illness.
>
> (p. 36)

> In gratifying this "mature" wish of childhood, there is also in the analytic situation, as in childhood, an acceptable form of love which, in an economic sense, may well contribute importantly to the incentive for mastery of unneutralized and unelaborated erotic and destructive drives.
>
> (p. 50)

The next quotation had a particularly strong impact:

> Whereas purely technical or intellectual errors can, in most instances, be corrected, a failure in a critical juncture to show the reasonable human response, which any person inevitably expected from another on whom he deeply depends, can invalidate years of patient and largely skillful work.
>
> (p. 55)

The historical reasons why Freud felt compelled to use the metaphor of the surgeon was no longer relevant to the post-Second World War generation of psychoanalysts.

Unlike most of the modifiers of Freud, Winnicott was always grateful to Freud, recognizing that, without him, the whole process of psychoanalysis would never have come into existence. But historically speaking he was the most radical modifier of Freud's work. In Winnicott's classic paper of 1953, *Transitional Objects and Transitional Phenomena*, the revolutionary nature of his discovery was not readily apparent; one could still classify that paper as an extension of Freud's work (Bergmann 1993b). When Winnicott went on to emphasize the central role of playing (Winnicott 1971), even though he used the word metaphorically he moved psychoanalysis beyond Freud.

> Psychotherapy takes place in the overlap of two areas of playing, that of the patient and that of the therapist. Psychotherapy has to do with two people playing together. The corollary of this is that where playing is not possible then the work done by the therapist is directed towards bringing the patient from a state of not being able to play into a state of being able to play.
>
> (p. 38)

Beyond Freud's horizon is also Winnicott's second idea: "The reason why playing is essential is that it is in playing that the patient is being creative" (p. 54). Even more directly, in the spirit of Romanticism, is the following statement by Winnicott:

> It is creative appreciation more than anything else that makes the individual feel that life is worth living ... compliance carries with it a sense of futility for the individual and is associated with the idea that nothing matters and that life is not worth living. In a tantalizing way many individuals have experienced just enough creative living to recognize that for most of their time they are living uncreatively, as if caught up in the creativity of someone else, or of a machine.
>
> (p. 65)

Another American modifier whose work is relevant to the topic under discussion is George Klein. Metapsychology reached its highest status in the United States during the Hartmann period and no analyst rivaled David Rapaport as the interpreter of chapter 7 of the *Interpretation of Dreams* (Bergmann 2000). The most brilliant among Rapaport's students was George Klein, who, in two chapters in his book *Psychoanalytic Theory: An Exploration of Essentials* (1976), declared metapsychology superfluous. Klein was not alone. He was supported by Benjamin Rubenstein, Charles Fisher, Roy Schafer, Robert Holt and others.

Klein did not mince words.

> The existence of two theories – the two cultures of psychoanalysis – is, I believe, a historical aberration traceable to Freud's philosophy of science. Freud's philosophy assumed: (1) concepts of purposefulness and meaning are unacceptable as terms of scientific explanation; (2) an acceptable explanation must be purged of teleological implications; (3) that regularities described with purposivistic concepts will ultimately be explained through purely psychological models, which disclose the causes of which the purpose principle is simply a descriptive expression.
>
> Freud's drive reduction model itself (into which Rapaport [1951] tried to encompass all psychoanalytic conceptions) is more appropriate to a rat than to a human.
>
> My own objection to the thermodynamic model of psychoanalysis, as well as the contemporary counterparts vying to replace it, is not their inherent implausibility; more to the point is that they are simply irrelevant to the clinical psychoanalytic enterprise.
>
> (p. 47)

> Let there be no mistake: psychoanalysts are theorists not on the "how" but on the "why" of behavior. Undeniably, some psychoanalysts are profitably engaged in "how" research; but you may note that they work outside of the psychoanalytic situation, in the university or medical laboratory.
>
> (p. 55)

This quote shows how well Klein understood Freud, but also how strong his feelings ran. Freud's philosophy is dismissed as an aberration.

Klein called Freud's his adherence to the "Brücke Oath" his historical aberration. He also added the pertinent observation that when Freud discarded his "Project" he was dissatisfied with his own achievement, though not with its objective: in chapter 7 of *The Interpretation of Dreams* the same objective was sought.

To my knowledge, the first psychoanalyst to question Freud's philosophy was Heinz Kohut (1977):

> Freud took the ultimate step that could still be taken by "objective science": he investigated the inner life of men including – and especially – his own. But – and here lies the crucial issue – he gazed at men's inner life with the objectivity of an external observer.
>
> (p. 67)

We should note that for Kohut gazing at man's inner life with the objectivity of the external observer is no longer a praise of Freud, but rather a criticism. Nevertheless, he was not willing to give up the claim that psychoanalysis was a science. In a letter to a colleague, Kohut (1980) wrote:

> All empirical sciences belong to one of two categories: there are, on the one hand, the sciences that base themselves on extrospection and vicarious extrospection, and there are, on the other hand, the sciences that are based on introspection and vicarious introspection (empathy). To the first category belong the physical and biological sciences, to the second the psychological sciences, par excellence psychoanalysis, the science of complex mental states.
>
> (p. 457)

In Kohut's view the human being strives to achieve a sense of cohesiveness and purpose. The infant first acquires a sense of body unity. Then, with further maturation, he acquires a cohesive self and becomes his own center of volition. Unlike Freud, Kohut saw the idealization of the parents and the repetition of this idealization in the transference as a positive sign. Such an idealization, if not traumatically interrupted, will endow the future adult with a sense of purpose and meaning. And, at the same time, Kohut visualized that a human being throughout his life span remains dependent on the support of self-objects. A self-object is another human being needed to support the cohesion of the self. When I differentiate the woman I love from the woman I cannot live without, the second woman is the self-object. The concert of the autonomous individual, so dear to the philosophers of the Enlightenment, became irrelevant to Kohut.

Peter Gay, in his biography of Freud, quoted Anna Freud as saying that Freud was not musical. He occasionally went to a few operas, but never to a concert. This is rather striking considering the fact that Vienna was, in the eyes of many, the musical capital of Europe. Kohut (1977) had this to say about Freud's relationship to music:

> It was his personality that determined his preference for the content of thought, for the clearly defined and the definable; it was his personality that made him shun the areas of contentless forms and intensities and unaccountable emotions.
>
> (p. 294)

Somewhat apologetically, Kohut added:

> In general I feel that Freud's limitation vis-à-vis the experience of music, while clearly of deep significance, should not be evaluated as a defect, but as a characteristic feature of his personality, a personality defined by the need for steadfast predominance of rationality.
>
> (p. 295)

In a letter, Freud once complained that Einstein had the support of a long series of predecessors, from Newton onward, while he had to "hack every step in my way through a tangled jungle alone." This powerful metaphor expresses how Freud felt about his life work.

Psychoanalysis was born at the crossroads between the rational philosophy of the Enlightenment and Romanticism. It seems to me unlikely that it could have emerged at any other point in history. In his philosophy Freud remained loyal to the Enlightenment and grateful for the liberation it gave to the Jews. But as a person he was strongly attracted to Romanticism and had to wage an inner struggle against it. Psychoanalysis was not a discovery, but a creation, and it therefore had to carry, for a long period of time, the stamp of its creator. It is a question whether the history of ideas will agree with him that psychoanalysis represents the attempt of natural science to conquer the inner world of men.

The persistence of different schools within psychoanalysis and the vehemence of the discussions that sometimes takes place is further proof that we cannot live up to the demands of rational discourse and rational behavior demanded by the philosophy of the Enlightenment and our own collective ego ideal. The ideas of the Enlightenment governed Freud's philosophy to the end of his life, but this belief was not transferred to the next generations. Are we a group of technicians, like builders of bridges; or physicians who "minister to a mind diseased" (*Macbeth*, Act V, Scene III) who need no common philosophy? The history of psychoanalysis presented raises these questions.

Freud would have felt that he was endangering the scientific status of psychoanalysis if he acknowledged his interest in Romantic philosophy. His discovery of the power of the unconscious and the inability to obtain mastery over it undermined the optimism of the Enlightenment. However, by promising to enlarge the area of consciousness, psychoanalysis gave the optimism of the Enlightenment a new chance.

The diversity among the schools of psychoanalysis has given its history a new urgency. When Freud wrote *On the History of the Psycho-Analytic Movement* (1914c), he could explain all defections and modifications as a resistance to psychoanalysis. It was a powerful argument in its own day and tended to consolidate the psychoanalytic movement around Freud with a feeling of sectarian superiority over all modifiers and defectors. Historically speaking, it was based on a premise of the Enlightenment, that there is only one truth and many falsehoods. We live in a different cultural climate today.

Note

1 An earlier version of this paper was read in 1999 before the Berlin Psychoanalytic Society as the Karl Abraham Lecture, and also as the 2000 Freud Anniversary Lecture before the New York Psychoanalytic Society in April 2000.

References

Balint, M. (1968) *The Basic Fault: Therapeutic Aspects of Regression*. London: Tavistock Publications.

Bergmann, M.S. (1976) Moses and the Evolution of Freud's Jewish Identity. In *Judaism and Psychoanalysis*, ed. M. Ostow. New York: Ktav Publishing House, 1982, pp. 115–141.

Bergmann, M.S. (1993b) Reflections on the History of Psychoanalysis. *Journal of the American Psychoanalytic Association* 41: 929–955.

Bergmann, M.S., ed. (2000) *The Hartmann Era*. New York: Other Press.

Bernfeld, S. (1944) Freud's Earliest Theories and the School of Helmholtz. *Psychoanalytic Quarterly* 13: 341–362.

Bowra, C.M. (1950) *The Romantic Imagination*. London: Oxford.

Cassirer, E. (1932) *Die Philosophie der Aufklärung* (*The Philosophy of the Enlightenment*). Princeton: Princeton University Press, 1951.

Chapelle, D (1993) *Nietzsche and Psychoanalysis*. Albany, NY: State University of New York Press.

Clark, K. (1973) *The Romantic Rebellion: Romantic versus Classical Art.* New York: Harper & Row.
Erikson, E.H. (1959) *Identity In the Life Cycle: Psychological Issues*, vol. 1, no. 1. Madison, CT: International Universities Press.
Ellenberger, H. (1970) *The Discovery of the Unconscious: The History and Evolution of Dynamic Psychiatry.* New York: Basic Books.
Fenichel, O. (1945) *The Psychoanalytic Theory of Neurosis.* New York: W.W. Norton & Co., Inc.
Freud, S. (1892–93) A Case of Successful Treatment by Hypnotism: With Some Remarks on the Origin of Hysterical Symptoms Through "Counter-Will." S.E. 1: 115–128.
Freud, S. (1895) A Project for a Scientific Psychology. S.E. 1: 283–397.
Freud, S. (1900) The Interpretation of Dreams, Part I and Part II. S.E. 4–5: 1–625.
Freud, S. (1910b) Leonardo da Vinci and a Memory of His Childhood S.E. 11: 63–137.
Freud, S. (1910c) The Future Prospects of Psychoanalytic Therapy. S.E. 11: 141–151.
Freud, S. (1910e) "Wild" Psycho-Analsis. S.E. 11: 219–228.
Freud, S. (1912c) Recommendations to Physicians Practising Psycho-Analysis. S.E. 12: 111–120.
Freud, S. (1913a) The Theme of the Three Caskets. S.E. 12: 291–301.
Freud, S. (1914c) On the History of the Psycho-Analytic Movement. S.E. 14: 7–66.
Freud, S. (1915c) Thoughts for the Times of War and Death. S.E. 14: 273–300.
Freud, S. (1919a) Lines of Advance in Psycho-Analytic Therapy. S.E. 17: 157–168.
Freud, S. (1919b) The Uncanny. S.E. 17: 219–256.
Freud, S. (1920) Beyond the Pleasure Principle. S.E. 18: 7–64.
Freud, S. (1924a) The Economic Problem of Masochism. S.E. 19: 157–170.
Freud, S. (1925c) An Autobiographical Study. S.E. 20: 7–74.
Freud, S. (1927a) The Future of an Illusion. S.E. 21: 3–56.
Freud, S. (1933) New Introductory Lectures on Psycho-Analysis. S.E. 22: 1–182.
Freud, S. (1940) An Outline of Psycho-Analysis. S.E. 23: 141–207.
Hynal, A. (1988) *Controversies in Psychoanalytic Methods: From Freud to Ferenczi and Michael Balint.* New York: New York University Press.
Jung, C.G. (1910) *C.G. Jung Letters, Volume I, 1906–1950*, eds G. Adler and A. Jaffe. Princeton, NJ: Princeton University Press, 1973.
Jung, C.G. (1918) *The Role of the Unconscious.* In *The Collected Works, Volume Ten: Civilization in Transition*, 2nd edition, eds H. Read, M. Fordham, G. Adler, trans. R.F.C. Hull. Routledge: London.
Kaufmann, W.A. (1950) *Nietzsche: Philosopher, Psychologist, Antichrist.* Princeton: Princeton University Press.
Klein, G. (1976) *Psychoanalytic Theory: An Exploration of Essentials.* New York: International Universities Press.
Kohut, H. (1977) *The Restoration of the Self.* New York: International Universities Press.
Kohut, H. (1980) Two Letters. In *Advances in Self Psychology*, ed. Goldberg, A.. New York: International Universities Press.
Loewald, H. (1960) On the Therapeutic Action of Psychoanalysis. *International Journal of Psychoanalysis* 41: 16–33.
Mann, T. (1922). Freud's Position in the History of Modern Thought. In *Past Masters.* New York: Knopf, 1933.
McGuire, W., ed. (1974) *The Freud/Jung Letters. The Correspondence Between Sigmund Freud and C. G. Jung*, trans. R. Manheim and R.F.C. Hall. Princeton: Princeton University Press.
Menninger, K.A. (1958) *Theory of Psychoanalytic Technique.* New York: Basic Books.
Nelson B., ed. (1957) *Freud and the 20th Century.* New York: Meridian Books.
Nunberg, H. and Federn, E. (1962) *Minutes of the Vienna Psychoanalytic Society, Volume I: 1906–1908.* New York: International Universities Press.
Nunberg, H. and Federn, E. (1967) *Minutes of the Vienna Psychoanalytic Society, Volume II: 1908–1910.* New York: International Universities Press.

Praz, M. (1970) *The Romantic Agony*. New York: Oxford University Press.
Stone, L. (1961) *The Psychoanalytic Situation: An Examination of its Development and Essential Nature*. New York: International Universities Press.
Strenger, C. (1989) The Classic and the Romantic Vision in Psychoanalysis. *International Journal of Psychoanalysis* 70: 593–610.
Vermorel, M. and Vermorel, H. (1986) Was Freud a Romantic? *International Review of Psychoanalysis* 13: 15–37.
Waelder, R. (1929) The Inference of Psychoanalysis on the Outlook on Life of Modern Man. In *Psychoanalysis, Observation, Theory, Application. Selected Papers of Robert Waelder*, ed. S.A.G. Guttman. New York: International University Press, 1976.
Winnicott, D.W. (1971) *Playing and Reality*. London: Tavistock.

CHAPTER 9

THE DUAL IMPACT OF FREUD'S DEATH, AND FREUD'S DEATH INSTINCT THEORY, ON THE HISTORY OF PSYCHOANALYSIS[1]

This paper is submitted for public consideration with the feeling that it is both important and likely to arouse controversy. I also have a feeling of "belatedness" that this topic should have been discussed much earlier at some international congress, and the failure to do so has handicapped the development of psychoanalysis. What I am suggesting is that we submit the psychoanalytic movement and some important aspects of its history to psychoanalytic scrutiny.

We often hear it said that one of the striking features that determined both the nature and the history of psychoanalysis is the fact that it was created and built by one man. To my knowledge we have never asked ourselves to examine the implications of this fact. It may even be that this subject has the status of a taboo subject. One is tempted to cite the many contributions of other creative analysts to our field to deny this fact. One of the unexpected consequences may be that no leader was permitted to emerge as the next spokesperson for psychoanalysis as a whole, and if a significant contender arises he or she can only be of equal significance to Freud to a limited number of followers who then form a school named after that leader; Kleinians, Lacanians and Kohutians come to mind. Those who do not follow have a tendency to blame the new leader for creating controversies and disturbing the unity of psychoanalysis. One can speak of a certain historical irony that it was Freud who discovered the significance of the Oedipus complex and at the same time also created a movement that could not resolve its oedipal strivings towards its founder.

After Freud's death psychoanalysis faced a choice between two alternatives: to remain frozen at the point where Freud left it and becoming an orthodoxy, or to make progress at the cost of breaking up into schools in conflict with each other. As it happened both approaches were tried at the same time. If I am right, the breakup of psychoanalysis into different schools often at war with each other had to happen because after Freud was disappointed in Jung, he never designated a successor. The sociology of psychoanalysis was such that no other analyst could replace Freud as a leader. However, the author of *Totem and Taboo* (1913b) must have known that to leave the succession to a band of brothers was hazardous. Freud died without leaving his heirs any guidelines as to how he visualized psychoanalysis would grow and develop after his death.

As to the dispute between Freud and Jung, the tendency was to blame Jung until 1964, when Winnicott showed that the autobiography of Jung demonstrated that his psychic structure was psychotic rather than neurotic and Freud had nothing of value to contribute to Jung. In retrospect we can also see that Freud's offer to Jung that he be the Joshua to bring psychoanalysis into the promised land, while Freud was its Moses, was not as flattering to Jung as it seemed. Freud implied that Jung, being "Aryan" rather than "Semitic" and being a professor at a highly respected university, would do for psychoanalysis what Freud, the marginal Jew, could not. It is therefore not surprising that Jung opted to be his own Moses.

In ordinary science there is usually a clear line of demarcation. Certain problems have been solved by the techniques of this science, and another set of problems have absorbed the attention of investigators and are now the subject of study. When Freud died such a line of demarcation was not present. We were dependent on creative individuals to determine the direction of further development in psychoanalysis.

Even in Freud's lifetime the boundaries of the discipline were never clear. It was always up to Freud to declare what was within the borders of psychoanalysis and what was not. The records of the Vienna Psychoanalytic Association leave us no doubt that it was Freud's prerogative to define what psychoanalysis is or is not. On February 1, 1911, Adler was speaking to the group on what he considered the "masculine protest" present in all women, without exception (Nunberg and Federn 1974). It evoked Freud's rebuke: "In point of fact, however, Adler's writings are not a continuation upward, nor are they a foundation underneath; they are something else entirely. This is not psychoanalysis" (p. 146). In their remarks the assembled disciples showed that they did not understand that at this moment the boundaries of psychoanalysis were being defined for the first time.

To advance further, I suggest that we look at the state of psychoanalysis at the moment of Freud's death. Freud died on September 23, 1939. War was declared on September 1, 1939. We have in our possession one prominent psychoanalyst's reaction to Freud's death. I am referring to the publication of Otto Fenichel's 119 circular letters. Circular letter 61, dated October 15, 1939, is the first letter written to the secret group of recipients after Freud's death. Fenichel's appraisal of the survival of psychoanalysis was pessimistic. He believed that Psychoanalytic International was held together only by the personal binding of its members to Freud. He foresaw the danger of its disintegration after his death; Europe appeared paralyzed and the US was succumbing to the danger of the popularization of psychoanalysis.

From London, Fenichel reported:

> Most of us have no patients at the moment, for everybody is busy with more urgent matters. I think as doctors we will get other work very soon. Dorothy Burlingham reported that Melanie Klein and Isaacs attacked her about a child analysis case, specifically about the "internal object" even though it had nothing to do with the subject. The Viennese complain that no productive discussions are possible.

Fenichel feared that the difference between "sexual" and "aggressive" drives was going to give way to the "good introjected object" and the "bad introjected object" under the rising power of the object relations theorists. Fenichel was also worried about the growing influence of Sandor Rado in the US.

If these dire predictions did not materialize, and Psychoanalytic International did survive, it is due that the fact that psychoanalysis after Freud's death did not expel what I call "the modifiers," a new type of psychoanalyst. In the fall of 1991, in my plenary address to the American Psychoanalytic Association (Bergmann 1993b),

I suggested that contributors to psychoanalysis fall into three categories: heretics, modifiers and extenders.

> The heretics, rare in recent years but prevalent in Freud's lifetime, were typically close to Freud for some time, made important contributions, and then bolted to start their own schools. They include Adler, Stekel, Jung, Rank, and Wilhelm Reich. During Freud's lifetime there were only heretics and extenders. Modifiers appeared after Freud's death when no one, not even Anna Freud, could lay claim to being the only heir to Freud's legacy.
>
> (p. 930)

Unlike the heretics, the modifiers also formed their own schools, but had no wish to resign or be expelled from the International. The modifiers, like the heretics, are also charismatic figures evoking both idealization and controversy. Extenders of psychoanalysis usually apply psychoanalysis to areas not yet explored; they are appreciated by their colleagues, become training psychoanalysts, and evoke no controversy. After Freud's death it was no longer possible to rebel against him and become a heretic. All a successor can do is modify one component or another of his work.

The modifier first emerged out of the controversial discussion between Anna Freud and her followers, and Melanie Klein and her disciples (King and Steiner 1991). Following the model of her father, Anna Freud tried to get the Kleinians expelled, but the British Psychoanalytic Society refused to give her the mantle of her father and once one modifier (Klein) was allowed to remain, others were more easily tolerated. Anna Freud's argument is well worth citing as an example of orthodoxy.

> Though the idea of an open forum for psychoanalytic teaching may seem tempting at a first glance, I personally doubt whether it could be carried out effectively and whether the result would not fall far short of the intentions, would not in effect turn out to be similar to institutes like the Tavistock Clinic with all their well-known shortcomings. If such a teaching procedure had been adopted from the beginning of psychoanalytic development psychoanalysis of the present day would include the theoretical and technical teachings of, for instance, Stekel, Adler, Jung, Rank, etc.
>
> (p. 633)

In her zeal, Anna Freud overlooked the possibility that the views of these heretics can be presented in a course on the history of psychoanalysis, explaining how these heresies came about without upsetting or confusing the candidate; and if it should turn out that a candidate finds any of the heretics enumerated congenial, the risk is better than orthodoxy based on withholding information about past controversies. My experience as a teacher of the history of psychoanalysis has convinced me that familiarity with old controversies, and why they emerged, contributes significantly to the maturity of the student of psychoanalysis.

But the problem goes deeper. Freud fundamentally changed his mind about his work twice in his life. The first instance was between the 1895 publication of the Breuer and Freud *Studies on Hysteria* and his own *The Interpretation of Dreams* in 1900. When these changes took place and the hypnotic-cathartic method was abandoned in favor of free association, Freud was a neurologist in private practice and no one else was affected by the change. There was, as yet, no band of followers and no International to be persuaded to adopt a new theory.

Due to the courage of Marie Bonaparte in defying Freud's wishes to destroy the Freud-Fliess correspondence, we have an excellent record of how this first transition took place (Masson 1985). Of particular interest is Freud's October 15, 1897 letter to Fliess, in which he reports:

> I have found, in my own case too, [the phenomenon of] being in love with my mother and jealous of my father, and I now consider it a universal event in early childhood. If this is so, we can understand the gripping power of Oedipus Rex.
> (Masson 1985, p. 272)

Thus the centrality of the Oedipus complex was first announced. Actually, in his self-analysis, Freud discovered only mild derivatives of his own Oedipus complex; its full discovery was possible only because Freud was acquainted with Sophocles' *Oedipus Rex* and Shakespeare's *Hamlet* (Bergmann 2001). The central role of the Oedipus complex as the organizer of infantile sexuality took a long time to emerge. When Freud was analyzing the Wolf Man, he realized that the Oedipus complex exists in its positive form when the parent of the same gender is the subject of murderous hostility, and the parent of the opposite sex is the object of sexual desire – but the Oedipus complex can also take a negative form when the parent of the same sex becomes the object of sexual desire, and the opposite parent the object of hostility. I will add an observation of my own: in those cases where the two are of the same approximate strength, any decision becomes difficult and every decision is followed by regret.

Transference analysis has familiarized us with the fact that at different times the same analyst can represent father, mother, sibling or grandparent. Less well known is the fact that this can also happen in real life, as the following example will illustrate. A young woman met and married a much older divorced man who was the father of children. The marriage began on a father transference, with the wife as the preferred child over his children. Slowly she discovered that this man had feminine traits that reminded her of her mother. A hostile maternal transference followed.

The contrast between the topographic and the structural point of view

The situation was very different when the next important change took place in Freud between 1920 and 1923. The transition from the topographic to the structural point of view took place in two books, *Beyond the Pleasure Principle*, where the death instinct was introduced, and *The Ego and the Id*, where the new tripartite division of the psychic apparatus was formulated. In the United States the change is described as shifting from the topographic to the structural point of view, while in Europe it is called a change from the first topographic to the second topographic model.

When these later changes were introduced in the 1920s there was already an organized psychoanalytic movement and the adherents of this movement were won over to psychoanalysis by the topographic point of view. So far as we know these psychoanalytic pioneers were entirely satisfied with the topographic point of view but were now confronted with the fact that the creator of this paradigm demanded a radical revision. It is hardly surprising that they reacted with bewilderment.

The task a psychoanalyst must perform under the topographic model was much simpler and it was correspondingly more pleasurable to be a psychoanalyst. The enemy was repression, directed particularly against the wishes of the Oedipus complex, and while the repression was necessary during childhood, Freud thought its task could be taken over and faced by the now more mature ego, without the need to repress. There are forces within the analysand that the therapist counts upon for assistance: the dynamic unconscious is pushing upward in dreams and slips of the tongue. Free association helps reach the unconscious; spontaneous childhood memories emerge and transference manifestations make the past reappear in the present. Once the unconscious was made conscious the topographic psychoanalyst could trust the ego of the analysand to do the rest. Relatively little help over a relatively short period of time is all that was necessary. Termination was clear-cut when the most important repressed wishes of childhood, particularly the specific oedipality of the patient, has been made conscious.

Under the structural model everything was more difficult, victory much less certain, and the demand on the psychoanalyst much heavier. Repression was no longer the main enemy; it was seen as just one of the many defenses of the ego and a relatively privileged defense easier to deal with than denial, projection or reaction formation. Because it interfered less in the capacity of the ego to test reality, under the widening scope of psychoanalysis the unwelcome discovery was made that too many patients use other defenses than repression, defenses that are less susceptible to modification by psychoanalysis.

Furthermore, under the structural point of view the impact of the death instinct was much harder to combat and the repetition compulsion was a more tenacious adversary. Intrapsychic conflict could not be eliminated; it could only be significantly modified. The point of termination was much harder to determine and the results less likely to be as permanent as was hoped (Bergmann 1997, 2005).

Up to 1920 conflict was conceptualized as taking place between the sexual drive and self-preservation; after 1920 the conflict was visualized as taking place between Eros, the life instinct, and Thanatos, the death instinct. Instead of the division of unconscious, preconscious and conscious, Freud introduced the intersystemic conflict between ego, id and superego. A new force, hitherto unnoticed – the repetition compulsion – was formulated as a new, formidable force working against the effort to cure the analysand. The repetition compulsion appears in the child's play when a traumatic experience is abreacted in play. Transference reactions are also due to the repetition compulsion. The power of the repetition compulsion, first described in *Beyond the Pleasure Principle* (1920), was thought to operate outside the parameters of the pleasure principle.

The ego protects itself against invasion by the unconscious and the repressed id by forming anticathexes (Freud 1920, p. 178) but in spite of this protective shield the repressed unconscious finds ways of overcoming the anticathexes through dreams, transference manifestations and parapraxes. In analysis, by free-associating, knowledge of the unconscious strengthens the weakened ego. Two further discoveries came from the structural phase: the discovery of the power of the unconscious sense of guilt as opposing the work of the analysis, and the fact that trauma becomes transformed into a powerful repetition compulsion.

From the topographic point of view Freud reaffirmed the demand that the analysand pledge to obey the "fundamental rule" that he or she say everything that comes to mind, without censorship. The fundamental rule was, however, more at home in the topographic than the structural point of view. The structural psychoanalyst knew, or at least should have known, that no patient can obey the fundamental rule until close to the end of the analysis. For the analysand the fear of the superego and the fear of losing the analyst's love will not allow the verbalization of complete candor.

When Freud introduced the death instinct into psychoanalysis it was only partially based on data obtained from clinical evidence. Freud derived the death instinct out of an assumption that everything that lives has to die and return to its earlier inorganic state. Because the inanimate preceded the animate, everything animate retains the "wish" to return to the inanimate state.

The ego treats the demand of infantile sexuality as it treats dangers coming from the external world, and even the sexual impulses of puberty can be treated like dangers from the external world, which the ego represses. One of the significant features of the superego, as formulated by Freud, is that it has its own contact with the repressed id. The superego knows what the ego has repressed and it punishes the person not only for conscious acts and thoughts, but also for the wishes that have undergone repression and consequently are unknown to the ego. The superego shows its power by creating a sense of guilt based on the information the superego has obtained by its direct contact with the id.

Freud's *Inhibition, Symptoms and Anxiety*, written in 1925, two years after *The Ego and the Id*, is a difficult but very interesting book because in it Freud, often uncertain, examines the implications of the new world he has discovered. The tripartite division of the id, ego and superego opened Freud's eyes to new sets of data. Inhibition could now be described as the restriction of an ego function. Certain ordinary ego functions, such as playing the piano or walking, can become eroticized and when this happens their function will become impaired. Freud then illustrated this point with a famous metaphor, "like a maidservant who refuses to go on cooking because her master started a love affair with her" (Freud 1925d, p. 89). The same ego, whose weakness was stressed in *The Ego and the Id*, was seen in 1925 as significantly stronger because it can give the anxiety signal. The aim of psychoanalytic treatment now became centered on helping the patient suffering from overwhelming anxiety to learn to use anxiety as a signal, and protect the ego from succumbing to anxiety states or forming phobias.

Freud then made the interesting observation that danger in the situation depended on what developmental phase one is in. The danger of earliest infancy is overstimulation, from which the caring adult must protect the infant. When the infant acquires the knowledge that the breast is not permanently available and not part of her or himself, the danger becomes withdrawal of love. When the oedipal stage is reached and the father's superiority is recognized the fear, at least for the boy, becomes castration. Finally, once the child recognizes the power of social relationships, the fear becomes the fear of the superego. Because previous stages of development are never fully overcome, all these fears can remain active to various degrees.

After the publication of *Inhibition, Symptoms and Anxiety* in 1925, something no one had expected happened: Freud lost much of his interest in psychoanalysis as a method of curing mental illness and turned to a broader interest in the future of civilization.

In the 1935 postscript to *An Autobiographical Study* (1925c), Freud himself noted some important changes.

> [S]ince I put forward my hypothesis of the existence of two classes of instinct (Eros and the death instinct) and since I proposed a division of the mental personality into an ego, a super-ego, and an id, I have made no further decisive contributions to psycho-analysis.
>
> (p. 72)

He then offered the following explanation:

> My interest, after making a lifelong *détour* through the natural sciences, medicine and psychotherapy, returned to the cultural problems which had fascinated me long before, when I was a youth scarcely old enough for thinking.
> (p. 72)

Freud then went on to say that the conflicts in cultural development were the same as the conflict between ego, id and superego that he studied in individuals.

I assume that the twin discoveries of the death instinct and the power of the repetition compulsion may have been traumatic for Freud and that the turning away from clinical psychoanalysis to a broader interest of the future of civilization became urgent for him. He was no longer sure that human civilization would survive; the therapeutic efforts of psychoanalysis seemed small by comparison with the danger the power of the aggressive drive posed. It is even more daring on my part to assume that unconsciously the psychoanalytic movement understood that its founder had left it to deal with larger and more pressing issues facing humankind. In *Analysis, Terminable and Interminable* (1937a), when Freud once more became interested in clinical psychoanalysis, his tone was more guarded and less optimistic.

> Everyday experience, however, teaches us that in a normal person any solution of an instinctual conflict only holds good for a particular relation between the strength of the instinct and the strength of the ego. If the strength of the ego diminishes, whether through illness or exhaustion, or from some similar cause, all the instincts which have so far been successfully tamed may renew their demands and strive to obtain substitutive satisfactions in abnormal ways.
> (pp. 225–226)

In 1927 Freud wrote *The Future of an Illusion*, in 1930 *Civilization and its Discontents* appeared, and close to the end of his life he published *Moses and Monotheism* as his personal reaction to the rise of anti-Semitism that followed Hitler taking power in Germany and later Austria. These books were interesting but in my view they must have suggested, unconsciously if not consciously, that after the formulation of the structural point of view Freud was no longer interested in psychoanalysis as a therapeutic movement. When Freud published *The New Introductory Lectures on Psychoanalysis* in 1933 they did not have much to say to the practitioner, as Freud himself noted. Some chapters were repetition of familiar data, while others, like the chapter on dreams and occultism, must have sounded puzzling – as did Freud's claim that psychoanalysis is not a point of view on life itself or, as he put it, psychoanalysis only shares the *Weltanschauung* of science. In retrospect this disclaimer sounds particularly strange when we remember that in both books a definite philosophy of life was represented.

Both *The Future of an Illusion* (1927a) and *Civilization and its Discontents* (1930) clearly show the impact of the structural point of view on Freud's thinking. In *The Future of an Illusion* Freud pointed out that "every individual is virtually an enemy of civilization" and "civilization has to be defended against the individual" (p. 6). Civilization in turn rests on a compulsion to work, and the renunciation of instinct (p. 10). Due to the formation of the superego the external coercion becomes internalized. Freud derived the need for a god from the need of the helpless child for a protective father. Religion is an illusion that failed to make its believers happy. It is the universal, obsessive neurosis of humanity (p. 43). Because Freud believed that humanity would, at some future time, outgrow the need to believe in a god, *The Future of an Illusion* belongs to the Enlightenment period of history. He concludes with a beautiful affirmation.

> The voice of the intellect is a soft one, but it does not rest till it has gained a hearing. Finally, after a countless succession of rebuffs, it succeeds. This is one of the few points on which one may be optimistic about the future of mankind, but it is in itself a point of no small importance. And from it one can derive yet other hopes.
>
> (Freud 1927a, p. 53)

> Since we are prepared to renounce a good part of our infantile wishes, we can bear it if a few of our expectations turn out to be illusions.
>
> (p. 54)

Since this book was written we have seen a number of attempts to create societies that are not based on belief in a god. They resulted in a "cult of personality." Freud's hopes that humanity will outgrow the need for an omnipotent god have not materialized.

Civilization and its Discontents (1930) opens with a discussion between Freud and Romain Rolland about the latter's ego-feeling as a basis for religion, which Freud explained in a very interesting way.

> originally the ego includes everything, later it separates off an external world from itself. Our present ego-feeling is, therefore, only a shrunken residue of a much more inclusive – indeed, an all-embracing – feeling which corresponded to a more intimate bond between the ego and the world about it.
>
> (p. 68)

In some people this early all-embracing ego feeling persists side by side with the "more sharply demarcated ego feelings of maturity" (p. 68). This persistent feeling of childhood is what Rolland calls "oceanic feeling," which he considers the basis of religion.

Freud then cites a famous statement by Goethe: "He who possesses science and art also has religion; but he who possesses neither of those two, let him have religion!" (fn, p. 74). Freud then concludes ruefully, "One feels inclined to say that the intention that man should be 'happy' is not included in the plan of 'Creation' " (p. 76). Unhappiness and suffering come from three directions: our own body, doomed to decay; from the external world that refuses to grant our wishes; and from our relations to other individuals (p. 72). Freud observed:

> The feeling of happiness derived from the satisfaction of a wild instinctual impulse untamed by the ego is incomparably more intense than that derived from sating an instinct that has been tamed.
>
> (p. 79)

Civilization and its Discontents was published only three years before Hitler seized power and yet Freud wrote that it was impossible for us to imagine what a victim of the Holy Inquisition or a Jew awaiting a pogrom felt, and concluded, "It seems to me unprofitable to pursue this aspect of the problem any further" (p. 89).

The enmity that Freud assumed to exist between the individual and society led him to raise the question of whether some societies allowed for more personal freedom than others. Freud assumed that Christianity, advocating universal love, led to a greater hostility towards the non-believer than was expressed by the Romans – who did not build their society on such an assumption and could afford to be more tolerant towards other religions (p. 114). Freud feared that as civilization advanced, the happiness of individuals would diminish because as more wishes became satisfied their guilt would be bound to increase (p. 134).

Politically more important were Freud's observations on communism. He questioned communism's basic assumption that humans were wholly good but private property had corrupted their nature. Under this theory, if private property were abolished all hostility would disappear. To Freud this was an illusion. Aggressiveness was not created by property; it was there before property became important. Humans do band together but then their hostility has to be directed outward. Freud wondered what the Soviets would do after they had wiped out the bourgeoisie (p. 115). (Since these lines were written, history has answered the question via the Moscow trials in the 1930s, and Stalin's terror campaigns.) Up to the discovery of the death instinct and the role of aggression, psychoanalysis was in alliance with forces operating for social change. With this book the psychoanalytic movement became more conservative.

In many ways the two books, written three years apart, are very similar. They are both based on Freud's new recognition of the role of aggression and the death instinct, but in other ways they are very different. *The Future of an Illusion* still belongs to the hopeful literature of the Enlightenment, but this cannot be said about the pessimism that dominates *Civilization and its Discontents* (1930). The first book ended with the affirmation of the voice of the intellectual; the second one ends thus:

> I have not the courage to rise up before my fellow-men as a prophet, and I bow to their reproach that I can offer them no consolation; for at bottom that is what they are all demanding – the wildest revolutionaries no less passionately than the most virtuous believers.
>
> (p. 145)

Taken together, in these two books Freud demonstrated that knowledge of psychoanalysis resulted in a definite philosophy of life or, as he preferred to call it, a *Weltanschauung*. Equally important was that psychoanalysis was no longer confined to a technique of therapy but leads to a new understanding of the world we live in.

The posthumously published *An Outline of Psycho-Analysis* (1940) is of special interest in this context because Freud demonstrates his struggle between the topographic and the structural point of view. Freud returned to reconsider the technique of psychoanalysis. Under the structural point of view the dream was reformulated as a "psychosis of short duration in a state of sleep" because in the dream the ego temporarily gives up its alliance with reality. Pathology was reformulated as a state in which the ego was so weakened as to make the fulfillment of its tasks impossible. The ego's task was formulated to reconcile the demands of reality, id and superego (p. 172).

If we read the *Outline* with some care the whole complex structure of psychoanalysis can be formulated succinctly. Freud has a developmental theory: under favorable conditions a normal child will go through three stages of development before reaching maturity. Every child will go through a period of infantile sexuality, which culminates in reaching a particular form of the Oedipus complex. Again, under normal conditions these oedipal wishes cannot find fulfillment. Next a latency period will ensue and this oedipal sexuality will undergo repression or even dissolution (Freud 1924b). In adolescence a new wave of sexuality will take over, which, under favorable conditions, will be directed to new objects that are no longer subject to the oedipal taboo and lead to adult sexuality. The inherent propensities of the human species will not take place if traumatic events occur, such as the seduction of the child by adults, separation from or death of a parent, and many more. Sometimes there will be no latency and the oedipal attachment will not result.

The *Outline* also determines the work of the therapist. The therapist uncovers both the infantile sexuality and the traumatic events that did not allow the expected developments to take place. The therapeutic intervention should enable the analysand to know what the infantile sexuality was like, what specific points of fixation hampered development, and how development becomes possible again.

What I have said is all to be found in the *Outline* but not as succinctly as I have formulated it and it has not been made available as clearly to the student of psychoanalysis. There is also much that is obsolete in the *Outline*, where Freud went astray. I will give only one example. On page 197 Freud says:

> in psychology, unlike physics, we are not always concerned with things which can only arouse a cool scientific interest. Thus we shall not be very greatly surprised if a woman analyst who has not been sufficiently convinced of the intensity of her own wish for a penis also fails to attach proper importance to that factor in her patients. But such sources of error, arising from the personal equation, have no great importance in the long run.

This prediction did not come true and is not likely to come true. Every psychoanalysis is limited not only by the limitations of the analysand but also by the blind spots of the analyst. Unique and non-repeatable events are also subject to scientific study but they offer special difficulties.

The psychoanalyst and the weakened ego of the analysand band together into a pact. The patient's ego promises complete "candor" to say everything that comes to mind without censorship, and the analyst promises "strictest discretion" and makes available his or her special knowledge. However, psychoanalysis is only productive if the analysand has an ego capable of entering into a productive alliance with the therapist. Psychotics and borderline patients do not have an ego with sufficient coherence and cannot profit from analysis. This led Freud to privilege the neuroses. Later on this restriction to working only with neuroses led to controversy about the widening scope of psychoanalysis, as the effort to extend psychoanalytic help to more disturbed patients was called.

Freud contrasted the two theories. Staying within the topographic model, he reiterated:

> The symptoms of neuroses are, it might be said, without exception either a substitutive satisfaction of some sexual urge or measures to prevent such a satisfaction; and as a rule they are compromises between the two, of the kind that come about in accordance with the laws operating between contraries in the unconscious.
>
> (Freud 1940, p. 186)

However, only a few lines later he introduces the structural point of view: "most of the urges of sexual life are not of a purely erotic nature but have arisen from alloys of the erotic instinct with portions of the destructive instinct" (ibid.). Still on the same page, after this hesitation Freud makes one of the most important formulations of developmental psychoanalysis, that an ideal human development consists of three different phases: the phase of infantile sexuality that culminates in one or another type of the Oedipus complex; the period of latency that leads to the weakening or even to the abolishing of the Oedipus complex (Freud 1924b); and the reawakening of sexuality in adolescence, now directed away from the objects of infantile sexuality towards non-incestuous objects. "External experiences" such as sexual seduction by an older person, or coming upon the primal scene – in addition to other traumatic experiences – delay this ideal development, resulting in either prolonging the oedipal attachment, neurosis or perversion.

The three stages of development – infantile sexuality culminating in the Oedipus complex, the latency period that succeeds in repressing the Oedipus complex, and sexuality re-emerging in adolescence and now directed towards new and non-incestuous individuals free from the incest taboo – are characteristic of human development and are not otherwise found in the animal kingdom. Even if they are only rarely achieved in real life they give the therapist a developmental map. The therapist studying a patient can determine where a fixation point has taken place and then find ways to help his patient overcome the point of arrest and restart new development.

Unfortunately Freud did not include in the scheme Ferenczi's significant observation (1929) that this development will not take place unless the child is lovingly received into the world. Spitz's observations on hospitalism (1945, 1946) further demonstrated that the human infant needs not only physical care but also love to combat the wish to die. That is why the need to love and be loved remains essential throughout the life cycle. I am not implying that Freud stated all that I said in these paragraphs, as clearly as my summary suggests, but all that I said was implicit in Freud's last formulation.

There is much in the *Outline* that is valuable, but there is also much that further understandings have shown to be outdated. It is a difficult task for the beginner to separate the wheat from the chaff and unfortunately there is no authorized guideline to help students accomplish this double task.

Freud's views on the death instinct were criticized by the analysts and others who believed that social conflicts, and particularly class conflicts, were not identical with the intrapsychic conflicts of the individual. The analysts who were also Marxists had particular difficulties with Freud's death instinct since it assumes that aggression is part of human nature and eternal peace will not take place even if capitalism is overthrown. In Fenichel's "A Critique of the Death Instinct" (1935) he maintained that the clinical facts of depression and the existence of the superego do not compel us to assume the existence of the death instinct. Fenichel agreed with Freud's clinical observations, but agreed only that

> primitive instinctual life has powerful destructive coloring; that this coloring is maintained throughout the "vicissitude of turning against the ego, and is reinforced in every libidinal regress." The clinical facts do not, however, posit anything concerning the genesis of this coloring. They say nothing about this destructiveness having been originally directed against one's own ego.
>
> (p. 369)

I doubt that the substitution of the much more vague term "coloring" for Freud's "death instinct" was of much help, but Fenichel was right that Freud's interpretation of the clinical facts to mean that a death instinct exists was a very daring step and cast a dark cloud over the future of civilization. The Second World War, the Holocaust, the atomic bomb, and the danger to the earth's climate, all point to the fact that Freud was wiser than Fenichel.

The argument about the death instinct had important clinical consequences. Fenichel was afraid that analysts who believe in the death instinct and who encounter masochism and self-punishment in their patients will assume that they have reached unanalyzable primary biological facts rather than search for determining experiences in the patient's life (p. 370). Reading Fenichel's circular letters further confirms how agitating the question of the death instinct was. Fenichel was a prominent psychoanalyst and there must have been others who shared his anxieties. Fenichel also thought that the strong suicidal tendency of depression is less directed at the self and more directed at the introjected object.

In my 2005 paper I emphasized that the death instinct has a major impact on termination, which can never be eliminated completely. We cannot predict whether some future traumatic events – such as the death of a loved one, or a reversal of fortune – will not once more reactivate the death instinct and require another analysis. Every termination is only a termination within a certain set of circumstances. At best we can only speak of a balance of forces that may or may not endure once circumstances have significantly changed.

In the 1930s, individual analysts began to respond to the idea of the death instinct. In 1930 Paul Federn wrote a paper on the reality of the death instinct in which he suggested that melancholia is the most direct expression of the death instinct. In *Mourning and Melancholia* (1917a) Freud described suicide wishes as internalized aggression at first directed outward and now directed inwardly. After the 1920 reformulation of the dual instinct theory the sequence was reversed: masochism, under the death instinct, was given priority and the direction of the aggression to the outside world was seen as an attempt to deflect the death instinct toward the outside world. In 1935 Eduardo Weiss, a pupil of Federn, wrote the paper *The Death Instinct and Masochism*, and in 1930 Bernfeld and Feitelberg also published a paper on *Entropy and the Death Instinct*.

Ferenczi's paper *The Unwelcome Child and the Death Instinct* (1929) was a significant milestone, for it not only gave Freud's death instinct clinical relevance but also gave it an object relationship. Had Freud been able to recognize its significance the rift between Freudians and object relationists may never have taken place. Ferenczi did not reject the death instinct but cast it into its clinical setting. The human baby, unlike lower animals, is not born with a strong wish to live; it must be welcomed to the world with love and, so to speak, coaxed into finding a life worth living. When, for whatever reason, the child is not welcomed, it will prefer not to fight to stay alive and at times even long for death. Traumatic events, pain, illness and the infirmity of old age all diminish the zest for life. Freud thought that in the absence of traumatic events the normal child will go through three phases of development: infantile sexuality, latency, and the awakening of adult sexuality in adolescence. However, none of these expected developments can take place unless the child receives this desire to live from the mother's love, to counteract the death instinct. Freud's dual instinct theory can be seen as a challenge to the therapeutic community, given a parental libidinal deficit that can make the child feel unwelcome. Can we therapists undo this deficit?

Ferenczi's paper transformed Freud's death instinct theory from metapsychological speculation into a clinical entity. However, in the *Outline* Freud did not include the need to be welcomed into the world as necessary for the child to strive. The 1945 and 1946 papers by Spitz on hospitality confirmed Ferenczi's finding, but Ferenczi's name does not appear in Spitz's bibliography.

From a historical perspective it is striking that only Melanie Klein and her disciples, over a long period of time, were able to incorporate the death instinct and make clinical use of the concept. Klein herself (1957) interpreted envy of the breast and the desire to spoil it as a manifestation of the death instinct. It is the working of the death instinct within the individual that is experienced as a fear of annihilation. Rosenfelt (1971) showed how the death instinct manifests itself in virulent forms of severe narcissistic conditions. These narcissistic patients attempt to escape the struggle between their destructive and libidinal impulses by killing their loving and dependent self and identifying themselves with the narcissistic-destructive part of the self, which gives them a sense of superiority and self-admiration. Kernberg's extensive writings on narcissism (1970, 1974c, 1974d) were written under Rosenfelt's influence. Segal (1993) observed that "confrontation with the death instinct, in favorable circumstances, mobilizes the life instinct" (p. 57). What these favorable circumstances are was not defined. However, what is striking in the cases she presented is how often the patients felt they could get rid of their inner deadness by killing the therapist. Segal also emphasized the close connection between envy and the death instinct.

The last paper in the series is Kernberg's 2009 paper. Here he proposed that the death drive is not a primary one, but rather "represents a significant complication of aggression as a major motivational system" and therefore "is useful as a concept in the clinical realm" (p. 1018). "Insecure attachments" contribute to the activation of negative affect, "while traumatic experiences in infancy contribute to self-destructive tendencies." If we examine Kernberg's position historically we will note that he replaced Freud's concept of drive with a special object relations theory.

In this historical context I see Andre Green's famous paper *The Dead Mother* (1983) as descending from Ferenczi, even though Green does not mention Ferenczi among those who had an influence on his concept. Green isolated a common clinical entity that had hitherto escaped notice: a maternal depression that takes place before the child has reached the necessary degree of independence from the mother. Such a mother had been a loving mother until she herself suffered a severe trauma that suddenly "transformed her into a distant figure, loveless, practically inanimate." The result is the triangle of mother, child, and the object of the mother's bereavement, which the child will try in vain to replace. Ferenczi's unwelcome child never had a vivid mother to receive her or him gladly; Green's child had such a mother until she herself was deprived of an object she needed.

In historical terms Ferenczi transposed Freud's death instinct into an object relations theory, but its limitations were that it made the mother responsible for a particularly strong death instinct, leaving open whether the death instinct can become particularly strong through other combinations of forces. In my experience with suicidal patients I could not always find that the child was unwelcome, but there was always a difficult fit between the needs of the child and the capacities of the mother.

I have earlier discussed how the Kleinians incorporated Freud's death instinct theory into their clinical work. By contrast American ego psychology, under the leadership of Hartmann, reacted very differently. The tone was set by Hartmann, Kris and Loewenstein in 1949.

> We do not propose to discuss the reasons that suggested to Freud the assumption concerning "life" and "death" instincts may have for the unification of

> psychoanalytic propositions. In *Beyond the Pleasure Principle* [Freud] refers to questions to be discussed and probably to be decided within biology proper.
>
> (pp. 10–11)

These lines were written sixty years ago but no biologist has been tempted to investigate this issue. For better or worse Freud's death instinct theory has remained a psychoanalytic controversy.

The authors then discuss Fenichel's view of the death instinct as laid out in his 1945 *The Psychoalaytic Theory of Neurosis* and conclude that Fenichel had "a genuine discomfort in the fact of Freud's far-reaching constructions." On the other hand, because I had data at my disposal not available to these earlier psychoanalysts, I concluded that it was Fenichel's political commitment that prevented him from accepting Freud's death instinct. It seems to me more likely that they themselves experienced the discomfort they attributed to Freud.

More surprising was Anna Freud's acceptance of this point of view in her 1949 paper *Notes on Aggression After Reviewing Klein's Point of View*. Anna Freud concluded, "Other analysts, in America and Europe, the author among them, hold the view that the co-existence of the two opposing instinctive forces in themselves is not sufficient to produce mental conflict" (pp. 69–70).

Arlow and Brenner's book *Psychoanalytic Concepts and the Structural Theory* (1964) was pivotal. To use a phrase coined by Arlow, neither of them was "apostolic," meaning that they no longer knew Freud face-to-face. They were strongly in favor of the structural theory over the topographic one and they opposed the idea that they saw as prevalent: that the two points of view, the topographic and the structural models, can be used interchangeably (p. 3). They regarded the structural theory as the more satisfactory of the two. Like Hartmann *et al.* (1949), they bypassed any discussion of the death instinct.

> It is thus impossible to discuss the topographic and the structural theories of the mental apparatus without frequent reference to the instinctual drives, and in particular to mental energies which derive from the drives. However, we shall not attempt any detailed discussion of the origin of the instinctual drives, or their nature, or of their classification. Such a detailed discussion is not essential for the purpose of our present work.
>
> (p. 7)

Unlike Fenichel, who frankly opposed the reformulation, Arlow and Brenner reinterpreted it.

The two most important chapters in this book were chapter 9, "Dreams and the Structural Theory," and chapter 10, "The Psychopathology of the Psychoses." Dream interpretation was the strong point of the topographic point of view as was the interpretation of psychoses. Looking at these two from a structural point of view was therefore particularly important. In their reformulation of dream theory Arlow and Brenner (1964) concluded:

> The dream work consists of an interplay, often a very complicated one, though at other times quite simple, among id, ego, and superego of which the final result is the manifest dream.
>
> (p. 122)

In this reformulation the dream lost its privileged position. An attempt to give back its special position, in opposition to this point of view, was undertaken by

Greenson in 1970. As to the understanding of the psychosis the authors felt that Freud's concept of regression of ego functions explained the clinical phenomena of the psychoses better than the topographic explanation of libidinal decathexes and pathological recathexes (Arlow and Brenner 1964, p. 154).

> It seems more accurate to speak of defensive disturbances in various ego functions in psychosis rather than to consider a break with reality or a loss of object relations.
>
> (p. 157)

Arlow and Brenner's book received a critical review from Hans Loewald in *Psychoanalytic Quarterly* (1966). Loewald was not an orthodox psychoanalyst. His 1960 article *On the Therapeutic Action of Psychoanalysis* was a path-breaking article. In his review he stated:

> In this book I am afraid, more issues are closed than opened, more answers given than questions raised and discussed in the spirit of scientific inquiry. This book gives an air of finality. In the authors' view issues are settled, concepts well defined and precise, problems well understood and in no need for further inquiry, but that many of them are neither as clear-cut nor as simple and one dimensional as they are represented.
>
> (p. 432)

Loewald found the book too simple for the experienced analyst and too dogmatic for the beginner. Their rendering of the topographic theory "was reduced to a scheme more right and final than it actually was" (p. 435). While I agree with Loewald's criticism, I also feel that he did not see this book within the proper historical context, as an attempt to deal with the painful challenge that Freud's structural reformulation inflicted on this generation of psychoanalysts, and therefore missed its historical significance.

By eliminating both the death instinct and the power of the repetition compulsion, while retaining the theory of conflict between ego, id and superego, Arlow and Brenner provided a simplified and far more optimistic version of the structural point of view.

Arlow and Brenner, in my interpretation, were modifiers of the structural point of view. It is conceivable that their slant on Freud's structural theory protected American psychoanalysis from Freud's pessimism and was more congenial to American culture. What they failed to do was to reflect Freud's thinking correctly and therefore they made the understanding of the history of psychoanalysis more difficult. The idea that its founder had deserted psychoanalysis for cultural interests and was pessimistic about its efficacy was too much to bear; it had to be denied. Denial, however, as psychoanalysts know, is a very costly defense, often requiring projection to support it. I argue that psychoanalysis had no choice but to break up into groups that suspect each other of denying Fraud's patrimony, and I hope I am right that this traumatic event has to be faced in order to give us a better understanding of our history and to correct controversies.

Moving another generation forward, I come to Andre Green's *Key Ideas for a Contemporary Psychoanalysis* (2005). Green made the truly heroic attempt to write a book bringing Freud's outline up to date. The accusation of oversimplification, of smoothing out all the wrinkles of the structural phase, cannot be directed at his book. Quite the contrary, the difficulties and contradiction of what he calls the second topographic point of view have been presented fully. Much that he says in the book is valuable, as, for example, when he points out that classical analysis privileged the neuroses at the expense of other mental illnesses, and that contemporary psychoanalysis must address its efforts to the far more numerous borderline individuals and psychotics. In addition, he states that classical psychoanalysis demanded much more time by its emphasis of four to five hours a week, while contemporary conditions demand that we work with less frequent visits. I would also add to this list that Freud privileged the analysand's remembrances over the analysand's acting, and we should accept the two forms of "remembering" with neutrality.

As to the way Green understood the working of the death drive, he emphasized negative narcissism: destruction through disinvestment. When the "disobjectilizing function" is applied to the "objectilizing process itself" disinvestment undoes in the short term what investment had succeeded in constructing. These are admittedly complex terms but they state clearly that the death drive is based on the human capacity, under duress, to take back what the psychic apparatus has previously invested in. The dead mother syndrome so central to Green's thinking is achieved by such a disinvestment in a mother that while she was inwardly alive she was heavily invested with the child's libido (p. 222). A patient suffering from "negative narcissism" shows little interest in winning the love of the therapist. To have reformulated the death drive into terms of withdrawal and decathexis was a considerable achievement by Green.

Green has also been one of the most important modifiers active today, and in his book he asks us to accept many of his modifications. If my analysis in this communication is correct, these two tasks cannot be combined. To reread the *Outline* and point out what has proven important, and to differentiate it from what must be discarded because the new data do not support it, is a valuable task of psychoanalytic historical criticism. One either makes demands of a modifier or one is interested in pointing out where Freud could not go further, and by doing so forward psychoanalysis as a whole; in my view one cannot successfully pursue the two tasks simultaneously.

In chapter 5 Green emphasized that the ego is unconscious of its own defenses (p. 69) and therefore a less reliable ally in our work than we would like to believe. The idea leads me to a different conclusion. The ego's unconsciousness of its own defenses is quite different from what Freud previously considered to be the unconsciousness of the Oedipus complex. The unconscious of the early Freud is a dynamic force: it pushes its way upward toward the conscious in dreams, parapraxies or symptoms; the countercathectic forces of the ego hold the unconscious back. The ego's defenses show no similar capacity or desire to push themselves upward; if they are unconscious they are unconscious in a radically different way than the "repressed unconscious." If the defenses are unconscious to the ego, as Green observed, they are not part of the dynamic unconscious. They do not appear in dreams, are not likely to betray themselves in parapraxes, and appear in transference only as a non-specific resistance. The patient almost never helps the therapist to uncover them; they can be discovered only because they block analytic progress.

Summary

Since I range over a rather large territory in this presentation I will summarize my main points. I claim that the very way Freud created psychoanalysis made it impossible for it to continue to grow and develop as a unified movement after his death. Unlike other sciences, psychoanalysis had no way of differentiating its basic findings from what is yet to be discovered. I then reintroduced my differentiation between heretics, modifiers and extenders, claiming that after Freud's death there was less opportunity for heritics and more space for modifiers. I assigned a crucial role to the fact that Anna Freud did not succeed in expelling the Kleinians.

In the second part of the paper I presented the view of those who made use of Freud's death instinct theory and those who opposed it. Many analysts preferred to ignore dealing with it rather than state their opposition. My presentation was biased in favor of those who chose to work with the death instinct as a clinical reality, highlighting Ferenczi's construction. I made the claim, so far as I know never made before, that Freud's death instinct theory had a traumatic impact on the psychoanalytic movement because it greatly limited the belief in the curative power of our therapeutic work and added the problem that after his announcement of the dual instinct theory Freud withdrew his interest in psychoanalysis as a method of cure.

I believe that the creativity of psychoanalysis will improve if we face this difficult chapter in our history.

Note

1 First published as Martin S. Bergmann (2011), "The Dual Impact of Freud's Death and Freud's Death Instinct Theory on the History of Psychoanalysis," *The Psychoanalytic Review*: 98 (5): pp. 665–686. Reprinted by permission of Guilford Press, Inc.

References

Arlow, J. and C. Brenner (1964) *Psychoanalytic Concepts and the Structural Theory*. New York: International Universities Press, Inc.

Bergmann, M.S. (1993b) Reflections on the History of Psychoanalysis. *Journal of the American Psychoanalytic Association* 41: 929–955.

Bergmann, M.S. (1997) Termination: The Achilles Heel of Psychoanalytic Technique. *Psychoanalytic Psychology* 14: 163–174.

Bergmann, M.S. (2001) The Leap from the Studies on Hysteria to the Interpretation of Dreams. In *Storms in Her Head*, eds M. Dimen, and A. Harris. New York: Other Press.

Fenichel, O. (1935) A Critique of the Death Instinct. In *Collected Papers*, 1st Series, eds Fenichel, H. and Rapaport, D., 1953, 363–372.

Fenichel, O. (1945) *The Psychoanalytic Theory of Neurosis*. New York: W.W. Norton & Co., Inc.

Ferenczi, S. (1929) The Unwelcome Child and His Death Instinct. In *Final Contributions to the Problems and Methods of Psychoanalysis*, ed. Balint, M. New York: Basic Books, 1955, 102–107.

Freud, A. (1949) Notes on Aggression After Reviewing Klein's Point of View. In *The Writings of Anna Freud. Volume IV 1945–1956. Indications For Child Analysis and Other Papers*. New York: International Universities Press, 1968.

Freud, S. (1917a) Mourning and Melancholia. S.E. 14: 237–260.

Freud, S. (1920) Beyond the Pleasure Principle. S.E. 18: 7–64.

Freud, S. (1924b) The Dissolution of the Oedipus Complex. S.E. 19: 173–179.

Freud, S. (1925c) An Autobiographical Study. S.E. 20: 7–74.

Freud, S. (1925d) Inhibition, Symptoms and Anxiety. S.E. 20: 77–175.

Freud, S. (1927a) The Future of an Illusion. S.E. 21: 3–56.

Freud, S. (1930) Civilization and its Discontents. S.E. 21: 57–145.

Freud, S. (1937a) Analysis, Terminable and Interminable. S.E. 23: 211–253.

Freud, S. (1940) An Outline of Psycho-Analysis. S.E. 23: 141–207.
Green, A. (1983) The Dead Mother. In *On Private Madness*. New York: International Universities Press, 1986.
Green, A. (2005) *Key Ideas for a Contemporary Psychoanalysis: Misrecognition and Recognition of the Unconscious*. New York: Routledge.
Hartmann, H., Kris, E. and Loewenstein, R. (1949) Notes on the Theory of Aggression. *Psychoanalytic Study of the Child* 3: 9–36.
Kernberg, O. (1970) Factors in the Psychoanalytic Treatment of Narcissistic Personalities. *Journal of the American Psychoanalytic Association*, 18: 51–85.
Kernberg, O. (1974c) Contrasting Viewpoints Regarding the Nature and Psychoanalytic Treatment of Narcissistic Personalities: A Preliminary Communication. *Journal of the American Psychoanalytic Association*, 22: 255–267.
Kernberg, O. (1974d) Further Contributions to the Treatment of Narcissistic Personalities. *International Journal of Psychoanalysis*, 55: 215–240.
Kernberg, O. (2009) The Concept of the Death Drive: A Clinical Perspective. *International Journal of Psychoanalysis* 90: 1009–1035.
King, P. and Steiner, R. (1991) *The Freud-Klein Controversies 1941–45*. New York: Tavistock/ Routledge.
Klein, M. (1957) *Envy and Gratitude and Other Works*. New York: Basic Books.
Loewald, H. (1960) On the Therapeutic Action of Psychoanalysis. *International Journal of Psychoanalysis* 41: 16–33.
Masson, J.M., ed. (1985) *The Complete Letters of Sigmund Freud to Wilhelm Fliess 1887–1904*. Cambridge, MA: The Belknap Press of Harvard University Press.
Nunberg, H. and Federn, E. (1974) *Minutes of the Vienna Psychoanalytic Meeting, Volume III: 1910–1911*. New York: International Universities Press.
Rosenfelt, H. (1971) A Clinical Approach to the Psychoanalytic Theory of the Life and Death Instincts: An Investigation into the Aggressive Aspects of Narcissism. *International Journal of Psychoanalysis* 52: 169–178.
Segal, H. (1993) On the Clinical Usefulness of the Concept of Death Instinct. *International Journal of Psychoanalysis*, 74: 55–61.
Spitz, R.A. (1945) Hospitalism – An Inquiry into Genesis of Psychiatric Conditions in Early Childhood. *Psychoanalytic Study of the Child* 1: 53–74.
Spitz, R.A. (1946) Hospitalism: A Follow-up Request. *Psychoanalytic Study of the Child* 2: 113–17.

CHAPTER 10

THE JEWISH AND GERMAN ROOTS OF PSYCHOANALYSIS AND THE IMPACT OF THE HOLOCAUST[1]

The Holocaust is an event in world history, an important event in the twentieth century, a terrible century that is just coming to a close. But it is also an event in German history that has to be faced and an event in Jewish history that has to be mastered. I and a group of colleagues spent ten years studying the effect of the Holocaust on its victims and their children. One of the painful events we had to face was that the Holocaust is transmitted by the survivors to their children and even to the third generation. In that book we also included a chapter on the children of Nazis and we made the discovery that came as a surprise to all of us: that children of Nazis who knew about the participation of their parents in the Holocaust often identified themselves with the Jews and feared that they would be annihilated by their parents should they show signs of any weakness.

Beyond the Jewish tragedy we all were forced to recognize that given certain social circumstances – such as a national humiliation, unemployment, and loss of religious and humanistic scruples – a democratic society did the equivalent of suicide by allowing an evil genius embodying the frustrations of many socially powerless people to gain power. Once in absolute control, he and his associates plunged the world into a devastating war. Were it not for the grace of God and the fact that so many European atomic scientists found refuge on these shores, the atomic bomb could have been discovered in Germany with results none of us dare imagine.

We psychoanalysts have learned to differentiate between at least three attitudes toward trauma: (1) The trauma has never been mastered, the Holocaust remains for its victim the only psychologically real event. One remains Hitler's victim for the rest of one's life. For such people, the Holocaust is forever in danger of returning. They think of a refuge somewhere in middle America and keep flight tickets ready just in case. These are admittedly extreme examples, but we have encountered them. (2) Under ordinary circumstances, the Holocaust has been successfully relegated to the past, but the past has not been mastered. It threatens to return. An example would be as follows: a refugee woman driving beyond the speed limit is followed by an officer. Without awareness, the officer becomes a Nazi. She steps on the gas to escape for her life and thus transforms a simple punishment into a much more severe one. (3) The Holocaust is denied. It never happened. We hear continuously of books appearing and denying the unbearable historical events. Denial, however, as the psychoanalyst Robert Waelder (1951) has found, is a weak defense and it has to be buttressed by a stable but dangerous paranoid defense. If the Holocaust cannot be denied it is because Jews and communists are perpetrating the lie that it did take place.

By comparison with these major issues, our symposium and exhibit is only a small event, but it reminds us that the Holocaust is also a part of psychoanalytic history. And we psychoanalysts must make sure that we have recorded it correctly without distortions or false idealizations, for any distortion of the past is conducive to recreation of the myth and is dangerous to our reality testing.

The Jewish roots of psychoanalysis

It is a historical fact that the creator of psychoanalysis was an Austrian Jew and the first circle of Freud's disciples were Jews. The first Gentile "converts" to psychoanalysis were psychiatrists in Bergholzi, a mental hospital in Zurich under the leadership of Bleuler and Jung. Freud was elated about this conquest of psychoanalysis. In his correspondence with Karl Abraham in 1908 (Abraham and E.L. Freud 1965) we read:

> Please be tolerant and do not forget that it is easier for you than it is for Jung to follow my ideas, for in the first place you are completely independent, and then you are closer to my intellectual constitution because of racial kinship, while he, as a Christian and a pastor's son, finds his way to me only against great inner resistances. His associations with us is the more valuable for that ... It was only by his appearance on the scene that psychoanalysis escaped the danger of becoming a Jewish national affair.
>
> (p. 34)

In his letter to Abraham, Freud assumes a great deal – namely that Jews inherently have less resistance to psychoanalysis than sons of pastors. That Judaism is a more rational religion was a theme made popular by Moses Mendelson. It was that version of Judaism that Freud's teachers transmitted to him. It ignored the mythological and mystical irrational parts also found in the Jewish religion. It was useful in comforting Abraham but I believe we will make a mistake in considering it a mature opinion of Freud's. The phrase "you are closer to my intellectual constitution because of racial kinship" shows that Freud thought that Jews show less resistance to psychoanalysis than others. In another letter, "our Aryan comrades are really indispensable to us, otherwise psychoanalysis would succumb to anti-Semitism." The differences between Freud and Jung went deeper than the differences between Gentile and Jew. Two months later he writes:

> I nurse a suspicion that the suppressed anti-Semitism of the Swiss that spares me is deflected in reinforced form upon you. But I think that we as Jews, if we wish to join in, must develop a bit of masochism, be ready to suffer. Otherwise there is no hitting it off. Rest assured that if my name were Oberhuber in spite of everything my innovations would have met with far less resistance.

On February 11, 1910, Jung wrote to Freud imploring him:

> To revive among the intellectuals the feeling for symbol and of myth and ever so gently to transform Christ back into the soothsaying God of the wine ... What infinite rapture and wantonness lie dormant in our religion, waiting to be led back to their true destination.
>
> (McGuire 1974, pp. 294–295)

It is not difficult to see that Jung is under the spell of Nietzsche's *The Birth of Tragedy Out of the Spirit of Music*. Two days later, Freud replied,

> You must not regard me as the founder of a religion. My intentions are not so far reaching ... I'm not thinking of a substitute for religion. This need must be sublimated.
>
> (McGuire 1974, pp. 294–295)

It is evident from this exchange of letters that under Jung's influence, psychoanalysis was in danger of severing its relationship to rational enlightenment and becoming a new religious movement. The period of friendship with Jung lasted between 1906–13, which was also Freud's most optimistic period. After the break with Jung, Freud became more self-consciously a Jew. However, when the First World War broke out, to our astonishment, for the time being at least, both he and Abraham were German nationalists, hoping for the victory of Germany.

If as a historian I look back at this early stage of psychoanalysis, I come to the conclusion that the defection of the Zurich group had a salutary effect. The attempt to make popular a tragic *Weltanschauung* created by a Jew behind a Gentile fig leaf was bound to fail and did not do credit to psychoanalysis. I am using the word *Weltanschauung* advisedly because in 1927 Freud rejected the idea that psychoanalysis is a *Weltanschaung* or even a philosophy. He felt that in its philosophical aspects it represents science only. But psychoanalysis is more than a therapy. It does lay claim to a philosophy of its own. After Jung's departure there were many creative analysts who were not Jews, but psychoanalysis did not attempt to deny its Jewish origins.

Who were those early disciples that gathered around Freud for the Wednesday night meetings? Fortunately the record of these meetings were preserved since 1906 (Nunberg and Federn, 4 vols, 1962–75). Many of these early adherents were physicians, but they included also a musicologist and a music critic, a philosopher and authors of popular books. To my knowledge they were all marginal Jews lacking in any Jewish cultural roots. On March 6, 1907, Alfred Adler, the future founder of individual psychology – but at the time still a member of Freud's inner circle – presented the case of a Russian Jewish student who had studied in an anti-Semitic *Gymnasium* and where in Adler's words the Jewish complex was very much in the foreground. This anti-Semitism was taking place in czarist Russia, far away, culturally speaking, from Austria. One cannot read this discussion today without being struck by the fact that the discussants carefully avoided any discussion of Jewish issues. (Freud's first biographer Willels (1931) does not discuss Freud's Jewish origins.)

What about Freud's own sense of Jewish identity? In 1976 I wrote what I believed to be the first paper on this topic. Since then a large literature has grown around the subject (Gay 1988; Rice 1990; Yerushalmi 1991). Almost all writers on the subject have cited a memory by Freud published in his *Interpretations of Dreams* (1900):

> I may have been ten or twelve years old, when my father began to take me with him on his walks and reveal to me in his talk his views about things in the world we live in. Thus it was, on one such occasion, that he told me a story to show me how much better things were now than they had been in his days. "When I was a young man," he said, "I went for a walk one Saturday in the streets of your birthplace; I was well dressed, and had a new fur cap on my head. A Christian came up to me and with a single blow knocked off my cap

> into the mud and shouted: Jew! Get off the pavement!" "And what did you do?" I asked. "I went into the roadway and picked up my cap," was his quiet reply. This struck me as unheroic conduct on the part of the big, strong man who was holding the little boy by the hand. I had contrasted this situation with another which befitted my feelings better: the scene in which Hannibal's father, Hamilcar Barca, made his boy swear before the household altar to take vengeance on the Romans. Ever since that time Hannibal had had a place in my fantasies.
>
> (p. 197)

This was obviously a decisive childhood memory that emerged in Freud's self-analysis. It contains the moment in which he lost his idealization for his own father and substituted a new ego ideal. Hannibal, although not a Jew, was a Semite and an enemy of Rome, which symbolized the Catholic Church.

Jacob Freud's story to his son should be understood in its historical context. Before the emancipation of the Jews in Germany, which occurred in 1809, they were prohibited from using public sidewalks and if a Gentile called out to a Jew "*Mach mores jud!*" the Jew had to take off his hat (Ewen 1948, p. 4). Full civil equality was granted to the German Jews in 1868, and Austria followed in 1869, when Freud was thirteen years old, some time after the incident reported.

In 1914, when Freud was visiting Rome, he stood before the Moses of Michelangelo in the church of San Pietro in Vincoli. There a new interpretation of that famous statue occurred to him. He saw Moses as "controlling his wrath and not about to break the tablets." He identified himself with Moses and attempted to sublimate his pain and anger about Jung's renegacy. This insight, we may assume, evoked in him a greater sympathy toward his father who also controlled his anger in the encounter with an anti-Semite.

In the preface to the Hebrew translation of *Totem and Taboo*, written in 1930, Freud said:

> No reader of [the Hebrew version of] this book will find it easy to put himself in the emotional position of an author who is ignorant of the language of the holy writ – as well as from every other religion – and who cannot take a share in nationalist ideals, but who has yet never repudiated his people, who feels that he is in his essential nature a Jew and who has no desire to alter that nature. If the question were put to him: "Since you have abandoned all these common characteristics of your countrymen, what is left to you that is Jewish?" he would reply: "A great deal, and probably its very essence." He could not now express that essence clearly in words; but some day, no doubt, it will become accessible to the scientific mind.
>
> (xv)

For Freud's thirty-fifth birthday his father, Jacob Freud, returned to him in a new binding the Philippson bible, the Bible that Freud read as a child, with a Hebrew dedication to his son. Rice and Yerushalmi take this as evidence that Freud could read Hebrew. I, on the other hand, believe that it shows that Freud's father was literate only in Hebrew.

Until recently the idea that psychoanalysis was a specific Jewish way of looking at the world would have been regarded as a sign of anti-Semitism. However, today many American Jewish analysts believe that there is at least a close affinity between psychoanalysis and Judaism. Ostow (1982) states:

> Both Judaism and psychoanalysis teach that salvation, though conceptualized differently, can be obtained by virtue of special knowledge. Judaism and psychoanalysis share marginality: Jews are considered socially marginal and psychoanalysis is considered academically marginal.

Ostow also believes that Freud's technique of free association has an affinity with the way the Jewish rabbis interpreted biblical text. The rabbis believe in four ways of interpreting the Bible: *Pshat*, the plain meaning of the text; *Remez*, hints of alternative implied meanings; *Drash*, a homiletic meaning; and finally *Sod*, the esoteric meaning. If I am not as persuaded by this argument it is because the fathers of the Church, St. Augustine for example, interpreted the Bible very differently – but in essence used this same technique of interpretation. Furthermore, to me the analogy between these techniques of interpretation and the technique of free association is not convincing. One can add that Freud, like the Jewish rabbis, put heavy emphasis on the role of memory, as already indicated earlier. What matters in this discussion is that Freud and his circle of assimilated Jews felt strongly about being Jews, but this feeling was not buttressed by any specific Jewish knowledge.

A most interesting connection between psychoanalysis and the Bible has been formulated by the French psychoanalyst Chasseguet-Smirgel (1984b). She contrasts the biblical creator of the world with the world that the Marquis de Sade had described. The famous Marquis advocated the abolishing of all differences. Thus, in his *One Hundred and Twenty Days*, he advocated marriage among children, costuming little boys as girls, and girls as boys. Similarly, a bishop in the guise of a woman marries a woman who plays the role of husband. In Chasseguet-Smirgel's interpretation, perversions are attempts to break down the barriers that separate men from women, child from adult, brother from sister, and the erogenic zones in one's body. All things revert to chaos, differences are abolished, murder is nothing more than transformation of matter, and everything is reduced to excrement.

By contrast, the God of the Bible separates light from darkness, and the earth from the ocean. In a beautiful passage, Jeremiah (chapter V, verse 22), states:

> Fear ye not me? Sayeth the Lord: Will ye not tremble at my presence, which have placed the sand for the bound of the sea by a perpetual decree, that it cannot pass it: and though the waves thereof toss themselves, yet can they not prevail; though they roar, yet can they not pass over it?

In keeping with this notion of separation, Leviticus 18, verses 6–18, gives a long list of incestuous relationships that are forbidden, beginning with, "None of you shall approach anyone that is near of kin to him to uncover their nakedness: I am the Lord." The list ends with, "Neither shalt thou take a woman as a rival wife to her sister to vex her, to uncover her nakedness, besides the other in her lifetime." The last prohibition is of particular interest since it is the very act that the patriarch Jacob committed when he married the two sisters Leah and Rachel.

To me it seems essential to differentiate between two aspects of the problems which are all too often confused. The first is the question of whether psychoanalysis as a discipline is derived from Jewish sources. Does it owe a cultural debt to Judaism? I believe that the answer is no. But this no must be qualified. True, there is no hard evidence as we have when we discuss the German influence of any direct Jewish influence on Freud. Nevertheless, Freud did say that even after religious and national aspirations have been given up, the very essence of Judaism remains. Here rational argument cannot play a decisive role. Chasseguet-Smirgel emphasized that the God of the Bible abhors incest as well as merger, thus making Judaism a non-symbiotic and non-incestuous religion. But there is also a Jewish religious term called "*Dvekut*" –which means cleaving unto God, a term very close to merger. A very different problem, sociological in nature, is whether psychoanalysis offered a way for assimilated Jews to find their way into the cultural mainstream, and here the answer must be yes. As Ostow put it, "Psychoanalysis offers an activity in which Jews struggling at the interface between the Jewish community and the non-Jewish world can express their conflicting needs." In this connection we might recall the ideas of a notable refugee from Germany, the psychoanalyst Kurt Lewin. He concluded that it is not the belonging to many groups that is the source of the difficulty – for we all belong to different groups – but the uncertainty of belonging. It is this uncertainty that has been referred to as Jewish marginality. A group, according to Lewin, is defined by interdependence rather than by similarity (K. Lewin 1948, pp. 179, 184). The Jews of Freud's circle were a community of fate rather than a community of faith.

If Freud was right – that the world had to wait for a Godless Jew to discover psychoanalysis, and that it is easier for Jews to find their way to psychoanalysis – it is the marginality that makes this possible. It is interesting that during an analysis the analyst becomes, for the analysand, a very important and sometimes even the most important object, but the analyst never shows up within the family circle. He remains at the margins of the analysand's life. If Jews are, as some people believe, particularly suitable for such occupations as psychology, psychiatry and anthropology, it is probably due to this marginality.

The German roots of psychoanalysis

Although Freud was born in Pribor, Czechoslovakia, and died in London, he spent all but his first years of life and his last year in Vienna, within the German cultural orbit. Freud was the product of the German *Gymnasium*. Quotations from Goethe, Schiller, Heine, Schelling, Nietzsche and Schopenhauer abounded. Goethe appears in Freud's dreams, and quotations from Goethe and Schiller occur spontaneously when Freud is free associating. When Freud analyzes slips of the tongue, he gives instances taken from Schiller's *Wallenstein*, *Don Carlos*, and *Die Raüber*.

In 1907 Freud was asked to comment on his ten favorite books and mentioned what he considered to be the most magnificent: Homer, Sophocles, Goethe's *Faust*, Shakespeare's *Hamlet* and *Macbeth*; then he included the most significant books: Yohan Weier, *Belief in Witches*, and Darwin's *Descent of Man*; favorite books, among which he included Milton's *Paradise Lost* and Heine's *Lazarus*; and finally, settling to ten good books, he included Mutatuly, *Letters and Works*; Kipling, *The Book*; Anatole France, *Sur la Pierre Blanche*; Zola, *Fecundite*; Merezhkovsky, *Leonardo da Vinci*; C.F. Meyer, *Huttens Letzte Tage*; Macauley, *Essay*; Gomperz, *Greek Thinkers*, and Mark Twain, *Sketches*. The list is a homage to Freud's universalism without language or national boundaries. The classical European past is alive to him. The authors are Dutch, English, French, American, Russian and Swiss. The only book that touches on Jewish issues is Heine's *Lazarus*.

Freud retained from the German classics many quotations that adorn his writings. For example, in *Studies on Hysteria* (Breuer and Freud 1985) he quotes Schillers' *The Bride of Messina*: "One countenance indeed shows before it happened and a different one shows the accomplished deed." In *Civilization and its*

Discontents (1930) Freud said "I took as my starting point a saying of the poet philosopher, Schiller, that 'hunger and love are what moves the world.' "

The influence of Goethe on Freud was, if anything, even greater. He decided to become a physician after hearing the poem on Nature, which at that time was attributed to Goethe. Wittels (1931), Freud's early biographer, reprinted this poem. It is far below the standards of Goethe, but Freud's contemporaries did not notice it. Freud was also the recipient of the Goethe prize, given by the city of Frankfurt, and on that occasion, Anna Freud, in the name of her father, delivered a short paper entitled *The Goethe Prize* (1930, p. 208).

In that address Freud drew many parallels between Goethe's insights and psychoanalysis. Of these the most striking is Goethe's line in the posthumously published poem to Charlotte von Stein.

> Ach du warst in Abgelbetten Zeiten
> meine Schwester oder meine frau.
>
> (Ahh! You were in times lived out long ago
> my sister or my wife.)

In an erudite study, the psychoanalyst and refugee Kurt Eissler (1963a) showed that Goethe's relationship to his sister was unusually close and incestuous. What Goethe labeled times "lived out long ago" psychoanalysis recognizes as referring to the early years of infancy.

A quote appears from Goethe on the very last page of the posthumously published *Outline of Psychoanalysis*. Freud was discussing there the formation of the superego as representing the world we inherit from our forebears. He quotes Goethe:

> Was du ererbet von deinen Vatern hast,
> Erwirb es, um es zu besitzen
>
> (What thou hast inherited from thy fathers,
> Aquire it to make it thine.)
> (Goethe's Faust, Part I, Scene 1)

These are almost the last lines we have from Freud's pen. It is indeed a most interesting statement for it contains a contradiction. We generally assume that what we inherit we need not acquire. However, Goethe believed – and Freud admired this belief – that the two are not opposed to each other, but what we inherit we must also acquire to make it our own.

As to Nietzsche's influence: in *On the History of the Psycho-Analytic Movement* (1914c) Freud said,

> I have denied myself the very great pleasure of reading the works of Nietzsche with the deliberate object of not being hampered in working out the impressions received in psychoanalysis by any sort of anticipatory ideas. I had therefore to be prepared – and I am so, gladly – to forego all claims to priority in the many instances in which laborious psychoanalytic investigation can merely confirm the truth which the philosopher recognized by intuition.

This passage has been criticized, and in my opinion rightly so, by Helmut Junker (1991). He was surprised to discover that Freud showed so little interest in his place in Western thought. One may also add that he did not do full justice to psychoanalysis because in the great discoveries that Freud made intuition played no smaller a role than it did in Nietzsche's work. Nietzsche anticipated Freud, when in his *Zarathustra* he recognized that many criminals feel guilty before they committed the crime; that is, they committed the crime out of a pre-existing sense of guilt. In 1916 Freud devoted a section of an essay to criminals out of a sense of guilt (Freud 1916–17b, p. 333). Nietzsche's superman, in Freud's own transvaluation of values, turned out to be the supreme narcissist who loves no one and treats everyone on a need gratification basis. Freud compared Nietzsche's superman with the father of the primal hoard (1921, p. 123).

By contrast to Nietzsche, Freud referred to Wagner only once (apart from associations of Freud's patients to Wagner's operas) in the Schreber case (1911, p. 68) where Freud made the significant observation that ideas of the end of the world occur in psychotics when there is a total withdrawal of attachment to people in the world. However, similar ideas can also take place in an overwhelming state of falling in love, when all of what Freud called cathexes pass over to the love object. He gave Tristan and Isolde as an example of such an overwhelming love.

In Wagner's *The Ring* a brother and sister perform incest on stage as an example of blissful love. To my knowledge, such a glorification of incest had never before been attempted in Western literature.

I would now like to present an example of a Freudian insight before Freud.

Let me bring you to the second act of *Tristan and Isolde* by Wagner. The couple has just been caught in flagrante by King Mark. The king is not angry at Tristan, but bewildered: "Where do loyalty and virtue flee when Tristan betrays?" Tristan replies, "What I did I cannot tell, what you are asking you will never find out." But after this disclaimer, Tristan provides the answer. When his mother died in childbirth, she exiled him to the current world where the sun shines. Now with Isolde, he will return to his mother's domain – the night devoid of sunlight. The explanation that he is ready to die because he wants to join his dead mother constitutes one of the great examples of a Freudian interpretation before Freud.

Had Freud listened carefully to Tristan and Isolde he would have discovered that when the lovers philosophized about overthrowing the tyranny of "the day" in favor of the kingdom of the night, they are in revolt against what Freud (1923b) described as being dominated by the superego.

It is of course well-known that Wagner was "The court musician" of Adolf Hitler, but so complex is this history that some of the great Freudian insights before Freud occur in the work of an anti-Semitic composer.

Freud particularly admired Heine's sarcasm. He often quoted Heine's remarks about philosophers: "With his nightcaps and the tatters of his dressing gown, he patches up the gaps in the structure of the universe." I will also remind you of the magnificent quote in Freud's paper on narcissism as to why God created the world, where Heine makes God say, "Illness was no doubt the final cause of the whole urge to create. By creating, I could recover; by creating, I became healthy" (Freud 1914d, p. 85). This citation comes from the last stanza of Heine's *Seven Songs of Creation*. They are humorous in nature and contain little that is profound. One wonders, therefore, how Freud kept these lines in memory and used them to such telling effect since the paper on narcissism is unquestionably one of Freud's most creative ones. It is a magnificent example of Goethe's statement that what we inherit we must acquire anew.

In *Civilizations and its Discontents* (1930, p. 110), Freud quoted Heine's remarks.

> Mine is a most peaceable disposition. My wishes are: a humble cottage with a thatched roof, but a good bed, good food, the freshest milk and butter, flowers before my window, and a few fine trees before my door; and if god wants to make my happiness complete, he will grant me the joy of seeing some six or seven of my enemies hanging from those trees.

What Freud admired here was the ease with which Heine could permit his hostile impulses to reach consciousness.

Freud also quoted Heine's complaint that "his religion was the plague dragged along from the Nile valley, the unhealthy beliefs of ancient Egypt." We can only speculate whether this remark – quoted in *Moses and Monotheism* – had given Freud the idea that Moses was an Egyptian. Freud not only took ideas from Heine; in my view Heine had a profound influence on Freud's style. This is not easy to prove; however, some examples taken from Heine's writings may be used as illustration. "I have given up the God of Hegel, or rather, the Godlessness of Hegel" (quoted in Ewen 1948, p. 213). We remember that Freud called himself a Godless Jew. "The poet, that overgrown child" (quoted in Ewen 1948, p. 221) recalls Freud's essay of 1908, *Creative Writers and Daydreaming* (1908b). Anyone familiar with the way Freud spoke about his impending death will note the similarity to the way Heine described his death to Alexander Dumas:

> You may no longer find me in my present apartment, 50 rue d'Amersterdam, and that I may have moved to another lodging, quite unknown to me – and I will not even be able to leave my new address with the porter in case tardy friends like you may ask for me. I have no illusion of my future residence. All I know is that you enter it through a drab and fetid passage, and this entrance displeases me in advance. In addition, my wife weeps whenever I talk of moving.
> (quoted in Ewen 1948, p. 226)

Heine died in 1857, the year Freud was born. He underwent baptism, while Freud only considered it and was dissuaded by Breuer (Bergmann 1976). Anyone who reads Heine's Hebrew melodies will know that baptism notwithstanding, he retained a deep attachment to Jewish lore and Jewish life which he expressed in such poems as *Princess Sabbath* and *Jehuda Ben Halevi*. There is no similar description in any of Freud's writings. Freud absorbed ideas from many writers but in my view he learned the most from Nietzsche. Nevertheless, Heine had the greatest influence on the formation of his personality. Style is an expression of the personality. In Heine the German and Jewish roots intermingled.

Psychoanalysis, in my opinion, emerged on the crossroads between the period of the Enlightenment and German Romanticism. As Fenichel (1941), one of the leading refugee psychoanalysts, said, "The subject matter of the psychoanalysis is the irrational. Its methodology, however, is rational." I believe that this synthesis between the Enlightenment and Romanticism constituted one of the important appeals of psychoanalysis. Psychoanalysis was created by a Godless Jew and originated in a circle of Jews; those from the first generation of emancipation who sought new ways of citizenship in a Europe that knew no national boundaries.

Epilogue: The encounter with National Socialism

In 1933 Freud's books were publicly burned. Jews were barred from participating in professional associations. On April 17, 1933, Boehm, a Gentile psychoanalyst, came to Vienna to ask Freud's blessing to replace Eitingon as president of the German Psychoanalytic Society. Kretschner resigned as the president of the International General Medical Society for Psychotherapy and was replaced by Jung, who was now an enthusiastic follower of Hitler. Jones (1953) reports that on December 1, 1933, he himself presided over a meeting of the Berlin Analytic Society "where the few remaining Jews volunteered to resign so as to save the society from being dissolved" (p. 186). Jones further reports that in January 1937, Boehm went once more to Vienna where he talked for three hours until Freud's patience gave out. Freud finally said,

> Quite enough! The Jews have suffered for their conviction for centuries. Now the time has come for our Christian colleagues to suffer in their turn for theirs. I attach no importance to my name being mentioned in Germany so long as my work is represented correctly there.

So saying, he left the room. Jones has done his utmost to exonerate himself and Freud from any complicity with National Socialism. Yet one cannot deny that both men tried to accommodate psychoanalysis into National Socialism. The accommodation failed, however; the fact that the International was willing to allow the German Psychoanalytic Society to remain within it if its Jewish members were to voluntarily resign rather than be expelled shows that psychoanalysis, too, shared in the spirit of accommodation to Hitler.

Anti-Semitism was endemic in Western culture. Restricted and expelled from some countries, the Jews found shelters in others, and thus survived. With the emergence of the Enlightenment – represented in Germany by writers like Lessing – and as the ideas of the French Revolution took hold, the Jews in the nineteenth century were emancipated and received equal rights. The euphoria of the French Revolution soon evaporated. The Congress of Vienna and the Holy Alliance restored the old legitimacy. Secular anti-Semitism became strong throughout the nineteenth century. On the other side of the ledger was the fact that Jews gained equal rights. Until the rise of Hitler, it had been hoped that eventually anti-Semitism would be overcome.

Psychoanalysis was one of the universalistic movements that emerged during this period of hope. Discovered by a Jew, supported by Jews, the language of psychoanalysis was a universal one. It emerged, as I have already said, at the crossroads between the rational beliefs of the Enlightenment and the interests of Romanticism in the morbid. The process of emancipation and the growth of a world based on order was reversed by a new and particularly violent form of anti-Semitism, culminating in Hitler's final solution. Fortunately for Western civilization, Hitler's Third Reich, proclaimed as intended to last one thousand years, lasted only a little over a decade. But we are still laboring over the impact of this catastrophe and the reversal of human values that took place. Hence this symposium.

Note

1 Originally published in Bergmann, M.S. (1995), "The Jewish and German Roots of Psychoanalysis and the Impact of the Holocaust," *American Imago*, 52: 243–259. Reprinted by permission of The Johns Hopkins University Press.

References

Abraham, H. and E. L. Freud, eds (1965) *A Psycho-Analytic Dialogue: The Letters of Sigmund Freud and Karl Abraham, 1907–1926*. New York: Basic Books.
Bergmann, M.S. (1976) Moses and the Evolution of Freud's Jewish Identity. In *Judaism and Psychoanalysis*, ed. M. Ostow. New York: Ktav Publishing House, 1982, pp. 115–141.
Breuer, J. and Freud, S. (1895) Studies on Hysteria. S.E. 2: 1–335.
Chasseguet-Smirgel, J. (1984b) *The Ego Ideal: A Psychoanalytic Essay on the Malady of the Ideal*. Trans. P. Barrows. New York: W.W. Norton.
Eissler, K. (1963a) *Goethe: A Psychoanalytic Study*, Vols. 1 & 2. Detroit: Wayne State University Press.
Ewen, F., ed. and trans. (1948) *Heinrich Heine, Self Portrait and Other Writings*. Secaucus, N.J.: The Citadel Press.
Fenichel, O. (1941) *Problems of Psychoanalytic Technique*, trans. D. Brunswick. New York: Psychoanalytic Quarterly.
Freud, Sigmund. (1911) Notes on an Autobiographical Account Case of Paranoia. S.E. 12: 9–82.
Freud, S. (1914d) On Narcissism: An Introduction. S.E. 14: 73–102.
Freud, S. (1916–17b) Introductory Lectures on Psychoanalysis, Part III. S.E. 16: 243–463.
Freud, S. (1921) Group Psychology and the Analysis of the Ego. S.E. 18: 69–143.
Freud, S. (1923b) The Ego and the Id. S.E. 19: 3–66.
Freud, S. (1930) Civilization and its Discontents. S.E. 21: 57–145.
Gay, P. (1988) *Freud: A Life for Our Time*. New York: W.W. Norton.
Jones, E. (1953) *The Life and Work of Sigmund Freud, Vol. I: The Formative Years and the Great Discoveries, 1856–1900*. New York: Basic Books.
Junker, H. (1991) *Von Freud in den Freudianern*. Tuebinqen: edition diskord.
Lewin, K. (1948) *Resolving Social Conflicts*. New York: Harper and Row Publishers.
McGuire, W., ed. (1974) *The Freud/Jung Letters. The Correspondence Between Sigmund Freud and C. G. Jung*, trans. R. Manheim and R.F.C. Hall. Princeton: Princeton University Press.
Ostow, M. (1982) Editor's Comment. In *Judaism and Psychoanalysis*, ed. Ostow, M. New York: Ktav Publishing House.
Rice, E. (1990) *Freud and Moses: The Long Journey Home*. New York: State University of New York Press.
Waelder, R. (1960) *Basic Theory of Psychoanalysis*. New York: International Universities Press.
Wittels, F. (1931) *Freud and His Time*. New York: Liveright.
Yerushalmi, Yosef H. (1991) *Freud's Moses*. New Haven: Yale University Press.

PART IV

APPLICATIONS

CHAPTER 11

FREUD'S THREE THEORIES OF LOVE IN THE LIGHT OF LATER DEVELOPMENTS[1]

Abstract

Evidence is presented that Freud developed three very different theories on love. These theories were not integrated into a coherent theory. In subsequent developments each theory had its own history. The paper discusses the history of the controversy on the genital character, the relation between love and gender identity, between love and narcissism, the hierarchical structure of the capacity to love, and the relation between love and object loss. The impact of some concepts such as symbiosis and the rapprochement subphase on the understanding of conflicts in loving is raised. While at present differences in emphasis make it difficult to build a coherent psychoanalytic theory of love, it is productive to bring divergent views in touch with each other. A unified theory of love based on psychoanalytic observations is suggested.

Freud approached the topic of love reluctantly, fearing to encroach on the poetic territory of gifted poets or philosophers like Plato and Schopenhauer. Not without irony he claimed that when psychoanalysis touches the subject of love its touch must be clumsy by comparison with that of the poets. In spite of this reluctance, I showed in a series of publications (1971, 1980 and 1982) that Freud contributed more to the understanding of love than anyone after Plato. In these publications I tried to disprove a widely held opinion– both outside and within psychoanalysis – that Freud, who changed our understanding of sexuality so fundamentally, had little or nothing to say about love. This opinion could be maintained only because Freud never unified his thinking on love along the lines of dream theory or the theory of sexuality.

Plato was the first to think systematically about the nature of love and to bring together contrasting views on this subject. Freud, as I showed elsewhere (Bergmann 1982), was influenced by Plato; we owe to Plato the concept, if not the word sublimation. The Greeks had two gods of love, Aphrodite and Eros, but these gods limited their concern to what we call falling in love. The maintenance of the marital bond, the Greeks assigned to the province of Hera. The Greeks would never have thought of confusing falling in love with the capacity to maintain prolonged marital fidelity. During the seventeenth century the emphasis shifted. Falling in love and maintaining the love tie within the marital bond became connected. Freud inherited this connection, but the cleavage is still evident. Some of his ideas pertain to falling in love, and others to the capacity to love.

Freud developed three distinct theories of love. The first followed the discovery of infantile sexuality in the *Three Essays on the Theory of Sexuality* (1905b). There, the crucial passage reads: "The prototype of every love relationship is the child sucking at his mother's breast. The finding of the love object is in fact a refinding" (p. 222). Human beings are unique in having a biphasic sexual history. During infancy, before the sexual drive becomes autoerotic, the child goes through a phase of sexual love toward the parent. During latency a split takes place separating passionate sexual feelings from the tender current; the former undergoes repression. During adolescence the two currents recombine and love is now directed toward a new, nonincestuous object. A failure of these currents to recombine will result in an incapacity to combine tender love with sexual desire. Freud discovered that most adults have a unique and individual precondition for loving; in neurosis this precondition can become narrow and repetitive. For example, the Wolf Man became enamored with any woman in the crouching position; this position had a special significance for him because this was the position of his mother during the primal scene. Freud's first theory of love was essentially a genetic theory.

Freud's second theory was associated with the discovery of narcissism (1914). Freud now postulated that not only the parent, but also the self, can be taken as a model for a love object. Narcissistic object choices can be mirror images of the self, past images of the self, or projections of one's own ego ideal. If one projects the ego ideal on the love object and love is reciprocated, the tension between the ego and ego ideal is eliminated as long as the state of being in love lasts. To the elimination of this tension Freud ascribed the sense of bliss evoked by love. Metapsychologically speaking, Freud saw love as a massive transformation of narcissistic libido into object libido. This transformation, as well as the projection of the ego ideal, explains the overestimation of the love object by the lover. Many lovers have reported that one of the greatest rewards of love is the sudden freedom from feelings of jealousy and envy.

Freud's third theory of love is found in the paper, *Instincts and their Vicissitudes* (1915a). It was the reading, and possibly the misreading, of this paper that was responsible for the widespread belief – cited earlier – that Freud confused love with sex. The paper is one of Freud's difficult essays, and it is difficult precisely because Freud himself was struggling for clarity. Freud now confronted the problem that many of his critics contended he never faced; namely, how sex, a drive, becomes love, an emotion. Freud recognized (1915a, p. 133) that "love refuses to be fitted into the scheme of instincts," that "love cannot be some kind of special component of the instinct of sexuality." He then proceeded to make the valuable suggestion: to regard loving as "the expression of the whole sexual current of feelings." However, he felt that such a designation did not clear up the difficulty. Freud was disturbed that love could not be conceptualized in terms of a simple duality, that it admitted three opposites; namely, loving and hating, loving and being loved, and loving and indifference. Since love cannot be explained as an instinct, Freud suggested that it be reserved for the relation of the total ego to its object. The term "total ego" was never clearly defined. Freud reached a startling conclusion: because love could not be derived from the sexual instincts, Freud concluded that the term could be applied only "after there has been a synthesis of all the components of instincts under the primacy of the genital and in the service of reproduction" (p. 138).

The conclusion did not follow from the premises.

If my reconstruction is correct, 1915 was Freud's last contribution to the understanding of love. In *Group Psychology and the Analysis of the Ego* (1921) and again in *Libidinal Types* (1931a), Freud elaborated on these findings: but no new contributions were made. Even though Freud's last theory made the shift from instinct to ego, Freud's three theories were formulated within the topographic frame of reference. By analogy to dream theory, the instigator of love is the prohibited oedipal wish; the person one actually falls in love with plays a role analogous to the day residue of the dream that awakens the dormant wish; that the similarity between the new love object and the old is not known to the lover testifies to the success of a force analogous to dream censorship. The topographic model was particularly well suited to explain "love at first sight" – when individuality and complex character of the love object play only a minor role. In falling in love at first sight, reality testing is at least to some degree excluded, in a way reminiscent of dream work. The dream-like quality that is typical of falling in love may be due to the absence of, or greatly diminished participation of, the reality-testing capacity of the ego.

The first psychoanalyst to see love from a structural point of view was Waelder, in his classic paper of 1930. To Waelder, love was an act of integration of a high order, a tribute to the ego's capacity to bring together harmoniously the wishes of the id, the demands of the repetition compulsion, the demands of the superego, and the claims of reality. The love object chosen must be sexually gratifying, connected unconsciously to love objects in the person's past, sufficiently admired to meet the approval of the ego ideal, and appropriate in meeting the demands of reality. By implication, when one of the partners to this "coalition" remains in opposition, love will become conflictual.

Until the 1970s love was of little interest to psychoanalysts. The general public learned about the psychoanalytic view of love mostly from former psychoanalysts who broke with Freud (Reik 1944, Fromm 1956). What brought about the renewal of interest in love was the growing debate on the nature of narcissism and the new insights into early infancy, such as concepts of object constancy, symbiosis, separation-individuation, and the self-object.

In recent years the field of love seems to be dominated by philosophers. Of these, Irving Singer's *The Nature of Love* (1984) and Roland Barthes's *A Lover's Discourse* (1978) are of particular interest. Since psychoanalysis does not have its own definition of love, it may be useful to recall definitions offered by philosophers. Schopenhauer (1858a) observed about love: "The quite special individuality of any person" (p. 536). Love, Schopenhauer defined as "this longing that closely associates the notion of endless bliss with the possession of a definite woman, an unutterable pain that this possession is unattainable" (p. 551).

In keeping with existential philosophy, Barthes (1978) avoids generalizations. He discusses love through well-selected aphorisms:

> "I encounter millions of bodies in my life; of these I may desire some hundreds; but of these hundreds I love only one. The other with whom I am in love designates for me the specialty of my desire.
>
> (p. 19)

Singer introduced into the discussion of love the differentiation between appraisal and bestowal. The real estate agent appraises the value of a house, but individual buyers and sellers add their personal bestowal, a private value of the house to them. Any psychoanalyst who deals with the world of single men and women knows the power of appraisal, where beauty, youth, education, wealth and success add value to the person. To such a "market appraisal," love adds a personal bestowal. It is love, therefore, that gives to men and women their value as individuals, beyond the social group to which they belong.

To be capable only of "appraisal" is to be incapable of loving. Carried to extremes, appraisal results in snobbishness. The descriptions of love by the philosophers I have quoted – and others could be added – however felicitously expressed, do not penetrate below the phenomenological surface; it remains to be seen if psychoanalysis as a depth psychology can do better.

To return to Freud, I have observed that each one of Freud's theories on love had its own line of development after Freud. I shall discuss these developments, however, in reverse order.

Love and genitality

In his paper on *Character Formation on the Genital Level of Libido-Development* (1924b), Abraham argued that a person's character can only be complete when the person's libido has reached the stage of genital object love. To reach this stage the person must first overcome his destructive hostile impulses, mistrust and avarice derived from the anal phase; the Oedipus complex must be subdued, narcissism overcome, and the dominance of the pleasure principle broken. Feelings of ambivalence toward the genital organs of the heterosexual partner have to give way to the capacity to enjoy sexual intercourse without inhibition. The genital character absorbs the best from all pregenital phases, from orality enterprise, and from anality perseverance (p. 415). The genital character does not disavow the instincts, but has them under control. Much that psychoanalysts will later assign to the ego is assigned by Abraham to the libido. Libido, if it is not interfered with by neurosis, was conceptualized as running a normal, predictable course toward genitality. Before he became a psychoanalyst, Abraham studied embryology; the inevitable biologically determined maturation of the libido was modeled after embryology. Frigidity and impotence were considered particularly detrimental because they dammed up the libido, preventing the unfolding of the genital character. Because homosexuals fail to reach the genital position, they were judged *ex definitio* as being incapable of loving.

Unfortunately, Freud's reaction to the concept of genital character is not known; Freud does not refer to it in his essay *Libidinal Types* (1931a), nor does the term appear anywhere in the *Standard Edition*. It does not play a role in the correspondence between Freud and Abraham.

Wilhelm Reich's (1929) *The Genital Character and the Neurotic Charact*er represents the next stage in the development of the concept of the genital character. The neurotic character is rigid because it has been formed on the basis of instinctual repression, which in turn gave rise to the character armor. Once a character trait has been established, Reich argued, the instincts need no longer be repressed, for the character trait has so modified the person's attitude toward his instincts that no further energy need be expended on repression. Character traits develop whenever a previously meaningful relationship leads to disappointment and is given up. Thus, character is achieved by the conversion of object libido into narcissistic libido. As we have seen in Freud's formulation, the very opposite process leads to falling in love. Unlike the neurotic character, the genital character has a superego that encourages sexuality, and libido flows freely into the sexual relationship.

Reich described the genital character as adhering to his sexual object not out of guilt or out of moral considerations, but out of a healthy desire for pleasure. The genital character can master polygamous desires if they are in conflict with his relations to the love object, without repression – but he can also yield to them if they disturb him. Such conflicts are solved in a realistic manner. However, the genital character does not always bow to reality for he is also capable of changing the environment. Because he is free of inhibitions, he can step outside of our neurotic civilization and face life without conformity (Reich 1929, p. 161).

Reich further argued that when there is no genuine transfer of the libido to the love object, sexual relations are experienced as insincere of fake, and there is disillusionment after intercourse. Fantasizing during intercourse about other sexual relations indicates that the transfer of the libido to the partner has not taken place. When this happens, a false idealization is often resorted to in order to defend against the breakdown of the illusion that one has found a satisfying partner (pp. 86–87).

Both Abraham's and Reich's formulations of the genital character had a Utopian ring, but Abraham's genital character was conceptualized in terms of object relations, while Reich's was narcissistic and politically revolutionary.

Today it is well known that Reich himself had a tragic life. In retrospect, it is not difficult to see that his concept of the genital character was an idealized self-representation; an attempt to maintain object ties threatened by psychic disintegration. However, in the 1920s he was a charismatic leader. In 1934 Reich severed his connections with psychoanalysis. His works were no longer taught, but his ideas lingered because they were incorporated into Fenichel's book (1945, p. 85).

Fenichel's own definition of love was a modest one. "One can speak of love only when consideration for the object goes so far that one's own satisfaction is impossible without satisfying the partner." Elsewhere in his book (p. 496), Fenichel defined the genital character in terms taken directly from Reich, except that he recognized what Reich did not: that the genital character is an ideal concept, not one found in real life. Unlike Reich's, Fenichel's authority remained high. It is therefore not an exaggeration to say that for a generation after Freud, the attainment of genitality was a major implicit goal of every psychoanalysis.

In 1947 the stage shifts from Fenichel and Reich to Balint. In his paper *On Genital Love*, without referring to Abraham or Reich by name, Balint observed that in psychoanalysis, genitality was defined essentially in negative terms: absence of oral greed, no wish to humiliate or devour the partner, no feelings of disgust for the sexual organs of the partner, no feelings of shame that one's penis is too small or that one's breasts are either too small or too large. In contrast to Abraham's and Reich's genital character, Balint drew attention to narcissistic personalities who are capable of genital orgasm but devoid of the capacity to love.

In another paper, Balint (1956) emphasized that in perversions, particularly among fetishists and transvestites, one finds a preference for orgasm with the aid of inanimate objects rather than with another person. The fetish is preferred because it is inanimate and always available, never needs to be taken into consideration, and makes no demands. Voyeurism and exhibitionism require the presence of other human beings, but not their cooperation. In these relationships the objects are exchangeable. The more primitive and infantile the psychosexual phase, the less are needs of objects taken into account. By contrast, genitality depends on the willingness and cooperative attitude of the partner. Genitality to Balint is not synonymous with genital love. Genital love becomes possible when genitality is associated with idealization, tenderness and a special form of identification.

The differentiation between genitality and genital love led Balint to draw a radical conclusion: genital love is a regressive phenomenon; it is our prolonged childhood that makes us susceptible to genital love and discontent with loveless genitality.

Balint saw genital love as a fusion of two nonharmonious elements: genital satisfaction and pregenital tenderness (Freud's two current theories revived):

> The reward for bearing the strain of this fusion is the possibility of regression periodically for some happy moments to an infantile stage of no reality testing, to the short-lived re-establishment of the complete union.
>
> (p. 137)

Love is to Balint not a natural emotion; it has to be taught. Culture compels the individual to fuse sex with love. Freud's ideas expressed in *Civilization and its Discontents* (1930) are applied by Balint to love. Balint suggested that man be looked upon as a retarded animal who, even in his mature years, remains under the sway of an infantile form of sexuality.

Neither Balint nor Reich could find good reason why two genital people should stay together in a prolonged or even a life-long relationship.

Handelsman (1965) showed that borderline or psychotic patients are capable of orgasm. Contrary to Reich's assumption, impotence and frigidity develop in a higher and more developed intrapsychic structure when there is conflict between superego, ego and id.

In 1968, at a meeting of the American Psychoanalytic Association, a symposium was held on "The Theory of Genital Primacy in the Light of Ego Psychology" (Berezin 1969, Ross 1970). In this symposium, Ross took the lead in questioning the connection between postambivalent object relations and the attainment of sexual orgasm. This was a significant turning point in the psychoanalytic understanding of love. Not that Freud had been entirely wrong; he was right in assuming that frigidity and impotence are associated with an inhibition in loving. But the reverse was not clinically demonstrable. Orgastic capacity and the capacity to love were no longer seen as synonymous.

The next significant contribution was a paper by Binstock (1973): he emphasized that in a happy heterosexual relationship each partner vicariously experiences the other in the act of love. Distinction between the sexes is not lost, but heightened; at the same time, remnants of bisexual needs are continuously projected on the partner, heightening one's own sense of gender identity. A similar identification cannot take place in homosexual love, and therefore the danger of confusion between self and object is greater for the homosexual. In Binstock's view, the person who feels that life without the partner is unthinkable, who prefers death to separation, has regressed to the state where boundaries of the self were lost. The celebrated *Liebestod* is not a sign of true love, but a sign of regression. Such relationships usually improve when the analysand in analysis recaptures the capacity to imagine that he or she can survive without the partner.

Freud discovered the ubiquitous presence of countergender wishes. As a technique of therapy, psychoanalysis has a dual purpose: to uncover the repressed "countergender wishes" and to increase the tolerance of the superego of the masculine wishes in women and the feminine wishes in men. When this has been achieved, falling in love becomes easier, and enables each partner to project countergender wishes on the other. Love can therefore be seen as the benign outcome of the bisexual conflict. Its bliss may consist, intrapsychically speaking, in freeing an individual from the need to repress countergender wishes.

Kernberg (1976) brought concepts derived from systems theory to the psychoanalytic literature on love. The key concept for Kernberg is, as it was for Waelder, integration. In Kernberg's view mature love is reached through a complex series of intrapsychic integrations. The emphasis on integration in turn makes it possible to construct a psychoanalytic diagnostic hierarchy for love different from that of Abraham. On the lowest rung of the ladder, he classified narcissistic personalities incapable of establishing either hetero- or homosexual object relations (p. 186). These narcissistic people fail in their attempts to love because they are consumed by envy and greed. They wish to devalue and spoil what they have conquered (p. 197).

In Kernberg's view, borderline personalities "whose sexuality is chaotic, polymorphous perverse, nevertheless have a better capacity than narcissistic personalities to invest their libido in others" because they are capable of idealization (p. 215).

The fourth group on Kernberg's ladder comprises neurotics whose object representations are coherent and separated from their self-representations. These people are capable of loving, but they cannot combine love with sexuality without feeling guilty because they have remained fixated at the oedipal level (p. 201). Freud dealt with this group in his papers on love.

Those capable of mature love, the final group in Kernberg's classification, have fully integrated their genital sexuality into a total capacity for object relations. Here tenderness expands into full sexual enjoyment. The partners have established a sense of identification with each other. The need to idealize has been transmuted into a mature commitment. In contrast to Freud, Kernberg finds that only in romantic adolescent love is the ego ideal projected. In mature love projection gives way to the sharing of ideals. Kernberg does not believe that mature love blurs the boundary between self and nonself. He states categorically: "There can be no meaningful love relationship without the persistence of the self, without firm boundaries of self which generate a sense of identity" (Kernberg 1980, p. 290).

In spite of many differences, Kernberg's mature love bears a resemblance to Abraham's genital character, and Arlow (1980) criticized it as Utopian – representing an ideal rather than a clinical reality.

The views on love of Klein and of those who followed her lead (Fairbairn and Winnicott) were framed within the model of genitality as the last phase of psychosexual development; but unlike the other authors their views are influenced to a great extent by the dual instinct theory and the significance of the aggressive drive as decisive for loving. They differentiate primitive or oral love from genital and mature love. Oral love has an aggressive aim and is unaffected by concern (Winnicott 1965, p. 22). Primitive love gives rise to splitting. In the well-known case of the ten-year-old Richard, M. Klein (1948, p. 365) found that by analogy to Freud's two current theories, Richard developed the dichotomy between the good breast-mother and the bad genital-mother who belongs to the father. The split interfered with Richard's capacity to reach the genital position.

Like Freud in 1905, Klein (1957) derived love from the infant's relation to the breast. If the breast is cathected with pleasure, it becomes the "good breast" and serves as the basis for the ego's capacity to love. The infant's feeling of bliss at being suckled is not only the basis for future sexual gratification, but for all human happiness. Gratitude is to Klein a major derivative of the capacity to love. Gratitude, in turn, makes possible the feeling of generosity. Idealization, which to Freud is one of the hallmarks of love, Klein sees as a defense against persecutory anxiety. Idealizations are unstable, and when they break down one love object has to be exchanged for another.

Fairbairn (1952) introduced a significant distinction when he suggested

> The important point about the mature individual is not that the libidinal attitude is essentially genital, but that the genital attitude is essentially libidinal ... It is in virtue of the fact that satisfactory object relationships have been established that true genital sexuality is attained.
>
> (p. 22)

By contrast, schizoid individuals experience their love as destructive. They have difficulty in expressing love because of deep anxiety, as expressed by Oscar Wilde in *The Ballad of Reading Gaol*: "Each man kills the thing he loves."

Love and narcissism

It will be recalled that Freud saw love and narcissism as antagonistic forces. This view was challenged by Van der Waals (1965). He noted that well-matched couples intuitively satisfy each other's narcissistic needs. When couples stay together, they find ways of modifying their respective narcissistic needs so that these become compatible with their relationship. (I have observed that in time the couple itself becomes a narcissistic unit. The disappearance of such a narcissistic bond within the couple, I have found, is often the prelude to a breakup.) Kernberg also believes that normal love increases both object and narcissistic libido (1980, p. 281). The depletion of narcissistic libido which Freud thought was characteristic of love is, in Kernberg's view, typical only in pathological love.

Grunberger (1979) finds that no object is sexually satisfying unless it also contributes to narcissistic enhancement. Every love relationship consists of an instinctual aspect mingled with an "elative gratification" of a narcissistic nature (pp. 223–224). Grunberger sees human beings as suffering permanently from a narcissistic wound. This wound manifests itself particularly in states of depression. Love heals this wound to some extent when the partner supplies the missing narcissistic enhancement.

Joffe and Sandler (1965) introduced the concept of "an ideal state of well-being." In this state, the object is seen primarily as a vehicle for the attainment of the ideal state of well-being. They believe that even after object constancy has been reached, the object is not loved for its own sake, but only as a vehicle for the attainment of the ideal state. Object love is a roundabout way to the attainment of the "ideal state of well-being." When a love object is lost, one experiences not only its loss, but also the loss of the object-complementary aspect of the self.

Bach (1980) highlighted difficulties some encounter in integrating love with self-feelings. He contrasts self-awareness with object awareness. Some people in the sexual act can feel either "all themselves" or "somebody's lover," but cannot integrate the two. Some are continuously plagued by self-observation, even at the moment of orgasm. In perversions one finds a denial of gender differences through fantasies of bisexuality. Conversely, simultaneous orgasm is so cherished because it celebrates the overcoming of the painful dichotomy of separateness.

I would like to stress the need of "narcissistic space" as a significant element in the functioning of a couple. To take an everyday experience: a man wishes to describe a trip he and his wife have taken, to visiting guests. His wife interrupts and describes the same trip with greater vivacity. The man feels left out. Or, the man is praised for a culinary feat which was in fact achieved by the wife. She feels deprived. In some cases one of the partners usurps a disproportionate share or even the total "narcissistic space" available to the couple. Deprivation of narcissistic space can lead to marital conflict and alienation.

Love and object loss

In 1971 I suggested that the symbiotic phase leaves a psychic residue in the form of a longing for merger, and this state of longing is re-evoked when one falls in love. It was this longing that Plato described so well over two-and-a-half thousand years ago. Bak's (1973) views on this subject are similar to mine. He writes: "Being in love is a uniquely human, exceptional emotional state, which is based on undoing of the separation between mother and child" (p. 6).

In 1971 I did not yet realize that yearning for the undoing of the separation can be achieved only when in one's own development one has reached a point where the wish to merge evokes neither fear of being devoured, nor fear of loss of identity. Love is fueled by symbiotic yearnings, but it can be realized without fear only when the separation-individuation subphases have been successfully accomplished. An analogous trend of thought applies to the Oedipus complex. Love can take place only when the earlier love for the incestuous object has been refound, but the refinding must be free from oedipal guilt.

Mahler's *rapprochement* subphase (1968) is of particular importance in understanding many difficulties in loving. Homer's *Odyssey* can be seen as the epic poem of this phase of development, with Penelope the ideal mother of the *rapprochement* subphase waiting for the errant husband-child Odysseus to come back. When this subphase has not been negotiated successfully, lovers repeat the need to leave and return, only to leave again, subjecting their partners to an infinite number of waiting tests. A typical reliving of the *rapprochement* subphase also takes place when a couple breaks up – the partners staying apart for some time, only to meet again, and this time experience an emotion far deeper than they have known during the first encounter – intrapsychically a symbolic resolution of the *rapprochement* subphase. The success of the refinding has enhanced the second meeting.

Bak (1973) stressed the connection between love and object loss. His point of departure was Freud's (1917a) statement: "In the two most opposed situations of being most intensely in love and of suicide the ego is overwhelmed by the object, though in totally different ways" (p. 252). In being in love, Bak observed, the self is overwhelmed by the "good object," and in suicide the self is overwhelmed by the "bad object"; in both instances the object has been taken into the self.

Bak saw love as midway between mourning and melancholia. In mourning the person who was loved has died; a real object is lost. In melancholia the loss is unconscious, intrapsychic and symbolic. In being in love, there is a real person in the real world, but the emotion of being in love is only in small part a response to that person. The urgency of love comes from the need to avoid experiencing object loss. To Bak love is a precarious state, for if the attempt to find a substitute for the lost person fails, love may turn into melancholia or suicide. Goethe's Werther is the outstanding example of such a love-suicide in literature.

Bak's approach to love was topographic. He assigned no role to the ego in falling in love. He did, however, add a universal precondition for loving: object loss. In Bak's view the personality of the beloved plays a subordinate role; what matters is that he or she be present at the time when the loss of the loved one takes place. We are all familiar with the bachelor or devoted daughter who marries shortly after the death of a parent, as does also the widower who remarries quickly, to the dismay of children and relatives.

Discussion

I have traced the history of Freud's three theories of love and concluded that all three were modified by subsequent developments, but none has lost validity.

The most enduring of Freud's contributions, the shibboleth that separates the psychoanalytic view on love from that of other disciplines, is the awareness of the link between adult love and love in infancy. The metapsychological aspects of this theory, postulated in terms of separation of currents and their remingling during puberty, has lost much of its appeal for it has turned out to be a metaphor with little explanatory value. The insight that all finding is refinding proved to be even richer than Freud had anticipated, for what we experience in childhood and the extent to which we work these experiences over become the model for our love life. Genital love may be a misnomer, as Balint thought, but without it most people fall back into depressive feelings, life loses its meaning, and it is difficult to maintain one's sense of uniqueness.

Love is not a psychoanalytic term, but neither is dream. Both are well-known normal states. Freud's investigation of dreams has yielded many dream terms specific to psychoanalysis as dream work, dream censor, or day residue. In the realm of love a number of terms emerged: precondition for loving, narcissistic love, genital love. However, a specific psychoanalytic formulation of the nature of love is yet to come.

Prerequisite for a unified psychoanalytic theory of love is the recognition that the so-called puzzle of love consists of a number of puzzles. These are interrelated but not identical.

The first question that demands an answer is why love is so central to human existence. The answer to this question is implicit in Freud's first theory. We need to love and be loved because our prolonged childhood has revealed us as dependent on parental love. The original mother-child dyad was of such overwhelming significance that we yearn to refind it. Even if current infant observations will modify Mahler's emphasis on symbiosis as an actual developmental phase, symbiotic yearnings will remain significant.

That the original dyad is subject to shock, stress and trauma, every analysis demonstrates. There is, therefore, not only yearning, but also fear of the return to infantile dependence.

The original tie to parents is very powerful and often results in fixation. During the stage of falling in love a major displacement from the original to the new love takes place. In the course of development not only objects, but also the self become cathected with love. Self-love may offer resistance to the intruding new love object, but negative narcissism manifesting itself in falling short of one's ego ideal also plays a role. Love can restore the balance.

Memories of yearnings to refind the blissful state of lack of intrapsychic conflict are necessary for falling in love, but much more is required to translate these wishes into an enduring relationship. The capacity to fall in love should not be confused with the psychosexual development that is the prerequisite for the capacity to sustain and translate into an enduring relationship such a state as falling in love.

Freud's views on love were directed backward toward infancy, but there is another force, a forward-looking one. It operates both in love in real life and in transference love. It consists in a hope that the lover will heal the wound inflicted by the less-than-good-enough early objects. That the lover should also be a healer is an important aspect of love. It contributes to making the healer lovable. That this task is often beyond the capacity of a lover gives love its sadness. When love takes place without the resolution of the ties to the parents, it lacks the vigor of a new chapter in love. The lover is experienced merely as a correction of the parents.

Freud believed that the process of refinding can consist only of refinding a physical similarity or character trait of one of the parents. This discussion has shown that the refinding process goes much deeper. If love is to be fulfilling, every important object in childhood must in some way be represented. When one of these objects has been excluded through repression, love is experienced as incomplete; then one needs more than one love object at the same time or in succession. From the point of view of the ego, love represents a triumph of the integrative function over the needs of the id for separate and conflict-laden refindings of the many love objects of childhood.

One of the best-known love poems in the English language, by Elizabeth Browning, opens with: "How do I love thee, let me count the ways." My own counting, less extravagant, is: refinding, hoping to find what was denied, idealization, and integration. I have stressed the connection between refinding and integration. I must now acknowledge the insight as a debt.

> Thou art the grave where buried love doth live,
> Hung with the trophies of my lovers gone,
> Who all their parts of me to thee did give;
> That due of many now is thine alone.
> Their images I loved I view in thee,
> And thou, all they, hast all the all of me.
> (Shakespeare, Sonnet 31)

Note

1 Originally published by Martin S. Bergmann (1988) as "Freud's Three Theories of Love in the Light of Later Developments," *Journal of the American Psychoanalytic Association*, 36: 653–672.

References

Abraham, K. (1924b) Character-Formation on the Genital Level of Libido-Development. In *Karl Abraham, Selected Papers* (Vol. 1: Selected Papers on Psychoanalysis). New York: Basic Books, 1953 pp. 418–501.

Arlow, J.A. (1980) Object Concept and Object Choice. *Psychoanalysis Quarterly* 44:109–133.

Bach, S. (1980) Self-Love and Object-Love: Some Problems of Self and Object Constancy, Differentiation, and Integration, In *Rapprochement*, ed. R. Lax, S. Bach and J. Burland. New York: Aronson, pp. 171–177.

Bak, R. (1973) Being in Love and Object Loss. *International Journal of Psychoanalysis* 54: 1–8.

Balint, M. (1947) On Genital Love. *International Journal of Psychoanalysis* 29: 34–40.

Balint, M. (1956) Perversions and Genitality. In *Perversions, Psychodynamics and Theory*, ed. S. Lorand. New York: Gramercy Books, pp. 16–27.

Barthes, R. (1978) *A Lover's Discourse*. New York: Hill & Wang.

Berezin, M.A. (1969) The Theory of Genital Primacy in the Light of Ego Psychology. *Journal of the American Psychoanalytic Association* 17: 968–987.

Bergmann, M.S. (1982) Platonic Love, Transference Love and Love in Real Life. *Journal of the American Psychoanalytic Association* 30: 87–111.

Binstock, W. (1973) Two Forms of Intimacy. *Journal of the American Psychoanalytic Association* 21: 543–557.

Fairbairn, W.R.D. (1952) *An Object Relations Theory of Personality*. New York: Basic Books.

Fenichel, O. (1945) *The Psychoanalytic Theory of Neurosis*. New York: W.W. Norton & Co., Inc.
Freud, S. (1905b) Three Essays on the Theory of Sexuality. S.E. 7: 135–245.
Freud (1915a) Instincts and Their Vicissitudes. S.E. 14: 117–140.
Freud, S. (1917a) Mourning and Melancholia. S.E. 14: 237–260.
Freud, S. (1921) Group Psychology and the Analysis of the Ego. S.E. 18: 69–143.
Freud, S. (1931a) Libidinal Types. S.E. 21: 217–220.
Fromm, E. (1956) *The Art of Loving*. New York: Harper & Row.
Grunberger, B. (1979) *Narcissism*. New York: International Universities Press.
Handelsman, I. (1965) The Effect of Early Object Relationships on Sexual Development. *Psychoanalytic Study of the Child* 20:367–383.
Joffe, W. and Sandler, J. (1965) Notes on Pain, Depression, and Individuation. *Psychoanalytic Study of the Child* 20: 394–424.
Kernberg, O.F. (1976) *Borderline Conditions and Pathological Narcissism*. New York: Aronson.
Kernberg, O.F. (1980) *Internal World and External Reality: Object Relations Theory Applied*. New York: Aronson.
Klein, M. (1948) *Contributions to Psychoanalysis*. London: Hogarth Press.
Klein, M. (1957) *Envy and Gratitude and Other Works*. New York: Basic Books.
Reich, W. (1929) The Genital Character and the Neurotic Character. In *The Psychoanalytic Reader*, ed. R. Fliess. New York: International University Press, 1948, 148–169.
Reik, T. (1944) *A Psychologist Looks at Love*. New York: Farrar & Rinehart.
Ross, N. (1970) The Primacy of Genitality in the Light of Ego Psychology. *Journal of the American Psychoanalytic Association* 18:267–284.
Van Der Waals, H.G. (1965) Problems of Narcissism. *Bull. Menninger Clin*. 29 243–274.
Waelder, R. (1930) The Principle of Multiple Function: Observations on Over-Determination. In *Selected Papers of Robert Waelder*, ed. S. A.G. Guttman. New York: International Universities Press, 1976, 68–83.
Winnicott, D.W. (1965) *The Maturational Processes and the Facilitating Environment*. New York: International University Press.

CHAPTER 12

ON THE INTRAPSYCHIC FUNCTION OF FALLING IN LOVE[1]

Abstract

Freud once planned a comprehensive "study of man's love life." Although only fragments of this project ever appeared in print, much of it can be reconstructed from Freud's letters and other sources. After tracing the evolution of Freud's thinking on this topic, the author proposes that there are five functions of the ego which are associated with falling in love. The bliss of falling in love is seen as the result of a revival of feelings that once belonged to the symbiotic phase of infancy. Other findings of Mahler are considered in terms of their significance for the understanding of love.

The term love lacks precision: we speak of love between mother and child, love of one's country, and love of knowledge. Theologians differentiate between sacred and profane love, Eros and Agape. Freud, and Plato before him, postulated that the plasticity of the libido is responsible for the many forms that love can take.

In this paper, I will deal only with sexual love, defined by Schopenhauer (1858a) as: "This longing that closely associates the notion of endless bliss with the possession of a definite woman, and an unutterable pain with the thought that this possession is not attainable" (p. 551). We need only enlarge this definition to read "man or woman" for it to remain valid.

I have shown earlier (Bergmann 1971) that this form of love alone has evoked a sense of fear and awe throughout recorded history. We delineate three groups of problems. The first should illuminate falling in love as a special ego state; the second should center on the problem of why a particular person is selected as a love object; the third should focus on the capacity to maintain a sustained love relationship with one person over a long period of time, with fidelity, maturity, and a preponderance of love over envy and aggression in the relationship.

Freud's concepts on love did not follow this sequence, although he dealt with each one of these categories. He became interested first in the question of whom one falls in love with. He then considered the state of falling in love primarily from a metapsychological point of view. He dealt last with the capacity for mature object relations.

My paper falls into three parts. In the first, I will retrace the steps that Freud took in the light of some new findings; in the second, I shall deal with the role of the ego in falling in love, a subject that Freud did not discuss; and third, I will attempt to show how Mahler's findings enhance our understanding of this topic.

The minutes of the Vienna Psychoanalytic Society (Nunberg and Federn 1962, 1967), together with the Freud/Jung correspondence (cf., McGuire 1974), offers an opportunity to observe at close range Freud's ideas on love as they evolved between 1906 and the outbreak of the First World War. The minutes of the meetings and his correspondence show that what appears to be an effortless creation of Freud's genius in his printed works was achieved only through an inner struggle. Freud never integrated his findings on love into a coherent theory. There is no equivalent to chapter 7 of *The Interpretation of Dreams* (1900) for the subject of love.

On November 28, 1906, Freud reported to the Vienna Society that he was planning "a study of man's love life" (Nunberg and Federn 1962, p. 66). In a more personal way he wrote to Jung from Rome on September 19, 1907, "When I have totally overcome my libido (in the common sense), I shall undertake to write a love life of mankind" (McGuire 1974, p. 89). Love, like the dream, belongs to normal psychology. It seems plausible that Freud thought that love, like the dream, would become a topic beyond psychopathology, to be illuminated by psychoanalysis.

At the same 28 November meeting of the Vienna Society, Freud was further quoted as saying:

> In the final analysis, the treatment accorded the child is decisive for his love life. People in love, for example, use for each other pet names by which they were called during childhood. Man becomes childish when he is in love ... Love is said to be irrational, but its irrational aspect can be traced back to an infantile source: the compulsion in love is infantile. Such a condition of love found a very beautiful expression in Goethe's Werther when young Werther enters the room and immediately falls in love with the maiden. He sees her buttering slices of bread and is reminded of his mother.
>
> (Nunberg and Federn, 1962, p. 66)

The scene in which Werther falls in love is richer in its nuances than Freud's summary would suggest. But if we read the actual text, there is no hint that Werther is reminded of his mother; it is Freud who is discovering that the woman one falls in love with reminds one of one's mother, while attributing his discovery to Goethe. This scene is rich in symbols. Werther comes upon the young woman dressed in white, holding a knife and a loaf of black bread. What impresses young Werther is the justice with which she distributes the evening bread to the children according to size and appetite. Significant, too, is her remark that the children will accept their evening meal from nobody else. She wields the "phallic" knife, belongs to another man, is pure, a feeder who plays no favorites, and no substitute for her is acceptable (an allusion to "object constancy") – a powerful combination conducive to falling in love.

It is not likely that the scene from Werther came to Freud's mind accidentally, for it is similar to the one depicted in Freud's (1899) own screen memory. Freud, too, fell in love at first sight. In Freud's case, also, the color of the girl's dress played a role, as did the fresh-tasting country bread and the woman (nurse) who wields the knife. It seems probable, then, that Freud had not yet discovered the mother figure behind his adolescent love when he analyzed his own screen memory, but rather that he completed the self-analysis when he came upon the scene of Werther's falling in love and attributed his own discovery to the idealized Goethe. The same fatal knife appeared again when Freud fell in love with his future wife, Martha. According to Jones (1953), "on this occasion, [Freud] was arrested by the sight of a merry maiden peeling an apple and chatting gaily at the family table ... That very first glimpse was a fatal one" (p. 103).[2]

Freud's (1905b) *Three Essays* already contained a theory of love derived from the diphasic nature of human sexuality. The mother is the first love-sexual object of the infant. During latency, the sexual drive is split into two currents: the sensuous and the tender. The sensuous undergoes repression while the tender remains conscious. During puberty, if all goes well, a new object replaces the old and the two currents are reunited. Thus, Freud said that "the finding of an object is in fact the re-finding of it" (p. 222). "Should these two currents fail to converge ... the focusing of all desire upon a single object, will be unobtainable" (p. 200). He went on to say that what is left over from the sexual relation to the first object "helps to prepare for the choice of an object and thus to restore the happiness that has been lost" (p. 222).

In addition to the *Three Essays* Freud's papers of 1910, 1912, 1914, 1915, 1917 and 1921, together with Abraham's papers of 1909 and 1913, represent the classical psychoanalytic literature on the subject of love.

Strictly speaking, only Freud's 1910d paper deals with the question of why a certain person or a given situation is conducive to falling in love. The later papers deal with the difficulty neurotics have in transferring their libido to nonincestuous objects; that is, with the split between love and sexual desire:

> impotence makes its appearance whenever an object which has been chosen with the aim of avoiding incest recalls the prohibited object through some feature, often an inconspicuous one ... Where they love they do not desire and where they desire they cannot love.
>
> (Freud 1912a, p. 183)

I believe that Freud came close to uncovering a basic contradiction at the core of all human love, but did not draw the ultimate conclusions. In any love relationship, the new love object must recall the old, but for this recall to result in happy love it must not reawaken incestuous guilt. After his betrothal, Tolstoy wrote, "I keep feeling as though I had stolen some undeserved illegal happiness that was not meant for me" (Troyat 1967). Here, a residue of guilt accompanies happy love; hence the poignancy of love, for every new love contains a triumphant overcoming of the incestuous barrier.

The correspondence with Jung further demonstrates that Freud frequently drew upon literature to enrich his insight into the nature of love. In a letter written to Jung in 1907 he explained Jensen's choice of Gradiva as a love object. Jensen's sister's foot was deformed; Gradiva was selected for the beauty of her gait. Memory alone would lead to the evocation of castration anxiety, and love results from this overcoming of the anxiety (McGuire 1974, p. 100; see also Freud 1906).

Freud went on to inform Jung:

> Our love objects form series, one is a recurrence of another (The Master of Palmyra) and each one is a reactivation of an unconscious infantile love, but this love must remain unconscious; as soon as it is aroused to consciousness, it holds the libido fast instead of guiding it onward, and a new love becomes impossible.
>
> (McGuire 1974, p. 100)

The Master of Palmyra mentioned in Freud's letter to Jung is a play in five acts by Adolf von Wilbrandt, published in 1889.[3] All but forgotten today, the play was well known to Freud's generation. It is a sentimental variant on the theme of Faust. The hero, a general of Palmyra living at the end of the Roman pagan era, is granted immortality. A woman companion is given the opportunity to return in every generation under a new guise, and become each time the beloved of the immortal hero. As his life continues, he finds himself alone in the increasingly strange Christian world and, in contrast to his earlier wish for immortality, he longs for death. The same woman appears for the last time and in her arms he finds the wished-for death.

I believe that *The Master of Palmyra* provided the stimulus not only for Freud's idea that love objects come in series but, probably, also for *The Theme of the Three Caskets*. There Freud (1913a) said:

> the three forms taken by the figure [are] of ... the mother herself, the beloved one who is chosen after her pattern, and lastly the Mother Earth who receives him once more. But it is in vain that an old man yearns for the love of woman as he had it first from his mother; the third of the Fates alone, the silent Goddess of Death, will take him into her arms.
>
> (p. 301)

If my reconstruction is correct, the *Three Caskets* paper, by its content as well as publication date, belongs to the series of papers on love and may represent Freud's personal feelings.

The idea that a man re-encounters in his love the same woman from infancy to death is so logically rooted in the Oedipus complex that one could easily believe that it was original to Freud. However, Ellenberger (1970) showed that it was a prevalent belief in the nineteenth century before Freud. He cited Nietzsche's aphorism: "Every man keeps in himself an image of the woman deriving from that of his mother, and according to the image he will be prone to respect or to despise women" (p. 708).

The unconscious equation of death and womb has a long tradition. Schopenhauer stated (1858a):

> If the universal mother carelessly sends forth her children without protection to a thousand threatening dangers, this can be only because she knows that, when they fall, they fall back into her womb where they are safe and secure.
>
> (p. 473)

Freud's 1910d paper on love was discussed on May 19, 1909, at the meeting of the Vienna Psychoanalytic Society. A striking difference between the two versions aroused my interest. The published paper opens with an apology for encroaching upon the territory of the creative writer in depicting the necessary conditions for loving. In the Minutes, a writer who was Freud's inspiration is cited:

> Another case of more deep-going prerequisite for love was recently related by Paul Lindau in a feuilleton in the Neue Freie Presse: a man, writing to his friend, tells him the story of his love affair, which he himself finds completely puzzling. The man, who, since his mother's death, had led an altogether solitary life, one day became engaged to a young girl, who was loveable in every respect. Accompanying her is a plain-looking girl, a close relative of hers, to whom he does not pay the slightest attention. One day,

> the young man rescues this [other] girl from the sea and when she, almost benumbed, is restored to life, he falls in love with her and [ultimately] marries her. To the psychoanalyst, there is nothing at all to question about this affair; for this man, the prerequisite for love is a [dead] body that one can love; in the man's introductory remarks, there is already the intimation that this refers to the dead mother.
>
> (Nunberg and Federn 1967, p. 238)

The feuilleton, entitled "The Resurrected One," appeared in the Neue Freie Presse in two installments on October 22 and 23, 1908 – eight months before the presentation to the Vienna Psychoanalytic Society.[4] The author Lindau, in the prologue, complained that he had never before experienced the insufficiency of psychology as strongly. "Our knowledge," he continued, "of the human psyche has not outgrown its baby shoes." ("Niemals habe ich das Unzulaengliche unserer Psychologie so empfunden wie jetzt. Unsere ganze Seelenkunde steckt noch in den Kinderschuhen.") It is easy to imagine how forcibly this sentence must have struck Freud. The author went on to describe an engagement to a worthy woman for whom he felt a great deal of sympathy but little passion. When he rescued the poor and plain-looking relative, he did not marry her as Freud's summary stated, but rather – for reasons he could not explain – broke off the engagement to the first woman. There is no reference to a "dead mother." If the rescued woman represented the mother, as Freud had postulated, her representative vetoed the marriage to another woman; although she herself did not meet the necessary precondition for loving, Lindau's account makes it clear that the original choice lacked the passion of love. Even before the rescue, the reporter was ambivalent. The feuilleton does not illustrate Freud's precondition of loving. Once more, as in the case of Werther, Freud credited another man with his discovery. In this instance he could do so only through a memory distortion.

The paper, *On Narcissism*, contained Freud's (1914d) second contribution to the problem of love. In it, he attempted to describe what happens when one falls in love. Expressed in current psychoanalytic vocabulary, Freud postulated that the libido with which the ego ideal and the wishful concepts of the self (Jacobson 1964) are cathected, can be projected. He delineated three stages in the development of narcissistic libido: during the first stage, the self (then called the ego) is the recipient of the total libido; parental criticism and the growing awareness of one's own shortcomings inaugurates the second stage – forcing the transfer of the libido from the self to the ego ideal; during the third stage, the ego ideal is projected and thus becomes what Freud called the sexual ideal. A person will then love "what he once was and no longer is, or ... what possesses the excellences that he never had" (p. 101).[5] From the storehouse of narcissistic libido Freud derived the overestimation so characteristic of many who are in love. He believed that neurotics particularly are in danger of impoverishing the self by excessive object cathexis.

In extreme cases, Freud added in 1921 (p. 113), "The object has, so to speak, consumed the ego." From 1914 on, Freud spoke of love increasingly in economic (quantitative) terms.

> the difference between an ordinary erotic object-cathexis and the state of being in love is that in the latter incomparably more cathexis passes over to the object and that the ego empties itself as if it were in favour of the object
>
> (Freud 1927b, pp. 164–165)

In *Instincts and Their Vicissitudes*, Freud (1915a) made his third contribution to the understanding of love. Loving, he stated, admits three opposites: loving-hating, loving-indifference, loving and being loved (p. 133). Love, Freud now emphasized, is not a characteristic of the instinct but rather of the total ego – meaning the self – toward the object (p. 137). In the early stages of libidinal development love is indistinguishable from hate. Love proper becomes synthesized under the supremacy of the genital phase (p. 138). In this context, the young child was not seen as capable of loving.

In his classic paper of 1924, Abraham traced a line of development from narcissism to object love, from preambivalence to ambivalence to postambivalence. Abraham's nosology in turn dominated psychoanalytic thinking until after the Second World War (see Fenichel 1945, p. 101).

It is evident that after 1914, Freud's understanding of love was based essentially on a metapsychological proposition that large quantities of libido can be transformed from narcissistic into object libido. Falling in love represents a transfer of libido from narcissistic to object libido, while in mourning the libido travels in the opposite direction.

Freud, therefore, conceptualized self-love as the antagonistic force to object love, with narcissistic object choice representing a compromise solution. In this context one may also see Kohut's self-object as a compromise between object and narcissistic love. If this basic postulate is called into question, either because of a general critique of metapsychology (Klein 1976), or when narcissism is conceptualized as being incapable of transformation into object libido – as in the work of Kohut (1971), 1977) – it follows logically that this aspect of Freud's theory of falling in love, too, will be called into question.

On the basis of Freud's paper on narcissism, Chasseguet-Smirgel (1976) formulated an intrapsychic explanation of love. She assumed a postoedipal yearning by the ego to be reunited with its ego ideal. Her view reinforces my belief that idealization is an integral part of falling in love. Lovers, temporarily or permanently, forfeit the autonomy of their intrapsychic structure by exchanging their ego ideal for another person. Unlike Freud, Chasseguet-Smirgel believes that love – including unrequited love – enriches rather than impoverishes the ego. Only in pathological love does the self feel impoverished, usually because the person does not believe that he or she deserves to be loved by the idealized object.

If, after falling in love, the partners become critical of one another, the happy union with the ego ideal ceases to exist and may be replaced by the re-emergence of a precursor of a new superego. The function of the superego itself in falling in love can be paradoxical. It can promote love when strictness evokes idealization; conversely, the partner's freedom from superego restraints may evoke love in those who have a harsh superego.

Freud's ideas on love were formulated within the topographic model. By analogy to dream theory, the unconscious wish evoking falling in love is the prohibited oedipal wish. The person one falls in love with is modeled after the day residue of the dream that awakens the dormant wish. The fact that the similarity between the new love object and the old is not known to the lover testifies to the success of a force analogous to the dream work. Dreaming and falling in love take place in a state of benign regression; normally, we expect no structural change to occur as a result of either.

The topographic model was particularly well-suited to explain love at first sight, when the individuality and complex character of the love object plays only an insignificant role. In falling in love at first sight, reality testing is excluded in a way that is reminiscent of dreams. The dreamlike quality that is typical of falling in love is due to the absence or the greatly diminished participation of the ego. The equation of dream and love is a familiar theme in poetry, as in these lines from *The Dream* by John Donne:

> Deare love, for nothing lesse than thee
> Would I have broke this happy dreame,
> It was a theame
> For reason, much too strong for phantasie,
> Therefore thou wak'dst me wisely; yet
> My dream thou brok'st not, but continued'st it,
> Thou art so thruth, that thoughts of thee suffice,
> To make dreames thruths; and fables histories;
> Enter these arms, for since thou thought'st it best,
> Not to dreame all my dreame, let's act the rest.

In some cases, one can observe that almost all the preparatory work of falling in love has taken place in fantasy before the encounter with the love object takes place. The encounter itself signals the displacement of these fantasies. One of my patients, disappointed in the woman he had chosen, ruefully observed, "When I fell in love I wrote the whole scenario myself and only later looked around for a cast of characters." Some can experience love with particular intensity when this relationship is isolated from everyday life and little is known about the real characteristics of the love object. Popular literature has idealized these brief encounters that take place shielded from the light of reality. Censorship in the topographic frame of reference is conceptualized as a passive barrier inhibiting the flow of libido, but incapable of initiating action of its own. This limitation does not apply to the ego after the reformulation of the structural point of view. Freud did not re-evaluate his views on love from the structural point of view. The ego plays no significant role in his views on love.

The first psychoanalyst to discuss love from the point of view of the ego was Waelder in his classic paper of 1930. The act of love he described as combining "physical gratification with a happy relationship. Fulfilment of the instinctual need, the deepest repetition impulse, a satisfaction of the demand of the superego, and the claims of reality are all contained therein" (p. 50). Thus, to Waelder, love represented an act of integration of a very high order. Balint (1948) suggested that love relationships can be differentiated from mere genital relationships because they include idealization, tenderness and a special form of identification. Altman (1977) stated that the ego imparts to love a sense of duration over time and the ability to endure frustration. I would stress five additional functions for the ego to perform, for in a felicitous falling in love there is no conflict between the need to refind, the need to bridge the gap between ego and ego ideal, and the forces of the ego. When these do not coincide, love is experienced as an intrapsychic conflict.

First, reality testing is one of the most important functions of the ego. Even though in falling in love the ego has lost much of its power, its first task is to observe the real qualities of the love object and to evaluate the future of the relationship. This task is particularly difficult, since falling in love is dominated by displacement and projection. The proverbial blindness of love is due to these mechanisms. The participation of the ego is experienced as a change from falling in love as a dream state, to experiencing the relationship as real. This transition is difficult for many lovers to make. On the other hand, when object choice is dominated by realistic ego considerations – talent, social position, health, or wealth – love is seldom experienced.

The second task I would assign to the ego is that of integration. Typically, the growing child has a number of love objects, mother, her substitutes, father, siblings, and so on. Under favorable conditions the object representations of these love objects become integrated and do not compete later on in life for supremacy. However, if there has been disharmony between these objects, their representations will tend to be at war with each other within the former child. The choice of the adult love object may be modeled on one of these early love objects, but love is richer if it can draw upon a significant number of them. In the topographic model, drawing on a number of significant objects of infancy takes place by chance through condensation. In the structural model, it is achieved by the integrative functions of the ego, working unconsciously.

Particularly when the early maternal functions were performed by more than one person, and when there was conflict between the original objects, the task of integration can be beyond the capacity of the ego. To resolve the intrapsychic strife, more than one love object will be sought at the same time or in rapid succession. Each object of infancy has remained cathected and demands its own refinding. There are other tasks of integration which the ego must perform. Bisexuality is a universal human endowment, but individuals differ in the strength of their respective masculine and feminine components, and they seek in the partner a corresponding mixture of the two components. Contradictory wishes may also be present. For example, the wish for the mirroring of the self in the love object is opposed to the wish to find the characteristics one lacks. The image of the mother or the father figure is not always a unified one and fragments of that image press for a separate refinding.

A third task of the ego is to counteract the force of the superego so that the love object does not succumb to the incest taboo, even though the similarities to the original incestuous love object are present.

A fourth task of the ego consists in counteracting the extreme demands of the id that insist on refinding the impossible, the replica of the longed-for symbiosis.

Finally, when one is under the pressure of the repetition compulsion and the new object has the same pain-evoking qualities that characterized the old, every effort will be made to transform the new object to conform to the original object before disappointment took place. It becomes the fifth task of the ego to find other solutions.

If the original objects were good enough, the refinding process can run more or less smoothly. For those who had unempathic or neglectful parents, the refinding process will lead to pathological object selection unless the ego intervenes. Thus, an already burdened ego is under pressure to direct the choosing of an object in opposition to infantile prototypes. The ego exercises a protective as well as anticipatory function. The beleaguered ego fails to observe the total personality of the love object and takes cognizance only of its opposition to the old. Even when the object is in fact different, under the pressure of the repetition compulsion the individual may succeed in eliciting responses characteristic of the defective parent (Lipin 1963). In an earlier paper (Bergmann 1971) I called this reactive type of object choice "counter-selection."

Attempts at counter-selection represent a vulnerable solution. Frequently the repetition compulsion opposes the efforts of the ego, and a state of conflict arises between the two opposing groups of wishes. Under such pressure, two love objects may be selected simultaneously, one representing counter-selection, the other the dangerous refinding. In such a situation, the person clings to the counter-selected object for safety, but seeks gratification with another, based on refinding.

In the earlier paper on love I suggested that the sense of bliss associated with falling in love has its origin in a state of longing (I dare not designate it as recall), however dim, of the feeling state of the symbiotic phase. It is from this phase that the lover ultimately derives the conviction that one person alone has it within his or her power to give or withhold the deepest satisfactions that would make the lover supremely happy or abysmally dejected. Following a similar thought, Bak (1973) saw the capacity to love as contingent on the separation of the self from the dual unity of mother and child. The aim of love is to undo this separation. Freud's refinding was the refinding of a person; what I am suggesting now is a refinding of a lost ego state.

John Donne must have intuitively grasped the symbiotic root of love when he wrote in *Aire and Angels*:

> Twice or thrice had I loved thee,
> Before I knew thy face or name;
> So in a voice, so in a shapeless flame.

Normally, derivatives of the symbiotic wish find expression in the desire of the lovers to be alone with each other and in the withdrawal of interest from the outside world. In happy love these wishes are experienced by both partners at approximately the same strength.

I have had an opportunity to observe a borderline woman whose symbiosis was unsatisfactory; she retained into adulthood longings for direct bodily contact with her mother. She was nevertheless capable of falling and even remaining in love for some time, but she could not tolerate the absence of her lover when he went to work. Her jealousy extended even to his musical instrument. Incapable of experiencing the symbiotic wishes selectively in certain moments in the sexual union, she vainly tried to recreate in adulthood a replica of the symbiotic phase. Jealousy is a complex affective state, as Freud described in 1922. To the well-known causes of pathological jealousy, I would add an unsatisfactory symbiosis. Countess Tolstoy was jealous of all her husband's premarital affairs, her jealousy extending even to the sexual encounters of his fictional characters (Troyat 1967).

Mahler's four subphases of separation-individuation, and particularly her concept of subphase inadequacy, throw a new light on much that is painful in the love life of adults. Failure in any of the separation-individuation subphases may later transform a new love object into one from whom one seeks liberation, and every new object is sought only as an escape from the clutches of the old. Those who suffer subphase inadequacy may counterselect, with the unconscious expectation that love can heal the deficiency. Thus a person whose symbiotic phase was abruptly terminated may select a clinging partner as a safeguard against the danger of abandonment, while at the same time finding the clinging burdensome. One of my patients aptly described the relationship with his woman friend as a mixture of "albatross and security blanket." The patient had been told by his mother that she could not control him outside the playpen, and he was sent directly, so to speak, from the playpen to the nursery, without a chance to experience the *rapprochement* subphase. Characteristically, he could not regulate distance between himself and his dependency object. He was entirely dependent on the coming and going of his woman friend.

Kohut (1977, p. 181) has drawn attention to Proust's narrator – in *The Remembrance of Things Past* – who does not love Albertine, but needs to keep her his prisoner. Subphase inadequacy, in my experience, leads to a sharp differentiation between needing and loving, with the two experienced as incompatible.

Mahler, in her writings, has not addressed herself to the question of the point of development at which the child becomes capable of experiencing love. She uses such terms as "the love object of the infant," "libidinal object constancy," and, when speaking of the earliest developmental stages, she describes "primitive identification taking place under the positive valence of love." This implies a type of love very early in life. In a passage particularly relevant for the purposes of this paper she speaks of "the image of the erstwhile 'good' symbiotic mother, whom we long for 'from the cradle on to the grave' " (1971, p. 416), and goes on to suggest that this image must in later development be blended with the "dangerous because potentially re-engulfing 'mother after separation.'" This good mother of symbiosis is identical to Freud's mother in *Three Caskets*, discussed earlier. The "good symbiotic mother" is refound in falling in love, while the engulfing "mother after separation" looms frequently behind lovers' discord. To these two "archetypes" I would add a third: the wished-for-mother of the *rapprochement* subphase, embodied in Penelope who loyally waits for her son-husband to return home even if her life is spent waiting.

Elsewhere Mahler and her co-workers (1975, pp. 97–98) discuss how, during the *rapprochement* subphase, the range of affects experienced by the toddler widens to include sadness, empathy, anger and disappointment. This is also the phase when the ambitendency described as "alternating desire to push mother away and cling to her" reaches its height. Now loyalty conflicts appear, people other than mother become important, and these new objects in turn threaten "the already toppling illusion of exclusive union with the mother" (p. 93). During the *rapprochement* subphase the "unspecific cravings" are transmuted into longing. In the state of longing, separateness is experienced for the first time. Longing marks the birth of love. For longing, as Spiegel (1966) has observed, will not be appeased by the need-satisfying object; it can only be dissipated by the constant object that is the true love object. Lovers seem to have known this secret all along, for they ask with trepidation, "Have you missed me?" There is no loving without missing, and when severe disappointment in the early love object results in an inhibition of longing, love cannot be experienced.

It is no accident that in the great love stories, lovers' meetings are usually of short duration and the longing for each other prolonged. Clinically, we sometimes discover that there is an unconscious preference for refinding the state of yearning at the expense of refinding the object. In Plato's *Symposium*, Socrates reminds those who would worship love as a god that love is a desire and only those who feel incomplete can love. The immortal gods are complete in their own self-love; they know no longing. The English word "want" designates both desire and feelings of insufficiency. Many languages – German, Spanish and Hebrew, for example – have two words that differentiate love from falling in love.

Popular literature has idealized the notion of remaining permanently in a state of falling in love. Great writers, however, have taken a different view. Emma Bovary is a literary monument to a prolonged state of falling in love and its inevitable doom. On a clinical level, Annie Reich (1953) has described masochistic women who remain in the state of falling in love for a long period, even though their love is based on primitive idealization and penis awe.

Kernberg (1974a, 1974b) has updated, as I see it, Abraham's (1924a) developmental point of view. Kernberg is influenced by systems theory and thus sees the capacity for mature love resulting from a progressive series of integrations. Ultimately, Abraham's concept of postambivalent love and Kernberg's concept of mature love have much in common, in that both theories hold that only those who have mature object relationships can experience love.

Kernberg considers falling in love and staying in love synonymous. I would suggest that these are two separate phenomena. In falling in love, only dim memories of the symbiotic phase are essential. To maintain a love relationship, considerable maturity is required. I agree with Altman (1977) that it is useful to differentiate between the capacity to experience the emotion of love and the capacity for mature object relations.

Finally, Kernberg (1977) believes "that there can be no meaningful love relation without the persistence of the self, without firm boundaries of the self that generate a sense of identity" (p. 95). Kernberg's emphasis on firm boundaries of the self and my focus on a refinding of the elements of the symbiotic phase can be reconciled if we realize that in falling in love feminine wishes in the man and masculine wishes in the woman are projected onto the partner, enhancing one's own gender identity and therefore the boundaries of the self.

The road from falling in love to enduring love involves the transmutation of the idealization into gratitude for the refinding and for the healing of earlier wounds. Love in my view has the following functions to fulfill:

1. To transfer the libido or the attachment from the infantile and incestuous objects to new, nonincestuous ones (see Eissler 1963a, chapter 6).
2. To integrate libidinal strivings originally attached to many objects of childhood into love for one person.
3. To add what was missing in the early relationships to objects. Love's potential to give to the adult what the child never had gives to it a powerful restitutional quality.
4. To return to the adults some of the feelings of bliss experienced in the symbiotic phase that had to be renounced in later developmental phases.

In loving and being loved, lovers give to each other a sense of uniqueness which only very few can find in other spheres of life. That all this may not always be possible creates the pain so many lovers experience.

On the basis of these findings, different types of the incapacity to love can be delineated. If the symbiosis has been interrupted by illness or desertion before it has reached its depth, or if too many hands have divided maternal functions, a depressive core will prevent refinding. If the ego ideal as a separate structure has not developed, and tension between ego and ego ideal is lacking, wishful images of the self (Jacobson 1964) predominate as they do in narcissistic personalities longing to fall in love. Finally, when the road back to the original object is blocked by later trauma, the ego's attempts at counter-selection will stand in the way of fully experiencing falling or remaining in love.

In a happy love relationship, I would suggest that three elements are harmoniously combined:

1. Refinding of the early love object simultaneously on a number of levels of development.
2. Improvement on the old object by finding what one has never had in childhood.
3. A certain amount of mirroring of the self in the beloved. The mirroring is sometimes transmuted into a mutual identification and a feeling of being understood in a special way by the beloved. Those who suffer from self-hatred will shun partners who remind them of themselves, or aspects of themselves, and therefore will not tolerate the mirroring that is part of any happy love.

The integration of these three elements makes love more than a repetition of the past. It makes love a new achievement of the integrative functions of the ego.

It appears that after a long period of separation and individuation – after the establishment of a sense of identity and firm ego boundaries – human beings still long, at least temporarily, to undo their separateness and to find their way back to a state of bliss they had known before individuation. Love takes place within the context of object relationships, but it is a phenomenon *sui generis* and not only a measure of maturity in object relations.

Notes

1 Symposium on Object Relations Theory and Love. This paper was also read before The New York Psychoanalytic Society, September 26, 1978; Drs Otto Kernberg and Theodore Shapiro were the discussants. First published as Martin S. Bergmann (1980), "On the Intrapsychic Function of Falling in Love, *Psychoanalytic Quarterly*, 49:56–77. © John Wiley & Sons, Inc. Reprinted by permission of John Wiley & Sons, Inc.
2 I am indebted to Dr. K.R. Eissler for drawing my attention to this episode.
3 I wish to thank Susanne Norenberg-Freymond, the librarian of Sils Baselgia, Switzerland, for locating this play for me.
4 I am indebted to Dr. Hugo Knoepfmacher for locating the original feuilleton in the Library of Congress.
5 A link may exist between the discovery of narcissism and the literature of the time. Two years before the appearance of Freud's paper on narcissism, Thomas Mann published *Death in Venice*. Never to my knowledge has narcissistic love for what one was, and no longer is, been sketched so sharply as in the love of the aging Aschenbach for the adolescent Tadzio. As did Freud's theme of *The Three Caskets*, Mann's novella portrayed love's affinity for death.

References

Abraham, K. (1924a) A Short Study of the Development of the Libido, Viewed in the Light of Mental Disorders. In *Karl Abraham, Selected Papers* (Vol. 1: Selected Papers on Psychoanalysis). New York: Basic Books, 1953, pp. 418–501.

Altman, L.L. (1977) Some Vicissitudes of Love. *Journal of the American Psychoanalytic Association* 25: 35–52.

Bak, R. (1973) Being in Love and Object Loss. *International Journal of Psychoanalysis* 54: 1–8.

Balint, M. (1947) On Genital Love. *International Journal of Psychoanalysis* 29: 34–40.

Bergmann, M.S. (1971) Psychoanalytic Observations on the Capacity to Love. In *Separation-Individuation: Essays in Honor of Margaret S. Mahler*, eds J.B. McDevitt and C.G. Settlage. New York: International Universities Press, Inc., pp. 15–40.

Chasseguet-Smirgel, J. (1976) Some Thoughts on the Ego Ideal. A Contribution to the Study of the "Illness of Ideality." *Psychoanalytic Quarterly* 45: 345–373.

Eissler, K. (1963a) *Goethe: A Psychoanalytic Study*, Vols. 1 & 2. Detroit: Wayne State University Press.

Ellenberger, H. (1970) *The Discovery of the Unconscious: The History and Evolution of Dynamic Psychiatry*. New York: Basic Books.

Fenichel, O. (1945) *The Psychoanalytic Theory of Neurosis*. New York: W.W. Norton & Co., Inc.

Freud, S. (1899) Screen Memories. S.E. 3: 303–322.

Freud, S. (1905a) Fragment of an Analysis of a Case of Hysteria. S.E. 7: 3–124.

Freud, S. (1905b) Three Essays on the Theory of Sexuality. S.E. 7: 135–245.

Freud, S. (1907) Delusions and Dreams in Jensen's "Gradiva." S.E. 9: 7–95.

Freud, S. (1912a) On the Universal Tendency to Debasement in the Sphere of Love. S.E. 11: 177–190.

Freud, S. (1913a) The Theme of the Three Caskets. S.E. 12: 291–301.

Freud, S. (1914d) On Narcissism: An Introduction. S.E. 14: 73–102.

Freud, S.(1915a) Instincts and Their Vicissitudes. S.E. 14: 117–140.

Freud, S. (1921) Group Psychology and the Analysis of the Ego. S.E. 18: 69–143.

Freud, S. (1925b) Some Psychical Consequences of the Anatomical Distinction between the Sexes. S.E. 19: 243–258.

Freud, S. (1927b) Humour. S.E. 21: 161–166.

Jacobson, E. (1964) *The Self and the Object World*. New York: International Universities Press.

Jones, E. (1953) *The Life and Work of Sigmund Freud, Vol. I: The Formative Years and the Great Discoveries, 1856–1900*. New York: Basic Books.

Kernberg, O.F. (1974a) Barriers to Falling and Remaining in Love. *Journal of the American Psychoanalytic Association* 22: 486–511.

Kernberg, O.F. (1974b) Mature Love: Prerequisites and Characteristics. *Journal of the American Psychoanalytic Association* 22: 743–768.

Kernberg, O.F. (1977) Boundaries and Structure in Love Relations. *Journal of the American Psychoanalytic Association* 25: 81–114.

Klein, G. (1976) *Psychoanalytic Theory: An Exploration of Essentials*. New York: International Universities Press.

Kohut, H. (1971) The Analysis of the Self: A Systematic Approach to the Psychoanalytic Treatment of Narcissistic Personality Disorders. *Psychoanalytic Study of the Child*, Monograph No. 4. New York: International Universities Press.

Kohut, H. (1977) *The Restoration of the Self*. New York: International Universities Press.

Lipin, T. (1963) The Repetition Compulsion and "Maturational" Drive-Representatives. *International Journal of Psychoanalysis* 44: 389–406.

Mahler, M.S. (1971) A Study of the Separation-Individuation Process and its Possible Application to Borderline Phenomena in the Psychoanalytic Situation. *Psychoanalytic Study of the Child* 26: 403–424.

Mahler, M.S., Pine, F. and Bergman, A. (1975) *The Psychological Birth of the Human Infant. Symbiosis and Individuation*. New York: Basic Books.

McGuire, W., ed. (1974) *The Freud/Jung Letters. The Correspondence Between Sigmund Freud and C. G. Jung*. Trans. R. Manheim and R.F.C. Hall. Princeton: Princeton University Press.

Nunberg, H. and Federn, E. (1962) *Minutes of the Vienna Psychoanalytic Society, Volume I: 1906–1908*. New York: International Universities Press.

Nunberg, H. and Federn, E. (1967) *Minutes of the Vienna Psychoanalytic Society, Volume II: 1908–1910*. New York: International Universities Press.

Nunberg, H. and Federn, E. (1974) *Minutes of the Vienna Psychoanalytic Meeting, Volume III: 1910–1911*. New York: International Universities Press.

Reich, A. (1953) Narcissistic Object Choice in Women. *Journal of the American Psychoanalytic Association* 1: 22–44.

Schopenhauer, A. (1858a) The Metaphysics of Sexual Love. In *The World as Will and Representation Vols. I, II*. Third Edition. Trans. E.F.J. Payne. New York: Dover Publications, 1966.
Spiegel, L.A. (1966) Affects in Relation to Self and Object: A Model for the Derivation of Desire, Longing, Pain, Anxiety, Humiliation, and Shame. *Psychoanalytic Study of the Child* 21: 69–92.
Troyat, H. (1967) *Tolstoy*. New York: Doubleday.
Waelder, R. (1930) The Principle of Multiple Function: Observations on Over-Determination. In *Selected Papers of Robert Waelder*, ed. S.A.G. Guttman. New York: International Universities Press, 1976, 68–83.

CHAPTER 13

PLATONIC LOVE, TRANSFERENCE LOVE, AND LOVE IN REAL LIFE[1]

Love, a powerful and puzzling emotion, has through the centuries evoked a wealth of images, metaphors and poetry, but seldom fostered the epistemological wish to discover its nature. The story of Cupid and Psyche, so often depicted in works of art, is of late origin (Apuleus), and therefore not a genuine myth. Nevertheless, it can be read as a cautionary tale, warning us that love will vanish if, like Psyche, driven by curiosity, we dare gaze upon its face.

Among the few who sought to solve the puzzle of love, Plato and Freud stand out as the two whose epistemological interest transformed our way of looking at it. Although more than two thousand years separate the two, they had much in common. Dodds (1951) described Plato as growing up in a social circle which took pride in settling all questions before the bar of reason. Plato believed that virtue (*arete*) consisted in rational living. This rational point of view was, during Plato's lifetime, challenged by events which would "well induce any rationalist to reconsider his faith" (Dodds 1951, pp. 214–215). Both Plato and Freud were deeply interested in exploring intrapsychic reality. Both interpreted dreams in a revolutionary manner. Plato was among the first to understand the dream (Bergmann 1966) not as a message from the gods, but as an intrapsychic event. Similarly, Freud insisted that the dream had an intrapsychic meaning. Both Plato and Freud were aware that incestuous wishes appear in dreams.

In Plato's time, under the impact of the rational philosophers, myths were gradually transformed into allegories. The Sophists called the Greek way of life into question. In the mythical view, the awe and mystery experienced by ancient man in the face of love were ascribed to the powers of a special god. Euripides describes love as "the breaths of Aphrodite" and the Bacchi as "frenzied with breaths from the god" (Onians 1954, p. 55). The power of love was experienced as the manifestation of power of the god of love, just as the god of fire was manifested in fire.

In the *Phaedrus*, Socrates and his companion find themselves on the banks of the river Illisus, where Boreas, the North Wind, is said to have carried off Orithyia. Socrates is asked whether he believes this myth. He replies cautiously,

> the wise are doubtful, and I should not be singular if, like them, I too doubted. I might have a rational explanation that Orithyia was playing with Pharmacia when a north gust carried her over the neighboring rocks, and this being the manner of her death she was said to be carried away by Boreas, the north wind … But to go reducing chimeras, gorgones, and winged steeds to rules of probabilities is [to Socrates] crude philosophy.

He has no leisure for such inquiries: he must first know himself. "To be curious about that which is not my concern while I am still in ignorance of myself would be ridiculous." Socrates then goes on to ask, "Am I a monster more complicated and swollen with passion than the serpent Typo, or a creature of gentler sort?"

This passage from *Phaedrus* has been quoted for many purposes. Cassirer (1946) made use of it to illustrate the relationship between myth and language. What is of importance in the current context is the connection between the loss of faith in myths and the command "know thyself." This connection goes beyond the superficial one stated by Socrates that he has no leisure for such pursuits, for as long as myths held sway over men's minds, man was not a puzzle to himself, and there was no inner need to know oneself.

For example, when Homer describes how Agamemnon compensated himself for the loss of his own mistress by robbing Achilles of his – an immoral act of greed that jeopardized the success of the Trojan War – he apologizes for his behavior by evoking the concept of Ate.

> Not I was the cause of this act, but Zeus, the Erinys who walk in darkness … they put wild Ate in my understanding on that day, so what could I do? Deity will always have its way.
>
> (quoted by Dodds 1951, p. 3)

In psychoanalytic parlance, we would say that man in the mythological era would project unacceptable id wishes on his god.

However, the fact that Agamemnon was overwhelmed by "Wild Ate" and acted as the instrument of divine power does not, in his own opinion, absolve him from responsibility, and he is willing to make amends.

In a similar manner, Helen was forced by Aphrodite to abandon home, husband and daughter for her passion for Paris, but this does not free her from feelings of guilt or mourning over the loss of her past life, as demonstrated when she laments to Priam,

> Before thy presence, father, I appear,
> With conscious shame and reverential fear,
> Ah! had I died ere to these walls I fled,
> False to my country, and my nuptial bed,
> My brothers, friends, and daughter left behind
> (*The Iliad*, Book III, trans. Alexander Pope)

When freed from Aphrodite's power, Helen scorns Paris and detests his bed, but under Aphrodite's command sweet desire for him overcomes her. Homer's heroes, therefore, live in a double world: one beyond their ego control and experienced as obedience to various gods; the other they experience as subject to their own ego and superego control.

By contrast to the Homeric Agamemnon, Socrates believes in the Daemon, an inner voice that warns him against evil and urges him toward the good. The waning of the mythological age is associated with a major advance in psychic internalization. Psychologically speaking, the accusation of impiety against the Olympians leveled against Socrates contained a kernel of truth.

Socrates was not the first to demand self-knowledge. Sophocles, born twenty-six years before Socrates, already made Oedipus proclaim,

Born thus, I ask to be no other man,
Than that I am, and will know who I am.

However, for Oedipus, self-knowledge is still external knowledge, and not the internal knowledge Socrates speaks of, which is close to insight. This moment in the evolution of human thought is also the moment when love for the first time appears as a puzzling emotion. Pre-Socratic man feared love as a destructive power of the god of love; post-Socratic man was puzzled by love.

Onians has noted that in Homer sexual love is described as a process of liquifying or melting. He speaks of "liquid desire." By contrast, hate is derived from freezing or stiffening (Onians 1954, p. 202). Dover (1978) stresses that to Homer, Eros meant desire. It could be desire for a drink or desire for a woman. In pre-Platonic Greece there was no word for love that precluded sexuality.

Plato's *Symposium* marks the transition from the mythical view on love to a philosophical one. Phaedrus, the first orator, praises the power of the god of love in mythological language. Love is a mighty god who inspires lovers to acts of unprecedented courage and devotion. The second orator, Pausanias, introduces a philosophical motif by differentiating between heavenly Aphrodite and common Aphrodite, a distinction which had a long history in Western thought. Other orators differentiate between honorable and vulgar love, between healthy and sick love. These differentiations were unknown when the mythical view prevailed. Socrates, the last speaker, presents a radically new view on love. He dethrones love by calling it the expression of a need, and only the needy can love. Love undoes this feeling of deficiency.

Homosexuality is not mentioned by Homer. It is generally believed that it was introduced as a quasi-official institution by the Dorians, who invaded Greece in the eleventh century; that is, about two hundred years after the events described in *The Iliad*. Homosexuality was glorified by the Dorians as contributing to martial valor. Echoes of this view are found in the *Symposium* when Phaedrus praises homosexual love as conducive to heroic deeds in battle, while Pausanias regards heterosexual love as common and earthly. However, homosexual love, too, should not be allowed to degenerate into sensuous love only. The objects of homosexual love in Greece were boys between the ages of twelve and sixteen; their lovers were usually men under forty-five. The boy (*eromenos*) was idealized for his beauty. The homosexual lover (*erastes*) was expected to elevate the *eromenos* through his wisdom and virtue. In reality, however, documents show that the *erastes* was all too often exploited by the *eromenos* and behaved masochistically (Flaceliere 1960; Dover 1978). In Plato's writing, desexualized love emerges gradually out of the idealization of homosexual love. Plato should, therefore, be regarded as the first to have conceived of sublimation.

In the *Symposium* two myths are told about love. Socrates told that when Aphrodite was born, a feast was held by the gods, and during this feast Resource was intoxicated and fell asleep. In this helpless state, Poverty seduced him and love was conceived.

As a son of Poverty, Eros is described as poor. He has neither shoes nor a house to dwell in. He sleeps on the bare ground under the open sky, and takes his rest on doorsteps. Like his mother, he is always in want. Like his father, he is a hunter of men, enterprising, scheming, and terrible as an enchanter, sorcerer and sophist.

The Socratic view on love has left a lasting imprint on Western thought. Panofsky (1939) traced the motif of the blind Cupid. We are so accustomed to the portrayal of the god of love as blindfolded that it comes as a surprise that Greek and Roman art never portrayed him as such. He appears blindfolded for the first time in the thirteenth century. "Blind Cupid," says Panofsky, "started his career in rather terrifying company. He belonged to night, synagogue, infidelity and death" (p. 111). The allegorical interpretation was most unflattering. "Cupid is nude and blind because he deprives men of their garments, their possessions, their good sense, and their wisdom" (p. 107). In spite of the contempt with which love is described in the Socratic allegory, the strange parentage of love does capture the paradoxical feelings many lovers have expressed of immense richness in the presence of their love, and dismal poverty when separated or abandoned.

The best known myth in the *Symposium* is told by Aristophanes. Primeval Man had two faces, four arms, four legs, two sexual organs, and could move freely forward or backward. There were three types of these primeval human beings, some were composed of two males, others of two females, and only a third were composed of men and women. These primeval humans were so powerful that they threatened the gods, and Zeus cut them into two, creating homosexual men, lesbian women and heterosexual couples. The reason why mankind was not annihilated is ascribed to the dependence of the gods on the sacrifices brought by man; a hostile oral dependence prevails.

> Each of us when separated, having one side only – like a flatfish – is but the indenture of a man, and he is always looking for his other half ... And when one of them meets with his other half, the actual half of himself, whether he be a lover of youth or a lover of another sort, the pair are lost in an amazement of love and friendship and intimacy, and will not be out of the other's sight, as I may say, even for a moment: these are the people who pass their whole lives together; yet they could not explain what they desire of one another. For the intense yearning which each of them has towards the other does not appear to be the desire of lover's intercourse, but of something which the soul of either desires and cannot tell, and of which she has only a dark and doubtful presentiment. Suppose Hephaestus, with his instruments, to come to the pair who are lying side by side and to say to them, "What do you people want of one another?" they would be unable to explain. And suppose further, that when he saw their perplexity he said, "Do you desire to be wholly one; always day and night to be in one another's company? for if this is what you desire, I am ready to melt you into one and let you grow together ..." There is not a man of them who when he heard the proposal would deny or would not acknowledge that this meeting and melting into one another, this becoming one instead of two, was the very expression of his ancient need. And the reason is that human nature was originally one and we were a whole, and the desire and pursuit of the whole is called love.
>
> (trans. B. Jowett).

The association between melting and love is not original to Plato. Sophocles praises love as omnipotent "for it melts its way into the lungs of those who have life in them" (Onians 1954, p. 37). Since the myth was ascribed by Plato to Aristophanes, the noted writer of comedies, there is some question whether he meant it to be taken seriously. We note that while the language is that of the mythical metaphor, the interest is philosophical: to differentiate love from sexual experience and to explain the longing that is such an integral part of loving. We should note the emphasis on preverbal experiences expressed by the phrase, "Dark and doubtful presentiment." Translated into psychoanalytic terms it expresses a feeling that emerges when an event, or a feeling state, in the present has established contact with an event, or a feeling state, belonging to the past without the past event becoming conscious. I assume it was no accident that Freud evoked the Platonic term "dim presentiment" when he wrote, "Following a dim presentiment, I decided to replace hypnosis by free association" (Freud 1914a, p. 19).

The myth told by Plato originated in India, but in his hand it underwent a typical Greek transformation.

> In the Upanishads, Purusa the primeval man looked around him and saw nothing but himself. At first, he said, "I am, and thus the word 'I' was born." He did not rejoice, and therefore one who is alone does not rejoice. He willed himself to fall into two separate pieces, and from these husband and wife were born. They united and from this mankind was born. She reflected, "How can he unite with me after engendering me from himself? For shame! I would conceal myself." She became a cow and he became a bull and united with her, and from them, all cattle was born: she became a mare and he a stallion, etc.
>
> (O'Flaherty 1975, p. 34)

In the Indian version, primeval man, like biblical Adam, is lonely. The cleavage is voluntary.

In the Greek version, the myth has been transformed by Plato to explain the puzzle of love. In Plato's version, primeval man lived in a state of narcissistic bliss, reminiscent of Freud's primary narcissism. Primeval man then committed the typical Greek sin of hubris, attempting to equal the gods. The cleavage and, by implication, love were his punishment.

The myth reappears with a reversed meaning when Dante enters the second circle of the Inferno reserved for carnal sinners whose crime was to subject reason to desire: those who died for love. There Francesca and Paolo appeared to Dante condemned never to separate. Francesca was married to Paolo's older crippled brother. The couple was apprehended in *flagrante delecto* by the husband-brother, who pierced them both with the same sword. In this version, eternal union is experienced as punishment. The lovers are physically merged, but have retained separate voices and separate individualities. The bliss of merger has become a source of torment. Freud's use of the Platonic myth is of interest. In the *Three Essays* (Freud 1905b) the myth is used as an introduction to the chapter on sexual aberration. It is called "A Poetic Fable" (p. 136). Freud does not refer to Plato by name. The myth is evoked a second time in *Beyond the Pleasure Principle* (1920), in the service of the idea that Eros in the form of a drive for union is active in all living beyond "the Kingdom of the Protista" (pp. 57–58).

As a young man, Freud used the Platonic myth with greater freedom to express his love to his fiancée. He wrote: "I am really only half a person in the sense of the old Platonic fable which you are sure to know, and the moment that I am not active my cut hurts me. After all, we already belong to each other" (E. Freud, 1960, Letter 17). This myth was often quoted by Romantic philosophers in the nineteenth century to demonstrate the fundamental bisexuality of human beings (Ellenberger 1970). The problem of bisexuality was prominent in Freud's thinking under the influence of Fliess, at the turn of the century.

Lewin (1952) suggests that it was no accident that this myth was told at a drinking party (*Symposium*). He sees the myth as based on denial of the attachment to the mother's body. In place of the mother, Plato put a narcissistically conceived brother and sister who could be said to be joined since they both came from the same womb and were nursed by the same breast. In his interpretation, the severing stands for weaning. Bradley (1967) interprets the myth as a primal scene fantasy, while I see it as an expression of symbiotic longing (Bergmann 1971).

While the myth can be interpreted on many levels, it is a poetic example of Freud's (1914b) description of narcissistic object choice. It has particular relevance to homosexual object choice where mirroring plays a significant role.

The Phaedrus is of interest from a psychoanalytic point of view for another reason; it contains the allegory of the charioteer. Each soul is divided into three parts: two horses and a charioteer. The right horse is white, with a lofty neck and aquiline nose. He loves honor, modesty and temperance. He needs no touch of the whip, being guided by admonition only. His companion is dark, with a short neck and flat face – a crooked and lumbering animal, a mate of insolence and pride, hardly yielding to the whip. When the charioteer beholds the vision of love, his soul is full of desire. The obedient steed under the government of shame holds back, while the other plunges forward. The opposing disposition of the two horses forces the charioteer to lose control. For a while, the dark horse wins. Eventually, the wild horse is tamed, and from now on the soul of the lover follows the beloved in modesty and holy fear. Freud did not refer to Plato when he used the rider and the horse as a metaphor for the ego and the id. However, Plato's allegory bears such a striking similarity to the tripartite division of the personality into superego, ego and id that his influence can be inferred. The allegory is a metaphorical description of the intrapsychic conflict which ends in the victory of desexualized love.

Plato's transcendental love is reached through the sublimation of homosexual love. Plato's metaphor is the ladder of love. Eros for wisdom is nobler than Eros for a beautiful youth. It is better to be in love with the qualities of a person than with his physical beauty. But the ultimate aim is to behold beauty itself. True to his Greek heritage, Plato equated beauty and goodness. The two were separated in Christian doctrine by Thomas Aquinas. The term "platonic love" – meaning desexualized love – was coined by Vicino, the leading neo-Platonist of the Renaissance. Thanks to Plato, the connection between divine and earthly love, between Eros and Agape, was never entirely lost. The neo-Platonists of the Renaissance differentiated three types of love: animal love (*amor bestiale*), human love (*amor humanus*), and divine love (*amor divinus*) (Panofsky 1969, p. 117).

In 1936 Marie Bonaparte acquired the by-now famous Fliess letters. Freud wished to destroy them. A most touching correspondence followed. The Princess wrote:

> You yourself, dear father, perhaps do not feel all your greatness. You belong to the history of human thought like Plato, we should say, or Goethe. What a loss for us, posterity, if the conversations with Eckermann had been destroyed, or the dialogues of Plato, these latter out of pity for Socrates, so that posterity would not learn that Socrates practiced pederasty with Phaedrus and Alcibiades? There can be nothing like that in your letters: Nothing, when one knows you, that could diminish you! and you yourself, dear Father, have written in your beautiful works against the idealization at all cost of great men.

In another paragraph of the same letter, she speaks of "this new and unique science, your creation, more important than the theory of ideas of Plato himself."

I shall make use of this letter to introduce the topic of Plato's influence on Freud – an influence which may have been more extensive than has hitherto been assumed. Freud's theory of the libido as well as the concept of sublimation can be better understood if we take Plato's influence into account. Before proceeding, I would like to emphasize that in Freud's hands, Plato's ideas underwent a radical transformation. Instead of a religiophilosophical system, Freud erected a secular and psychological one. He was influenced by Plato but was not a Platonist. Simon (1978) notes that both Plato and Freud used the person-within-a-person language. He believes the model derives from introspection when a person in conflict experiences different voices within him, counseling opposing actions (p. 203).

When Freud (1905b) summarized his understanding of love with the epigram, "All finding is refinding" (p. 202), he was echoing Platonic doctrine. However, what to Plato was the refinding of the prenatal bliss of the soul became to Freud the refinding in adult love of the infantile love object.

That Freud's concept of libido has much in common with Plato's Eros has been noted by Nachmanson (1915), Pfister (1921), and recently by Simon (1978). Nachmanson noted that the term "libido" is the Latin translation of the Greek "Eros." He deplored this Latinization, for had Freud retained the original Greek term, the historical connection between Plato and Freud would have been self-evident. Nachmanson also noted that the separation between drive and object so characteristic of Freud's metapsychology goes back to Plato.

Prior to 1920 Freud used the term Eros only in his biography of Leonardo da Vinci (1910b), where he said of Leonardo's drawings:

> So resolutely do they shun everything sexual that it would seem as if Eros alone, the preserver of all living things, was not worthy material for the investigator in his pursuit of knowledge.
>
> (p. 70)

Strachey remarks that the designation of Eros as the preserver of all living things antedates Freud's use of this term in *Beyond the Pleasure Principle* (1920) by ten years. After 1920 Freud no longer used the terms libido and Eros as synonymous.[2] The term Eros was used to designate the life force that combines organic substances into ever larger units. It is Eros that seeks to force and hold together portions of living substance and is therefore the opponent of the death instinct. In this new context libido is conceptualized as that aspect of Eros which is directly concerned with sexuality, although sexuality in the broad sense.

Freud acknowledges his indebtedness to Nachmanson in the preface to the fourth edition of the *Three Essays* (1905b).

> anyone who looks down with contempt upon psychoanalysis from a superior vantage point should remember how closely the enlarged sexuality of psychoanalysis coincides with the Eros of the divine Plato.
>
> (p. 134)

We note the choice of the word "coincides" rather than, as I would suggest, "influenced" by Plato's thought. There has been a reluctance on the part of psychoanalytic writers to admit that Freud was directly influenced by Plato. Jones (1953, p. 56) reports Freud as remarking in 1933 that "his knowledge of Plato's philosophy was very fragmentary." Jones adds, however, that Freud had been greatly impressed by Plato's theory of reminiscence. Simon (1978) also states that Freud was not particularly steeped in Plato (p. 201). Although this has been hitherto the unchallenged view, it is not convincing: not only did Freud read Greek, and use freely Greek myths and Greek terms, he also selected Gomperz's book *Greek Thinkers* as one of his ten "good" books (Eissler 1951). And Gomperz devoted a volume-and-a-half to Plato's thought.

I have stressed that Plato was the originator of the concept of sublimation. The term has an interesting history. It is derived from the Latin *sublimare*, a term used by chemists and alchemists during the Middle Ages, meaning "to raise into vapor in order to purify." It also acquired a metaphorical meaning. In the eighteenth century it was used by Goethe – according to Kaufmann (1950) – in the sense that human feelings and events cannot be portrayed on the stage in their original naturalness, but must be sublimated. According to Ellenberger (1970), the term was also used by Novalis and Schopenhauer, but as Kaufmann makes clear, the first to assign to sublimation a central psychological function was Nietzsche. He speaks of good actions as sublimated bad ones. He also speaks of the artist's sublimation of his impulses, and of sublimated sexuality. Nietzsche even spoke the language of psychoanalytic metapsychology when he said, "One brings about a dislocation of one's quanta of strength by diverting one's thoughts and play of physical forces into other channels" (Kaufmann 1950, p. 192). It is of interest to note that Nietzsche was mainly concerned with the sublimation of the will to power – in psychoanalytic language the sublimation of the aggressive drive – rather than the sublimation of the libido.

In Freud's writings, the term sublimation appeared for the first time in the Dora case (Freud 1905a).[3]

> The sexual life of each of us extends to a slight degree – now in this direction, now in that – beyond the narrow lines imposed as the standards of normality. The perversions are neither bestial nor degenerate in the emotional sense of the word. They are a development of germs all of which are contained in the undifferentiated sexual disposition of the child, and which, by being suppressed or by being diverted to a higher, asexual aim – by being 'sublimated' – are destined to provide the energy for a great number of our cultural achievements. (p. 50)

This is Platonic doctrine, but it has undergone modification. Culture is derived from suppression as well as sublimation of the pregenital perverse impulses, not the genital ones. Freud elaborated the concept of sublimation further in the *Three Essays* (1905b).

Historians of civilization appear to be at one in assuming that powerful components are acquired for every kind of cultural achievement by this diversion of sexual instinctual forces from sexual aims and their direction, to new ones – a process which deserves the name of "sublimation" (p. 178).

Plato derived gymnastics, agriculture, pottery, archery and poetry, as well as the art of the smith, directly from Eros. In a humorous vein, Rabelais' Pantagruel adds that Eros can even instruct brutes in arts that are against their nature, making poets out of ravens, jackdaws and chattering jays, parrots and starlings. He also makes poetesses out of magpies.

In *Leonardo* Freud (1910b) contrasts sublimation with repression. He notes that some people "pursue research with the same passionate devotion that another would give to his love" (p. 77).

> The sexual instinct is particularly well fitted to make contributions of this kind since it is endowed with a capacity for sublimation: that is, it has the power to

> replace its immediate aim by other aims which may be valued more highly and which are not sexual.
>
> (p. 78)

> the libido evades the fate of repression by being sublimated from the very beginning into curiosity and by becoming attached to the powerful instinct for research.
>
> (p. 80)

It is evident that Freud saw sublimation as an alternate route that the libido can follow, avoiding repression. In so doing, Leonardo could command energy not available to those who have to repress. While Freud's view on sublimation is significantly different from that of Plato, the emphasis on the higher value implicit in sublimatory activity shows the persistence of Platonic influence.

In the postscript to *Group Psychology and the Analysis of the Ego* (1921), Freud adds:

> Those sexual instincts which are inhibited in their aims have a great functional advantage over those which are uninhibited. Since they are not capable of really complete satisfaction, they are especially adapted to create permanent ties; while those instincts which are directly sexual incur a loss of energy each time they are satisfied, and must wait to be renewed by a fresh accumulation of sexual libido, so that meanwhile the object may have been changed ... On the other hand, it is also very usual for directly sexual impulsions, short-lived in themselves, to be transformed into a lasting and purely affectionate tie; and the consolidation of a passionate love marriage rests to a large extent upon this process.
>
> (p. 139)

Freud speaks of a marriage consummated out of a passionate falling in love (*Aus verliebter Leidenschaft geschlossne Ehe*), becoming consolidated by transformation into a tender tie only (*bloss zärtliche Bindung*). Freud (1923b) reiterated his belief in the permanence of aim-inhibited ties when he compared "the affectionate relations between parents and children, which were originally fully sexual" with "the emotional ties in marriage" of long duration, which also "had their origin in sexual attraction" (p. 258).

Princess Bonaparte reported that Freud told her that only platonic love is durable. On another occasion she quotes Freud as saying, "Culture has no worse enemy than woman and love." "Woman is certainly needed to continue a civilization, but she never ceases to threaten it." Some of these remarks are expressed in stronger language than what appears in his published writings, but in essence they are not different. To see woman as a threat to civilization is in harmony with Freud's (1925b) view that women, being castrated, do not have the same need to develop a superego as men do.

Freud's mistrust of sexual passion as a binding force can also be observed in the dark view he took of "first marriages of young women which they have entered into when they were most passionately in love." These passionate marriages come to grief from unavoidable disappointment while "second marriages," presumably less passionate, "turn out much better" (Freud 1931b, p. 234).

The conviction that tender feelings are transformed sexual feelings is at the core of Freud's theory of infantile sexuality. Better infant observations have made it more likely that the tender core of a child's feelings toward the mother is formed simultaneously with the sexual feelings associated with the erogenous zones. Already in 1947, Balint questioned this assumption. He noted that pregenital forms of love are not necessarily connected with tenderness, while genital love is genuine only when fused with tenderness. Like Plato, Balint believed that genital love only uses genital sexuality "as stock upon which to graft something essentially different" (p. 132). In his opinion, the prolonged emotional tie that lasts beyond genital satisfaction among partners represents the transference of devotion the child once experienced toward the parent. Loewald (1979) goes even further in stating that "an original intimate unity [between mother and child] is anterior to what is commonly called sexuality" (p. 765).

It is likely that the phenomenon of transference, so puzzling to Freud at the turn of the century, supplied the dynamic force for his inquiries into the nature of love. The Dora case (Freud 1905a) contains the first statement on the nature of transference beyond the early conceptualization in 1895, when transference was seen as resulting from false connections. Dora's premature termination of her treatment was retrospectively attributed by Freud to his failure to master the transference. We might add that at that time his understanding of love was rudimentary. He thought that Mr. K., a close associate of Dora's father – whose wife was her father's paramour – was an appropriate marriage partner for the nineteen-year-old girl. Today, due to our better understanding of adolescence, we can see both Mr. and Mrs. K. as Dora's adolescent displacement figures, standing for her parents. They offered Dora what Blos calls "a second chance" to displace and work out her positive and negative oedipal feelings with substitute parents. Freud interpreted to Dora that she summoned her love for her father as a defense against her love for Mr. K. At that time, he failed to understand that Mr. K.'s advances evoked in Dora an intrapsychic conflict precisely because he was so close to the original father image. His advances could not fail but evoke the incest taboo, forcing her to reject Mr. K. in spite of her love for him.

In the Dora case, Freud established for the first time a significant connection between transference and sublimation. He differentiated two types of transference, the first type differing from the original model "In no respect whatsoever, except for substitutions." These Freud called "Mere reprints." Other transferences have been subjected to sublimation and they resemble revised editions of the original (p. 116).

In 1915, Freud brought together his insights into the nature of transference and his understanding of love in real life. The problem that confronted him was how to treat a woman patient who openly declared she had fallen in love with the therapist. He advised the therapist to renounce his pride in having made a conquest, to recognize that the patient's falling in love was brought about by the analytic situation. Having mastered the countertransference, the therapist must be careful not to steer away from transference love, or repel it, but just as resolutely withhold any response to it. He must demonstrate to the patient that she fell in love at a time when particularly distressing events in her life were about to emerge. He must insist that falling in love is in the service of the resistance, and that demands for gratification have replaced the necessity of analytic work. In reading Freud's (1915b) paper, up to this point, one would conclude that transference love is by its very nature different from love in real life. However, toward the end, Freud makes a striking observation:

> I think we have told the patient the truth, but not the whole truth regardless of the consequences ... The part played by resistance in transference-love

> is unquestionable and very considerable. Nevertheless the resistance did not, after all, create this love; it finds it ready to hand, makes use of it and aggravates its manifestations. Nor is the genuineness of the phenomenon disproved by the resistance ... It is true that the love consists of new editions of old traits and that it repeats infantile reactions. But this is the essential character of every state of being in love. There is no such state which does not reproduce infantile prototypes. It is precisely from this infantile determination that it receives its compulsive character, verging as it does on the pathological. Transference-love has perhaps a degree less of freedom than the love which appears in ordinary life and is called normal; it displays its dependence on the infantile pattern more clearly and is less adaptable and capable of modification; but that is all, and not what is essential.
>
> (p. 168)

All love, according to Freud, "repeats infantile reactions." But transference love is dominated by the repetition compulsion to a greater degree than love in real life. Freud, whose writings on love antedate his discovery of the role of the ego, does not elucidate why this should be so. In an earlier paper (Bergmann 1980), I suggested that if the parent imagos form an unsatisfactory basis for object selection, love will evoke a conflict between object selection based on the infantile imagos and the forces of the ego which resist this painful refinding. In such a case, selection away from the infantile prototype represents a victory of the ego over the repetition compulsion.

When the parental representations have been particularly good, there will be no reason for the ego to veto the selection based on their model. When they have been particularly unsatisfactory, the ego may lack the strength to oppose the repetition compulsion and the new object will be a reprint of the old.

In the psychoanalytic situation the forces of the repetition compulsion are mainly responsible for the transference neurosis, while the forces of the ego, with the assistance of the analyst, are charged with maintaining the differentiation between the analyst and what is being projected or displaced upon him. The lover in real life has to repress or displace his negative feelings about the love object, while the analysand has the opportunity to work through, in the analysis, the negative transference. Schafer (1977) suggests that:

> Freud had not thought through something essential. He was in effect juxtaposing and accepting two views of the matter without integrating them. On the one hand, transference love is sheerly repetitive, merely a new edition of the old, artificial and regressive (in its ego aspects particularly) and to be dealt with chiefly by translating it back into its infantile terms. (From this side flows the continuing emphasis in the psychoanalytic literature on reliving, re-experiencing, and recreating the past.) On the other hand, transference is a piece of real life that is adapted to the analytic purpose, a transitional state of a provisional character that is a means to a rational end and as genuine as normal love.
>
> (p. 340)

Transference love is indeed repetitive as is, also, some of love in real life. It is not by itself adaptive. It is only the sublimation of this love with the aid of the analyst that makes it adaptive for the purposes of cure, when inquiry is substituted for gratification.

Transference love differs from love in real life in a significant way. During childhood, or even later, many anaylsands become disillusioned in their early love objects. This disillusionment leads to the building of defenses against loving. The reactivation and working through of these events liberates libido which can be invested in new objects or reinvested in the analyst. Love in real life can also to some extent undo earlier trauma, but it is more likely to succumb to the repetition compulsion. In real life many traumatized patients fall in love not with a person who reminds them of their parent, but with the person they hope will heal the wound the parental figures have inflicted. To fall in love with the rescuer or the person one has rescued is a frequent theme of romantic love. It is also an important source of transference love.

Transference love and love in real life, in Freud's view, draw upon the same libidinal sources, the same infantile imagos. But they take a different course. In real life, the infantile prototypes behind falling in love remain unconscious; while unconscious, they provide the energy for the new love. In the analytic situation, these early imagos are made conscious and thereby deprived of their energizing potential. The uncovering of the incestuous fixations behind transference love loosens the incestuous tie and prepares the way for a future love freed from the need to repeat oedipal triangulations. In the analytic situation the channels for the expression of concern and reciprocity from the analysand to the analyst are radically curtailed. Transference love thus becomes a special hothouse variety of love that makes fewer demands on object relations than love in real life. It is especially designed for the purpose of cure, but unsuitable for the meeting of the more mature needs of the analysand.

Conversely, in states of narcissistic depletion and when other fixations on early developmental stages dominate, transference love has the advantage of demanding less reciprocity from the analysand than love in real life. It is ultimately the inability of transference love to meet the adult needs of the analytic patient that propels him to redirect the libido freed through the analytic process to love objects in the real world.

The term transference connotes the therapeutic activation of all memories and feelings once associated with the parental figures. Of these, only a small and highly specific number of evocations are conducive to the emergence of transference love. The term "erotized transference" does not appear in Freud's writing.

Blum (1971) describes a woman who, early in analysis, developed an erotized transference. She rejected all interpretations related to the revival of the past and felt that she had fallen completely in love with the analyst. Blum observed that the sense of reality distorted in an erotized transference is due to the repetition of the altered sense of reality in masturbation, and the evocation of real memories of childhood seduction. Erotized transference is likely to develop when the parents were seductive in their behavior toward the child. It serves as a defense against the loss of the love object and is an act of restitution of the lost object. It is, therefore, not dependent on a similarity between analyst and parent. Strictly speaking, it connotes the refinding of an infantile threatening situation, not the refinding of an early infantile love object. Erotized transference, in addition to its defensive and regressive attributes, may also be an attempt to master trauma through repetition.

In my previous papers on love (Bergmann 1971, 1980), I suggested that the ability to love one person rests on the capacity of the ego to integrate love impulses coming from many early objects. Children raised by many hands will, as adults, find it particularly difficult to achieve such an integration. They will need more than one love object or love objects alternating in rapid succession. It may also happen that in the course of development the adult love object was based on one parental object, while the other had to be repressed. In the course of an analysis, the love feelings that underwent repression become liberated. Transference love will then be based on a new refinding. At times we can observe this integrative force at work in dreams when the dreamer is successful in making love with a figure that combines features of father and uncle or grandfather, or even father and mother.

In a historical perspective, Freud's twin discoveries that the transference feelings of his patients contained psychic energy that could be harnessed in the service of a treatment procedure that aimed at insight, and that the emotion of love could be subjected to analysis because it was based on the refinding of infantile love objects, is an astonishing example of a secular utilization of Plato's ladder of love. That love can be diverted from its natural course where it seeks gratification and mutuality and be pressed into the service of bringing about intrapsychic change confirms Plato's original insight into the plasticity of Eros.

Summary

Plato and Freud transformed our way of looking at love. In Plato's *Dialogues* one can trace the transition and transformation of the mythical view on love into philosophical conceptualizations. The waning of the mythical point of view created the demand for man to know himself, and love became a puzzle. Plato was the first to propose that erotic impulses can undergo sublimation to higher and desexualized aims. Freud was not a Platonist, but if we trace the history of certain ideas it becomes evident that Plato's influence on Freud went further and deeper than was assumed by previous psychoanalytic writers. Freud's conceptualization of the libido can be seen as a Latinized version of Plato's Eros. Some of the difficulties associated with the psychoanalytic use of the term "sublimation" go back to the Platonic origin of the term. Freud's conviction that tender and aim-inhibited love was a later transformation of sexual impulses also went back to Plato; as did his belief that aim-inhibited love endures longer than sexual love. Because erotic love impulses can be sublimated, transference love can be harnessed in the service of cure based on insight. Erotized transference is not based on the refinding of an early love object and therefore is less capable of yielding the therapeutic climate required for psychoanalytic treatment. Freud's treatment procedure confirms Plato's belief in the plasticity of Eros.

Notes

1 First published as Bergmann, M.S. (1982), "Platonic Love, Transference Love, and Love in Real Life," *Journal of the American Psychoanalytic Association*, 30: 87–111.
2 I am indebted to Dr. Harold Blum for drawing my attention to this.
3 Freud used the term "sublimation" earlier on in a letter to Fliess (Freud 1892–99, p. 249), but it had not yet acquired the full technical meaning he gave it in his polished writings.

References

Balint, M. (1947) On Genital Love. *International Journal of Psychoanalysis* 29: 34–40.

Bergmann, M.S. (1966) The Intrapsychic and Communicative Aspects of the Dream – Their Role in Psycho-Analysis and Psychotherapy. *International Journal of Psychoanalysis* 47: 356–363.

Bergmann, M.S. (1971) Psychoanalytic Observations on the Capacity to Love. In *Separation-Individuation: Essays in Honor of Margaret S. Mahler*, eds J.B. McDevitt and C.G. Settlage. New York: International Universities Press, Inc., pp. 15–40.
Bergmann, M.S. (1980) On the Intrapsychic Function of Falling in Love. *Psychoanalysis Quarterly* 49: 56–77.
Blum, H.P. (1971) Transference and Structure. In *The Unconscious Today: Essays in Honor of Max Schur*, ed. M. Kanzer. New York: International Universities Press.
Bradley, N. (1967) Primal Scene Experience in Human Evolution. *Psychoanalytic Study of Society* 4: 34–79.
Cassirer, E. (1946) *Language and Myth*. Trans. S.K. Langer. New York: Dover.
Dodds, E.R. (1951) *The Greeks and the Irrational*. Berkeley, CA.: University of California Press.
Dover, A.J. (1978) *Greek Homosexuality*. Cambridge: Harvard Univ. Press.
Eissler, K.R. (1951) An Unknown Autobiographical Letter by Freud and a Short Comment. *International Journal of Psychoanalysis* 32: 319–324.
Ellenberger, H. (1970) *The Discovery of the Unconscious: The History and Evolution of Dynamic Psychiatry*. New York: Basic Books.
Flaceliere, R. (1960) *Love in Ancient Greece*. New York: Crown.
Freud, E., ed. (1960) *Letters of Sigmund Freud*. New York: Basic Books.
Freud, S. (1892–99) Extracts from the Fliess papers. S.E. 1: 175–280.
Freud, S. (1905a) Fragment of an Analysis of a Case of Hysteria. S.E. 7: 3–124.
Freud, S. (1905b) Three Essays on the Theory of Sexuality. S.E. 7: 135–245.
Freud, S. (1910b) Leonardo da Vinci and a Memory of His Childhood S.E. 11: 63–137.
Freud, S. (1913a) The Theme of the Three Caskets. S.E. 12: 291–301.
Freud, S. (1914b) The Moses of Michelangelo. S.E. 13: 211–238.
Freud, S. (1920) Beyond the Pleasure Principle. S.E. 18: 7–64.
Freud, S. (1921) Group Psychology and the Analysis of the Ego. S.E. 18: 69–143.
Freud, S. (1923b) The Ego and the Id. S.E. 19: 3–66.
Freud, S. (1931b) Female Sexuality. S.E. 21: 223–243.
Freud, S. (1935) Postscript to *An Autobiographical Study*. S.E. 20: 71–74.
Joncs, E. (1953) *The Life and Work of Sigmund Freud, Vol. I: The Formative Years and the Great Discoveries, 1856–1900*. New York: Basic Books.
Kaufmann, W.A. (1950) *Nietzsche: Philosopher, Psychologist, Antichrist*. Princeton: Princeton University Press.
Lewin, B.D. (1952) Phobic Symptoms and Dream Interpretation. In *Selected Papers of B.D. Lewin*, ed. J.A. Arlow. New York: Psychoanalysis Quarterly, 1973.
Loewald, H. (1979) The Waning of the Oedipus Complex. *Journal of the American Psychoanalytic Association* 27: 751–775.
Nachmanson, M. (1915) Freud's Libido Theorie verglichen mit der Eroslehre Platos *Int. Z. Psychoanal.* 3: 65–83.
O'Flaherty, W.D. (1975) *Hindu Myths*. Baltimore: Penguin Books.
Onians, R.B. (1954) *The Origins of European Thought*. Cambridge, England: Cambridge University Press.
Panofsky, E. (1939) Blind Cupid. In *Studies in Iconology*. New York: Harper Torch Books, 1962.
Panofsky, E. (1969) *Problems in Titian*. New York: New York University Press.
Pfister, O. (1921) Plato als Vorlaufer der Psychoanalyze. *Int. Z. Psychoanal.* 7: 264–269.
Schafer, R. (1977) The Interpretation of Transference and the Condition of Loving. *Journal of the American Psychoanalytic Association* 25: 335–362.
Simon, B. (1978) *Mind and Madness in Ancient Greece*. Ithaca: Cornell University Press.

BIBLIOGRAPHY

Aarons, Z. (1965) On Analytic Goals and Criteria for Termination. *Bulletin of the Philadelphia Association for Psychoanalysis* 15: 97–109.

Abend, S.M. (1988) Unconscious Fantasies and Issues of Termination. In H.P. Blum, A.K. Richards and Y. Kramer, eds, *Unconscious Fantasy, Myth and Reality*. Madison, CT: International Universities Press.

Abraham, H. and E.L. Freud, eds (1965) *A Psycho-Analytic Dialogue: The Letters of Sigmund Freud and Karl Abraham, 1907–1926*. New York: Basic Books.

Abraham, K. (1909) The Significance of Intermarriage Between Close Relatives in the Psychology of the Neuroses. In *Clinical Papers and Essays on Psychoanalysis*. New York: Basic Books, 1955, pp. 21–28.

Abraham, K. (1913) On Neurotic Exogamy: A Contribution to the Similarities in the Psychic Life of Neurotics and of Primitive Man. In *Clinical Papers and Essays on Psychoanalysis*. New York: Basic Books, 1955, pp. 48–50.

Abraham, K. (1924a) A Short Study of the Development of the Libido, Viewed in the Light of Mental Disorders. In *Karl Abraham, Selected Papers* (Vol. 1: Selected Papers on Psychoanalysis). New York: Basic Books, 1953, pp. 418–501.

Abraham, K. (1924b) Character-Formation on the Genital Level of Libido-Development. In *Karl Abraham, Selected Papers* (Vol. 1: Selected Papers on Psychoanalysis). New York: Basic Books, 1953, pp. 418–501.

Adams, M.V. and J. Sherry (1991) Significant Words and Events. In *Lingering Shadows*, ed. A.M. Brown and S.A. Martin. Boston: Shambala.

Alexander, F. (1954) Psychoanalysis and Psychotherapy. *Journal of the American Psychoanalytic Association* 2: 722–733.

Alexander, F. and T.M. French (1946) *Psychoanalytic Therapy*. New York: Ronald Press.

Altman, L.L. (1977) Some Vicissitudes of Love. *Journal of the American Psychoanalytic Association* 25: 35–52.

Arlow, J.A. (1969) Unconscious Fantasy and Disturbances of Conscious Experience. *Psychoanalytic Quarterly* 38: 1–27.

Arlow, J.A. (1980) Object Concept and Object Choice. *Psychoanalysis Quarterly* 44: 109–133.

Arlow, J.A. (1991) Perspective on Freud's "Analysis Terminable and Interminable" after 50 Years. In *On Freud's "Analysis terminable and interminable,"* ed. J. Sandler. New Haven, CT: Yale University Press, pp. 73–88.

Arlow, J. and C. Brenner (1964) *Psychoanalytic Concepts and the Structural Theory*. New York: International Universities Press, Inc.

Bach, S. (1980) Self-Love and Object-Love: Some Problems of Self and Object Constancy, Differentiation, and Integration, In *Rapprochement*, ed. R. Lax, S. Bach and J. Burland. New York: Aronson, pp. 171–177.

Bader, M.J. (1994) The Tendency to Neglect Therapeutic Aims in Psychoanalysis. *Psychoanalytic Quarterly* 63: 246–270.

Bak, R. (1973) Being in Love and Object Loss. *International Journal of Psychoanalysis* 54: 1–8.

Balint, M. (1935) The Final Goal of Psycho-Analytic Treatment. In *Primary Love and Psycho-Analytic Technique*. New York: Liveright, 1953, pp. 188–199.

Balint, M. (1947) On Genital Love. *International Journal of Psychoanalysis* 29: 34–40.

Balint, M. (1956) Perversions and Genitality. In *Perversions, Psychodynamics and Theory*, ed. S. Lorand. New York: Gramercy Books, pp. 16–27.

Balint, M. (1968) *The Basic Fault: Therapeutic Aspects of Regression*. London: Tavistock Publications.

Balint, M. (1969) Trauma and Object Relationship. *International Journal of Psychoanalysis* 50: 429–437.

Barthes, R. (1978) *A Lover's Discourse*. New York: Hill & Wang.

Berezin, M.A. (1969) The Theory of Genital Primacy in the Light of Ego Psychology. *Journal of the American Psychoanalytic Association* 17: 968–987.

Berliner, B. (1958) The Role of Object Relations in Moral Masochism. *Psychoanalytic Quarterly* 27: 38–56.

Bergmann, M.S. (1963) The Place of Paul Federn's Ego Psychology in Psychoanalytic Metapsychology. *Journal of the American Psychoanalytic Association* 11: 97–116.

Bergmann, M.S. (1966) The Intrapsychic and Communicative Aspects of the Dream – Their Role in Psycho-Analysis and Psychotherapy. *International Journal of Psychoanalysis* 47: 356–363.

Bergmann, M.S. (1971) Psychoanalytic Observations on the Capacity to Love. In *Separation-Individuation: Essays in Honor of Margaret S. Mahler*, eds J.B. McDevitt and C.G. Settlage. New York: International Universities Press, Inc., pp. 15–40.

Bergmann, M.S. (1976) Moses and the Evolution of Freud's Jewish Identity. In *Judaism and Psychoanalysis*, ed. M. Ostow. New York: Ktav Publishing House, 1982, pp. 115–141.

Bergmann, M.S. (1980) On the Intrapsychic Function of Falling in Love. *Psychoanalysis Quarterly* 49: 56–77.

Bergmann, M.S. (1982) Platonic Love, Transference Love and Love in Real Life. *Journal of the American Psychoanalytic Association* 30: 87–111.

Bergmann, M.S. (1986) *The Anatomy of Loving*. New York: Columbia University Press.

Bergmann, M.S. (1987) *The Anatomy of Loving: The Story of Man's Quest to Know What Love Is*. New York: Columbia University Press.

Bergmann, M.S. (1988) On the Fate of the Intrapsychic Image of the Psychoanalyst After Termination of the Analysis. *Psychoanalytic Study of the Child* 43: 137–153.

Bergmann, M.S. (1989) Science and Art in Freud's Life and Work. In *Sigmund Freud and Art: His Personal Collection of Antiquities*, ed. L. Gamwell and R. Wells. New York: Harry M. Abrams, pp. 173–183.

Bergmann, M.S. (1991) Reflections on the History of Psychoanalysis: Plenary Address to the Fall Meeting of the American Psychoanalytic Association. *Journal of the American Psychoanalytic Association* 41: 929–955.

Bergmann, M.S. (1992) *In the Shadow of Moloch: The Sacrifice of Children and its Impact on Western Religions*. New York: Columbia University Press.

Bergmann, M.S. (1993a) Reality and Psychic Reality in Ernst Kris's Last Papers: An Attempt to Update his Findings. *Psychoanalytic Inquiry* 13 (4): 372–383.

Bergmann, M.S. (1993b) Reflections on the History of Psychoanalysis. *Journal of the American Psychoanalytic Association* 41: 929–955.

Bergmann, M.S. (1997) Termination: The Achilles Heel of Psychoanalytic Technique. *Psychoanalytic Psychology* 14: 163–174.

Bergmann, M.S. (1998a) Asking for Freud's Blessing. *The Modern Freudians: Contemporary Psychoanalytic Technique*, eds C. Ellman, S. Grand, M. Silvan and S. Ellman. North Vale, NJ: Jason Aronson.

Bergmann, M.S. (1998b) Ringen mit Freud: Sigmund Freud Vorlesung. Frankfurt A.M. *Zeitschrift fur Psychoanalitische Theory und Praxis*. Jahrgang 13. 1998.

Bergmann, M.S., ed. (2000) *The Hartmann Era*. New York: Other Press.

Bergmann, M.S. (2001) The Leap from the *Studies on Hysteria* to *The Interpretation of Dreams*. In *Storms in Her Head*, eds M. Dimen and A. Harris. New York: Other Press.

Bergmann, M.S. (2002) The Relevance of History to the Psychoanalytic Controversy on Homosexuality. In *The Annual of Psychoanalysis: Rethinking Psychoanalysis and the Homosexualities*, eds J.A. Winer and J.W. Anderson, Hillsdale, NJ: Analytic Press, 37–41.

Bergmann, M.S. and Hartman, F., eds (1976) *The Evolution of Psychoanalytic Technique*. New York: Basic Books.

Bernfeld, S. (1944) Freud's Earliest Theories and the School of Helmholtz. *Psychoanalytic Quarterly* 13: 341–362.

Bernfeld, S. and Feitelberg, S. (1930) Der Entropiesatz und der Todestrieb. *Imago* 61: 187–206.

Bibring, G. (1936) A Contribution to the Subject of Transference Resistance. *International Journal of Psychoanalysis* 17: 181–189.

Bibring, E. (1953) The Mechanism of Depression. In *Affective Disorders*, ed. P. Greenacre. New York: International Universities Press, pp. 13–48.

Binstock, W. (1973) Two Forms of Intimacy. *Journal of the American Psychoanalytic Association* 21: 543–557.

Bion, W. (1967) Notes on Memory and Desire. *Psychoanalytic Forum* 2 (3): 272–273.

Blanton, S. (1971) *Diary of My Analysis with Sigmund Freud*. New York: Hawthorn Books.

Blum, H.P. (1971) Transference and Structure. In *The Unconscious Today: Essays in Honor of Max Schur*, ed. M. Kanzer. New York: International Universities Press.

Blum, H. (1973) The Concept of Erotized Transference. *Journal of the American Psychoanalytic Association* 29: 61–76.

Blum, H.P. (1989) The Concept of Termination and the Evolution of Psychoanalytic Thought. *Journal of the American Psychoanalytic Association* 37: 275–295.

Bond, A., Franco, D. and Richards, A. (1992) *Dream Portrait: A Study of Nineteen Sequential Dreams as Indicators of Pretermination*. Madison, CT: International Universities Press.

Bowlby, J. (1960) Grief and Mourning in Infancy and Early Childhood. *Psychoanalytic Study of the Child* 15: 9–52.

Bowra, C.M. (1950) *The Romantic Imagination*. London: Oxford.

Bowra, C.M. (1957) *The Greek Experience*. New York: World Publishing Co.

Bradley, N. (1967) Primal Scene Experience in Human Evolution. *Psychoanalytic Study of Society* 4: 34–79.

Brenner, C. (1976) *Psychoanalytic Technique and Psychic Conflict*. New York: International Universities Press.

Breuer, J. and Freud, S. (1895) Studies on Hysteria. S.E. 2: 1–335.

Brunswick, R.M. (1928) A Supplement to Freud's "History of an Infantile Neurosis." *International Journal of Psychoanalysis* 9: 439–476.

Burlingham, M.J. (1989) *The Last Tiffany: A Biography of Dorothy Tiffany Burlingham*. New York: Atheneum.

Cassirer, E. (1932) *Die Philosophie der Aufklärung* (*The Philosophy of the Enlightenment*). Princeton: Princeton University Press, 1951.

Cassirer, E. (1946) *Language and Myth*, trans. S.K. Langer. New York: Dover.

Chapelle, D (1993) *Nietzsche and Psychoanalysis*. Albany, NY: State University of New York Press.

Chasseguet-Smirgel, J. (1976) Some Thoughts on the Ego Ideal. A Contribution to the Study of the "Illness of Ideality." *Psychoanalytic Quarterly* 45: 345–373.

Chasseguet-Smirgel, J. (1984a) *Creativity and Perversion*. New York: Norton.

Chasseguet-Smirgel, J. (1984b) *The Ego Ideal: A Psychoanalytic Essay on the Malady of the Ideal*. Trans. P. Barrows. New York: W.W. Norton.

Chasseguet-Smirgel, J. (1986). *Sexuality and Mind: The Role of the Father and the Mother in the Psyche*. New York: New York University Press.

Clark, K. (1973) *The Romantic Rebellion: Romantic versus Classical Art*. New York: Harper & Row.

Coen, S.J. (1981) Sexualization as a Predominant Mode of Defense. *Journal of the American Psychoanalytic Association* 29: 395–411.

Dewald, P.A. (1982) The Clinical Importance of the Termination Phase. *Psychoanalytic Inquiry* 2: 441–461.

Dicks, H.V. (1967) *Marital Tensions*. New York: Basic Books.

Dickinson, Emily (1890), eds T.W. Todd and Mabel Loomis, Poem IV.XXVII (p. 138) in: Higginson, *Poems by Emily Dickinson*. Boston: Roberts Brothers.

Dodds, E.R. (1951) *The Greeks and the Irrational*. Berkeley, CA: University of California Press.

Dover, A.J. (1978) *Greek Homosexuality*. Cambridge: Harvard University Press.

Edelson, M. (1986) Heinz Hartmann's Influence on Psychoanalysis as a Science. *Psychoanalytic Inquiry* 6: 575–600.

Eissler, K.R. (1951) An Unknown Autobiographical Letter by Freud and a Short Comment. *International Journal of Psychoanalysis* 32: 319–324.

Eissler, K.R. (1953) The Effect of the Structure of the Ego on Psychoanalytic Technique. *Journal of the American Psychoanalytic Association* 1: 104–143.

Eissler, K.R. (1958) Notes on Problems of Technique in the Psychoanalytic Treatment of Adolescents. *Psychoanalytic Study of the Child* 13: 223–254.

Eissler, K. (1963a) *Goethe: A Psychoanalytic Study*, Vols 1 and 2. Detroit: Wayne State University Press.

Eissler, K.R. (1963b) The Emotion of Amorousness and the Principle of Repetition. In *Goethe: A Psychoanalytic Study, Vol. I, 1775–1786*. Detroit: Wayne State University Press, pp. 656–668.

Eissler, K.R. (1971) Freud's Approach to the Analysis of Literary Works. In *Discourse on Hamlet and "Hamlet."* New York: International Universities Press, Inc., pp. 459–493.

Eissler, K.R. (1971) *Talent and Genius: The Fictitious Case of Tausk Contra Freud*. New York: Quadrangle.

Ellenberger, H. (1970) *The Discovery of the Unconscious: The History and Evolution of Dynamic Psychiatry*. New York: Basic Books.

Erikson, E.H. (1959) *Identity In the Life Cycle: Psychological Issues*, vol. 1, no. 1. Madison, CT: International Universities Press.

Erikson, E.H. (1962) Reality and Actuality. *Journal of the American Psychoanalytic Association* 10: 454–461.

Ewen, F., ed. and trans. (1948) *Heinrich Heine, Self Portrait and Other Writings*. Secaucus, NJ: The Citadel Press.

Fairbairn, W.R.D. (1952) *An Object Relations Theory of Personality*. New York: Basic Books.

Federn, P. (1930) The Reality of the Death Instinct. *Psychoanalytic Review* 19: 129–151.

Fenichel, O. (1935) A Critique of the Death Instinct. In *Collected Papers*, 1st Series, eds Fenichel, H. and Rapaport, D (1953), 363–372.

Fenichel, O. (1941) *Problems of Psychoanalytic Technique*, trans. D. Brunswick. New York: Psychoanalytic Quarterly.

Fenichel, O. (1945) *The Psychoanalytic Theory of Neurosis*. New York: W.W. Norton & Co., Inc.

Fenichel, O. (1998) *Rundbriefe 1938–1945* (2 vols), eds J. Reichmayr and E. Mühlleitner. Frankfurt, Germany: Stromfeld.

Ferenczi, S. (1924) *Thalassa: A Theory of Genitality*. New York: Psychoanalytic Quarterly.

Ferenczi, S. (1928) The Problem of Termination of the Analysis. In *Final Contributions to Problems and Methods of Psychoanalysis*, ed. Balint, M.. New York: Basic Books, 1955, 77–86.

Ferenczi, S. (1929) The Unwelcome Child and His Death Instinct. In *Final Contributions to the Problems and Methods of Psychoanalysis*, ed. Balint, M. New York: Basic Books, 1955, 102–107.

Ferenczi, S. (1933) Confusion of Tongues Between Adult and Child. In *Final Contributions to Problems and Methods of Psychoanalysis*, ed. Balint, M.. New York: Basic Books, 1955, 156–167.

Ferenczi, S. (1988) *The Clinical Diary of Sándor Ferenczi*, ed. J. Dupont. Cambridge, MA: Harvard University Press.

Ferenczi, S. and Rank, O. (1924) *Entwicklungsziele der Psychoanalyse: Zur Wechselbeziehung von Theorie und Praxis*. Leipzig: Internationaler Psychoanalytischer Verlag.

Ferenczi, S. and Rank, O. (1925) *The Development of Psychoanalysis*, trans. C. Newton. New York: Nervous and Mental Disease Publishing.

Firestein, S.K. (1969) Problems of Termination in the Analysis of Adults. *Journal of the American Psychoanalytic Association* 17: 222–237.
Firestein, S. (1978) *Termination in Psychoanalysis*. New York: International Universities Press.
Flaceliere, R. (1960) *Love in Ancient Greece*. New York: Crown.
Fleming, J. and Benedek, T. (1966) *Psychoanalytic Supervision*. New York: Grune & Stratton.
Freud, A. (1936) The Ego and the Mechanisms of Defense. In *The Writings of Anna Freud: Volume II 1936: The Ego and the Mechanisms of Defence*. New York: International Universities Press.
Freud, A. (1943) Memorandum. In *The Freud-Klein Controversies 1941–1945*, eds P. King and R. Steiner. London: Routledge, 1991, pp. 629–634.
Freud, A. (1949) Notes on Aggression After Reviewing Klein's Point of View. In *The Writings of Anna Freud. Volume IV 1945–1956. Indications For Child Analysis and Other Papers*. New York: International Universities Press, 1968.
Freud, A. (1954) The Widening Scope of Indications for Psychoanalysis. In *The Writings of Anna Freud. Volume IV 1945–1956. Indications For Child Analysis and Other Papers*: 356–376. New York: International Universities Press.
Freud, A. (1965a) The Concept of Developmental Lines. *The Psychoanalytic Study of the Child* 18: 245–265. New York: International Universities Press.
Freud, A. (1965b) *Normality and Pathology in Childhood, Writings* 6. New York: International University Press.
Freud, A. (1976) Changes in Psychoanalytic Practice and Experience. In *The Writings of Anna Freud, Vol. VIII: Psychoanalytic Psychology of Normal Development*: 176–185. New York: International Universities Press.
Freud, E., ed. (1960) *Letters of Sigmund Freud*. New York: Basic Books.
Freud, S. (1886–99) Pre-Psychoanalytic Publications and Unpublished Drafts. S.E. 1.
Freud, S. (1887–1904) *The Complete Letters of Sigmund Freud to Wilhelm Fliess, 1887–1904*, ed. and trans. J.M. Masson. Cambridge, MA: Harvard University Press, 1985.
Freud, S. (1892–93) A Case of Successful Treatment by Hypnotism: With Some Remarks on the Origin of Hysterical Symptoms Through "Counter-Will." S.E. 1: 115–128.
Freud, S. (1892–99) Extracts from the Fliess papers. S.E. 1: 175–280.
Freud, S. (1895) A Project for a Scientific Psychology. S.E. 1: 283–397.
Freud, S. (1898) Sexuality in the Aetiology of the Neuroses. S.E. 3: 261–285.
Freud, S. (1899) Screen Memories. S.E. 3: 303–322.
Freud, S. (1900) The Interpretation of Dreams, Part I and Part II. S.E. 4–5: 1–625.
Freud, S. (1901) The Psychopathology of Everyday Life. S.E. 6: 1–336.
Freud, S. (1905a) Fragment of an Analysis of a Case of Hysteria. S.E. 7: 3–124.
Freud, S. (1905b) Three Essays on the Theory of Sexuality. S.E. 7: 135–245.
Freud, S. (1905c) On Psychotherapy. S.E. 7: 257–268.
Freud, S. (1905d) Jokes and Their Relation to the Unconscious. S.E. 8: 9–236.
Freud, S. (1907) Delusions and Dreams in Jensen's "Gradiva." S.E. 9: 7–95.
Freud, S. (1908a) "Civilized" Sexual Morality and Modern Nervous Illness. S.E. 9: 177–204.
Freud, S. (1908b) Creative Writers and Day-Dreaming. S.E. 9: 141–153.
Freud, S. (1910a) Five Lectures of Psycho-Analysis. SE 11: 1–5.
Freud, S. (1910b) Leonardo da Vinci and a Memory of His Childhood S.E. 11: 63–137.
Freud, S. (1910c) The Future Prospects of Psychoanalytic Therapy. S.E. 11: 141–151.
Freud, S. (1910d) A Special Type of Choice of Object Made by Men (Contributions to the Psychology of Love I). S.E. 11: 165–175.
Freud, S. (1910e) "Wild" Psycho-Analsis. S.E. 11: 219–228.
Freud, S. (1911) Notes on an Autobiographical Account Case of Paranoia (*Dementia Paranoides*). S.E. 12: 9–82.
Freud, S. (1912a) On the Universal Tendency to Debasement in the Sphere of Love. S.E. 11: 177–190.
Freud, S. (1912b) The Dynamics of Transference. S.E. 12: 99–108.
Freud, S. (1912c) Recommendations to Physicians Practising Psycho-Analysis. S.E. 12: 111–120.
Freud, S. (1913a) The Theme of the Three Caskets. S.E. 12: 291–301.
Freud, S. (1913b) Totem and Taboo. S.E. 13: 1–161.

Freud, S. (1914a) Remembering, Repeating and Working Through. S.E. 12: 145–156.
Freud, S. (1914b) The Moses of Michelangelo. S.E. 13: 211–238.
Freud, S. (1914c) On the History of the Psycho-Analytic Movement. S.E. 14: 7–66.
Freud, S. (1914d) On Narcissism: An Introduction. S.E. 14: 73–102.
Freud, S. (1915a) Instincts and Their Vicissitudes. S.E. 14: 117–140.
Freud, S. (1915b) Observations on Transference-Love: Technique of Psycho-Analysis. S.E. 12: 159–171.
Freud, S. (1915c) Thoughts for the Times of War and Death. S.E. 14: 273–300.
Freud, S. (1916) Some Character Types Met With in Psychoanalytic Work. S.E. 14: 309–333.
Freud, S. (1916–17a) Introductory Lectures on Psychoanalysis, Parts I and II. S.E. 15: 9–239.
Freud, S. (1916–17b) Introductory Lectures on Psychoanalysis, Part III. S.E. 16: 243–463.
Freud, S. (1917a) Mourning and Melancholia. S.E. 14: 237–260.
Freud, S. (1917b) Transformations of Instinct as Exemplified by Anal Erotism S.E. 17: 127–33.
Freud (1918) The Taboo of Virginity (Contributions to the Psychology of Love III). S.E. 11: 193–208.
Freud, S. (1919a) Lines of Advance in Psycho-Analytic Therapy. S.E. 17: 157–168.
Freud, S. (1919b) The Uncanny. S.E. 17: 219–256.
Freud, S. (1920) Beyond the Pleasure Principle. S.E. 18: 7–64.
Freud, S. (1921) Group Psychology and the Analysis of the Ego. S.E. 18: 69–143.
Freud, S. (1922) Some Neurotic Mechanisms in Jealousy, Paranoia and Homosexuality. S.E. 18: 223–232.
Freud, S. (1923a) Two Encyclopaedia Articles. S.E. 18: 233–259.
Freud, S. (1923b) The Ego and the Id. S.E. 19: 3–66.
Freud, S. (1924a) The Economic Problem of Masochism. S.E. 19: 157–170.
Freud, S. (1924b) The Dissolution of the Oedipus Complex. S.E. 19: 173–179.
Freud, S. (1925a) Resistance to Psychoanalysis. S.E. 19: 212–222.
Freud, S. (1925b) Some Psychical Consequences of the Anatomical Distinction between the Sexes. S.E. 19: 243–258.
Freud, S. (1925c) An Autobiographical Study. S.E. 20: 7–74.
Freud, S. (1925d) Inhibition, Symptoms and Anxiety. S.E. 20: 77–175.
Freud, S. (1926) The Question of Lay Analysis. S.E. 20: 177–250.
Freud, S. (1927a) The Future of an Illusion. S.E. 21: 3–56.
Freud, S. (1927b) Humour. S.E. 21: 161–166.
Freud, S. (1930) Civilization and its Discontents. S.E. 21: 57–145.
Freud, S. (1931a) Libidinal Types. S.E. 21: 217–220.
Freud, S. (1931b) Female Sexuality. S.E. 21: 223–243.
Freud, S. (1932) My Contact with Josef Popper-Linkeus. S.E. 22: 218–224.
Freud, S. (1933) New Introductory Lectures on Psycho-Analysis. S.E. 22: 1–182.
Freud, S. (1935) Postscript to *An Autobiographical Study*. S.E. 20: 71–74.
Freud, S. (1937a) Analysis, Terminable and Interminable. S.E. 23: 211–253.
Freud, S. (1937b) Constructions in Psycho-Analysis S.E. 23: 257–269.
Freud, S. (1939) Moses and Monotheism. S.E. 23: 1–137.
Freud, S. (1940) An Outline of Psycho-Analysis. S.E. 23: 141–207.
Fromm, E. (1956) *The Art of Loving*. New York: Harper & Row.
Gay, P. (1988) *Freud: A Life for Our Time*. New York: W.W. Norton.
Gedo, J.E. and Goldberg, A. (1973) *Models of the Mind*. Chicago: University of Chicago Press.
Gill, M. (1954) Psychoanalysis and Exploratory Psychotherapy. *Journal of the American Psychoanalytic Association* 2: 771–797.
Gitelson, M. (1958) On Ego Distortion. *International Journal of Psychoanalysis* 19: 245–257.
Glover, E. (1955) *The Technique of Psychoanalysis*. New York: International Universities Press.
Glover, E., Fenichel, O., Strachey, J., Bergler, E., Nunberg, H. and Bibring, E. (1937) Marienbad Symposium on the Theory of the Therapeutic Results of Psychoanalysis. *International Journal of Psychoanalysis* 18: 125–189.
Goldberg, A. and Marcus, D. (1985) "Natural Termination": Some Comments on Ending Analysis Without Setting a Date. *Psychoanalytic Quarterly* 54:46–65.

Goldstein, J. (1982) The Hysteria Diagnosis and the Politics of Anticlericalism in Late Nineteenth-Century France. *Journal of Modern History* 54: 209–239.

Gomperz, T. (1896) *Greek Thinkers*, trans. L. Magnus. London: Murray.

Green, A. (1975) The Analyst, Symbolization and Absence in the Analytic Setting (On Changes in Analytic Practice and Analytic Experience). *International Journal of Psychoanalysis* 56: 1–22.

Green, A. (1983) The Dead Mother. In *On Private Madness*. New York: International Universities Press, 1986.

Green, A. (1999) On Discriminating and Not Discriminating Between Affect and Representation. *International Journal of Psychoanalysis* 80 (2): 277–316.

Green, A. (2005) *Key Ideas for a Contemporary Psychoanalysis: Misrecognition and Recognition of the Unconscious*. New York: Routledge.

Greenacre, P. (1954) The Role of Transference: Practical Considerations in Relation to Psychoanalytic Therapy. *Journal of the American Psychoanalytic Association* 21: 671–684.

Greenson, R. (1967) *The Technique and Practice of Psychoanalysis*. New York: International University Press.

Greenson, R. (1970) The Exceptional Position of the Dream in Psychoanalytic Practice. In *Explorations in Psychoanalysis*. New York: International Universities Press.

Grubrich-Simitis, I. (1991) *Freud's Moses-Studie als Tagtraum*. Weinheim: Verlag Internationale Psychanalyse.

Grunberger, B. (1971) *Narcissism*. New York: International Universities Press.

Gunderson, J.G. and Gabbard, G.O. (1999) Making the Case for Psychoanalytic Therapy in the Current Psychiatric Environment. *Journal of the American Psychoanalytic Association* 47: 679–703.

Guthrie, W.K. (1962) *The History of Greek Philosophy* (2 vols). Cambridge, England: Cambridge University Press.

Handelsman, I. (1965) The Effect of Early Object Relationships on Sexual Development. *Psychoanalytic Study of the Child* 20:367–383.

Hartmann, H. (1958) *Ego Psychology and the Problem of Adaptation*. New York: International Universities Press.

Hartmann, H. (1939) Psychoanalysis and the Concept of Health. In *Essays on Ego Psychology*. New York: International Universities Press, 3–18.

Hartmann, H. (1950) Comments on the Psychoanalytic Theory of the Ego. In *Essays on Ego Psychology*. New York: International Universities Press, 1964, 113–141.

Hartmann, H. (1959) Psychoanalysis as a Scientific Theory. In *Psychoanalysis Scientific Method and Philosophy*. New York: Washington Square Press, 3–37.

Hartmann, H. (1964) *Essays in Ego Psychology*. New York: International Universities Press.

Hartmann, H., Kris, E. and Loewenstein, R. (1949) Notes on the Theory of Aggression. *Psychoanalytic Study of the Child* 3: 9–36.

Hazo, R.G. (1967) *The Idea of Love*. New York: Praeger.

Hitschmann, E. (1952). Freud's Conception of Love. *International Journal of Psychoanalysis* 33: 421–428.

Horney, K. (1937) *Neurotic Personality of Our Time*. New York: Norton.

Hurn, H.T. (1971) Toward a Paradigm of the Terminal Phase: The Current Status of the Terminal Phase. *Journal of the American Psychoanalytic Association* 19: 332–348.

Hynal, A. (1988) *Controversies in Psychoanalytic Methods: From Freud to Ferenczi and Michael Balint*. New York: New York University Press.

Jacobson, E. (1957) Denial and Repression. *Journal of the American Psychoanalytic Association* 5 (1): 61–92.

Jacobson, E. (1959) The Exceptions: An Elaboration of Freud's Character Study. *Psychoanalytic Study of the Child* 14: 135–154.

Jacobson, E. (1964) *The Self and the Object World*. New York: International Universities Press.

Jacobson, E. (1967) *Psychotic Conflict and Reality*. New York: International Universities Press.

Jekels, L. and Bergler, E. (1949). Transference and Love. *Psychoanalytic Quarterly* 18: 325–350.

Joffe, W. and Sandler, J. (1965) Notes on Pain, Depression, and Individuation. *Psychoanalytic Study of the Child* 20: 394–424.
Jones, E. (1953) *The Life and Work of Sigmund Freud, Vol. I: The Formative Years and the Great Discoveries, 1856–1900*. New York: Basic Books.
Jung, C.G. (1910) *C.G. Jung Letters, Volume I, 1906–1950*, eds G. Adler and A. Jaffe. Princeton, NJ: Princeton University Press, 1973.
Jung, C.G. (1918) *The Role of the Unconscious*. In *The Collected Works, Volume Ten: Civilization in Transition*, 2nd edition, eds H. Read, M. Fordham and G. Adler, trans. R.F.C. Hull. Routledge: London.
Junker, H. (1991) *Von Freud in den Freudianern*. Tuebinqen: edition diskord.
Kaplan, A. (1957) Freud and Modern Philosophy. In *Freud and the 20th Century*, ed. Nelson, B.. New York: Meridian Books.
Kaufmann, W.A. (1950) *Nietzsche: Philosopher, Psychologist, Antichrist*. Princeton: Princeton University Press.
Keiser, S. (1953), A Manifest Oedipus Complex in an Adolescent Girl. *Psychoanalytic Study of the Child* 8: 99–107.
Kernberg, O. (1970) Factors in the Psychoanalytic Treatment of Narcissistic Personalities. *Journal of the American Psychoanalytic Association*, 18: 51–85.
Kernberg, O.F. (1974a) Barriers to Falling and Remaining in Love. *Journal of the American Psychoanalytic Association* 22: 486–511.
Kernberg, O.F. (1974b) Mature Love: Prerequisites and Characteristics. *Journal of the American Psychoanalytic Association* 22: 743–768.
Kernberg, O. (1974c) Contrasting Viewpoints Regarding the Nature and Psychoanalytic Treatment of Narcissistic Personalities: A Preliminary Communication. *Journal of the American Psychoanalytic Association*, 22: 255–267.
Kernberg, O. (1974d) Further Contributions to the Treatment of Narcissistic Personalities. *International Journal of Psychoanalysis*, 55: 215–240.
Kernberg, O.F. (1976) *Borderline Conditions and Pathological Narcissism*. New York: Aronson.
Kernberg, O.F. (1977) Boundaries and Structure in Love Relations. *Journal of the American Psychoanalytic Association* 25: 81–114.
Kernberg, O.F. (1980) *Internal World and External Reality: Object Relations Theory Applied*. New York: Aronson.
Kernberg, O. (2009) The Concept of the Death Drive: A Clinical Perspective. *International Journal of Psychoanalysis* 90: 1009–1035.
King, P. and Steiner, R. (1991) *The Freud-Klein Controversies 1941–45*. New York: Tavistock/Routledge.
Klein, G. (1976) *Psychoanalytic Theory: An Exploration of Essentials*. New York: International Universities Press.
Klein, M. (1948) *Contributions to Psychoanalysis*. London: Hogarth Press.
Klein, M. (1950) On the Criteria for Termination of a Psychoanalysis. In *Envy and Gratitude and Other Works*. New York: Delacorte, 43–47.
Klein, M. (1957) *Envy and Gratitude and Other Works*. New York: Basic Books.
Kohut, H. (1971) The Analysis of the Self: A Systematic Approach to the Psychoanalytic Treatment of Narcissistic Personality Disorders. *Psychoanalytic Study of the Child*, Monograph No. 4. New York: International Universities Press.
Kohut, H. (1977) *The Restoration of the Self*. New York: International Universities Press.
Kohut, H. (1980) Two Letters. In *Advances in Self Psychology*, ed. Goldberg, A.. New York: International Universities Press.
Kris, A. (1982) *Free Association: Method and Process*. New Haven, CT: Yale University Press.
Kris, E. (1951) Ego Psychology and Interpretation in Psychoanalytic Therapy. In *Selected Papers of Ernst Kris*. New Haven, CT: Yale University Press, 1975, 237–251.
Kris, E. (1956a) On Some Vicissitudes of Insight in Psychoanalysis. In *Selected Papers of Ernst Kris*. New Haven, CT: Yale University Press, 1975, 252–271.
Kris, E. (1956b) The Personal Myth: A Problem in Psychoanalytic Technique. In *Selected Papers of Ernst Kris*. New Haven, CT: Yale University Press, 1975, 272–300.

Kubie, L.S. (1968) Unsolved Problems in the Resolution of the Transference. *Psychoanaytic Quarterly* 37: 331–352.
Kuhn, T. (1962) *The Structures of Scientific Revolutions*. Chicago, IL: University of Chicago Press.
Lear, J. (1990) *Love and its Place in Nature: A Philosophical Interpretations of Freudian Psychoanalysis*. New York: Farrar, Straus & Giroux.
Lester, E. (1985) The Female Analyst and the Erotized Transference. *Journal of the American Psychoanalytic Association* 66: 283–293.
Lewin, B.D. (1950) *The Psychoanalysis of Elation*. New York: Norton.
Lewin, B.D. (1952) Phobic Symptoms and Dream Interpretation. In *Selected Papers of B.D. Lewin*, ed. J.A. Arlow. New York: Psychoanalysis Quarterly, 1973.
Lewin, K. (1948) *Resolving Social Conflicts*. New York: Harper and Row Publishers.
Lipin, T. (1963) The Repetition Compulsion and "Maturational" Drive-Representatives. *International Journal of Psychoanalysis* 44: 389–406.
Loewald, H. (1960) On the Therapeutic Action of Psychoanalysis. *International Journal of Psychoanalysis* 41: 16–33.
Loewald, H. (1962) Internalization, Separation, Mourning, and the Superego. *Psychoanalytic Quarterly* 31: 483–504.
Loewald, H. (1966) Review of Arlow and Brenner. *Psychoanalytic Quarterly* 35: 430–436.
Loewald, H. (1979) The Waning of the Oedipus Complex. *Journal of the American Psychoanalytic Association* 27: 751–775.
Loewald, H. (1988) Termination, Analyzable and Unanalyzable. *Psychoanalytic Study of the Child* 43: 155–166.
Mahler, M.S. (1966) Notes on the Development of Basic Moods: The Depressive Affect. In *Psychoanalysis – a General Psychology: Essays in Honor of Heinz Hartmann*, eds R.M. Loewenstein, L.M. Newman, M. Schur and A.J. Solnit. New York: International Universities Press, 152–168.
Mahler, M.S. (1967) On Human Symbiosis and the Vicissitudes of Individuation. *Journal of the American Psychoanalytic Association* 15: 740–763.
Mahler, M.S. (1968) *On Human Symbiosis and the Vicissitudes of Individuation*. New York: International Universities Press.
Mahler, M.S. (1971) A Study of the Separation-Individuation Process and its Possible Application to Borderline Phenomena in the Psychoanalytic Situation. *Psychoanalytic Study of the Child* 26: 403–424.
Mahler, M.S., Pine, F. and Bergman, A. (1975) *The Psychological Birth of the Human Infant. Symbiosis and Individuation*. New York: Basic Books.
Makari, G.J. (1991) German Philosophy, Freud, and the Riddle of the Woman. *Journal of the American Psychoanalytic Association* 39: 183–213.
Mann, T. (1922). Freud's Position in the History of Modern Thought. In *Past Masters*. New York: Knopf, 1933.
Masson, J.M., ed. (1985) *The Complete Letters of Sigmund Freud to Wilhelm Fliess 1887–1904*. Cambridge, MA: The Belknap Press of Harvard University Press.
McDougall, J. (1980) *A Plea for a Measure of Abnormality*. New York: International Universities Press.
McDougall, J. (1986) Eve's Reflection: On the Homosexual Components of Female Sexuality. In *Between Analyst and Patient*, ed. H.C. Meyers. Hillsdale, NJ: The Analytic Press.
McGrath, W.J. (1992) Freud and the Force of History. In *Freud and the History of Psychoanalysis*, eds T. Gelfands and J. Kerr, Hillsdale, NJ: Analytic Press, 79–97.
McGuire, W., ed. (1974) *The Freud/Jung Letters. The Correspondence Between Sigmund Freud and C. G. Jung*, trans. R. Manheim and R.F.C. Hall. Princeton: Princeton University Press.
Menninger, K.A. (1958) *Theory of Psychoanalytic Technique*. New York: Basic Books.
Miller, J.P. and Post, S.L., eds (1990) How Theory Shapes Technique: Perspectives on a Self-Psychological Clinical Presentation. *Psychoanalytic Inquiry* 10: 457–624.
Nachmanson, M. (1915) Freud's Libido Theorie verglichen mit der Eroslehre Platos *Int. Z. Psychoanal.* 3: 65–83.

Nagel, E. (1959) Methodological Issues in Psychoanalytic Theory. In *Psychoanalysis, Scientific Method and Philosophy*. New York: Washington Square Press, 38–57.

Nelson B., ed. (1957) *Freud and the 20th Century*. New York: Meridian Books.

Niehbuhr, R. (1957) Human Creativity and Self-Concern in Freud's Thought. In *Freud and the 20th Century*, ed. Nelson, B. New York: Meridian Books.

Novick, J. (1982) Termination: Themes and Issues. *Psychoanalytic Inquiry* 2: 329–365.

Nunberg, H. (1930) The Synthetic Functions of the Ego. In *Practice and Theory of Psychoanalysis*. New York: International Universities Press, 120–136.

Nunberg, H. (1951) Transference and Reality. *International Journal of Psychoanalysis* 32: 1–9.

Nunberg, H. (1955). *Principles of Psychoanalysis*. New York: International Universities Press.

Nunberg, H. and Federn, E. (1962) *Minutes of the Vienna Psychoanalytic Society, Volume I: 1906–1908*. New York: International Universities Press.

Nunberg, H. and Federn, E. (1967) *Minutes of the Vienna Psychoanalytic Society, Volume II: 1908–1910*. New York: International Universities Press.

Nunberg, H. and Federn, E. (1974) *Minutes of the Vienna Psychoanalytic Meeting, Volume III: 1910–1911*. New York: International Universities Press.

Oates, W.J. and O'Neil, E. Jr., eds (1938) *The Complete Greek Drama*. New York: Random House.

O'Flaherty, W.D. (1975) *Hindu Myths*. Baltimore: Penguin Books.

Onians, R.B. (1954) *The Origins of European Thought*. Cambridge, England: Cambridge University Press.

Orens, M. (1955) Setting a Termination Date: An Impetus to Analysis. *Journal of the American Psychoanalytic Association* 3: 661–665.

Ostow, M. (1982) Editor's Comment. In *Judaism and Psychoanalysis*, ed. Ostow, M. New York: Ktav Publishing House.

Panofsky, E. (1939) Blind Cupid. In *Studies in Iconology*. New York: Harper Torch Books, 1962.

Panofsky, E. (1969) *Problems in Titian*. New York: New York University Press.

Person, E.S. (1985) The Erotic Transference in Women and in Men: Differences and Consequences. *Journal of the American Academy of Psychoanalysis* 13: 159–180.

Pfister, O. (1921) Plato als Vorlaufer der Psychoanalyze. *Int. Z. Psychoanal.* 7: 264–269.

Pine, F. (1990) *Drive, Ego, Object, and Self: A Synthesis for Clinical Work*. New York: Basic Books.

Plato. *The Dialogues of Plato*, trans. B. Jowett. New York: Random House, 1937.

Praz, M. (1970) *The Romantic Agony*. New York: Oxford University Press.

Rangell, L. (1954) Similarities and Differences Between Psychoanalysis and Dynamic Psychotherapy. *Journal of the American Psychoanalytic Association* 2: 734–744.

Rank, O. (1924) *The Trauma of Birth*. New York: Harcourt, Brace and Company.

Rapaport, D. (1951) The Autonomy of the Ego. In *Collected Papers*, ed. Gill, M.M. New York: Basic Books, 1967, 357–367.

Rappaport, E. (1956) The Management of an Erotized Transference. *Psychoanalytic Quarterly* 25: 515–527.

Reich, A. (1953) Narcissistic Object Choice in Women. *Journal of the American Psychoanalytic Association* 1: 22–44.

Reich, A. (1958a) A Character Formation Representing the Integration of Unusual Conflict Solutions into the Ego Structure. In *Annie Reich: Psychoanalytic Contributions*. New York: International Universities Press, 1973, 250–270.

Reich, A. (1958b) A Special Variation on Technique. In *Psychoanalytic Contributions*. New York: International Universities Press, 236–249.

Reich, W. (1927, 1928) Report on the Seminar for Psychoanalytic Therapy. *Int. Ztschr. fr Arztliche Psychoanal.* 13: 241–244; 40: 438–440.

Reich, W. (1929) The Genital Character and the Neurotic Character. In *The Psychoanalytic Reader*, ed. R. Fliess. New York: International University Press, 1948, 148–169.

Reich, W. (1940) *The Function of the Orgasm*. New York: Orgone Institute Press.

Reik, T. (1935) *Der Überraschte Psychologe*. Leiden, Holland: A.W. Sijthoff's Uitgevers-maatschappij N.V.

Reik, T. (1944) *A Psychologist Looks at Love*. New York: Farrar & Rinehart.
Reik, T. (1948) *Listening with the Third Ear*. New York: Farrar, Straus & Co.
Reik, T. (1949) *Fragment of a Great Confession: A Psychoanalytic Autobiography*. New York: Farrar, Straus & Co.
Rice, E. (1990) *Freud and Moses: The Long Journey Home*. New York: State University of New York Press.
Ritvo, S. (1966) Correlation of a Childhood and Adult Neurosis. *International Journal of Psychoanalysis* 47: 130–131.
Riviere, J. (1936) On the Genesis of Psychical Conflict in Earliest Infancy. *International Journal of Psychoanalysis* 17: 395–422.
Rosenfelt, H. (1971) A Clinical Approach to the Psychoanalytic Theory of the Life and Death Instincts: An Investigation into the Aggressive Aspects of Narcissism. *International Journal of Psychoanalysis* 52: 169–178.
Ross, N. (1970) The Primacy of Genitality in the Light of Ego Psychology. *Journal of the American Psychoanalytic Association* 18:267–284.
Russell, B. (1930) *The Conquest of Happiness*. London: Allen & Unwin.
Russell, B. (1951) *The Autobiography of Bertand Russell*, Vol. 1. Boston: Little, Brown.
Sadow, L., Gedo, J.E., Miller, J., Pollock, G.H., Sabshin, M. and Schlessinger, N. (1968) The Process of Hypothesis Change in Three Early Psychoanalytic Concepts. *Journal of the American Psychoanalytic Association* 16: 245–273.
Sandler, J. and Dreher, A. (1996) *What Do Psychoanalysts Want? The Problem of Aims in Psychoanalytic Therapy*. London: Routledge.
Schafer, R. (1977) The Interpretation of Transference and the Condition of Loving. *Journal of the American Psychoanalytic Association* 25: 335–362.
Schopenhauer, A. (1858a) The Metaphysics of Sexual Love. In *The World as Will and Representation Vols. I, II*. Third edition. Trans. E.F.J. Payne. New York: Dover Publications, 1966.
Schopenhauer, A. (1858b) *The World as Will and Representation Vols. I, II*. Third edition. Trans. E.F.J. Payne. New York: Dover Publications, 1966.
Schimek, J.G. (1975) The Interpretations of the Past: Childhood Trauma, Psychical Reality, and Historical Truth. *Journal of the American Psychoanalytic Association* 23: 845–865.
Segal, H. (1993) On the Clinical Usefulness of the Concept of Death Instinct. *International Journal of Psychoanalysis*, 74: 55–61.
Simon, B. (1978) *Mind and Madness in Ancient Greece*. Ithaca: Cornell University Press.
Singer, I. (1984) *The Nature of Love*. Chicago: University of Chicago Press.
Spiegel, L.A. (1966) Affects in Relation to Self and Object: A Model for the Derivation of Desire, Longing, Pain, Anxiety, Humiliation, and Shame. *Psychoanalytic Study of the Child* 21: 69–92.
Spitz, R.A. (1945) Hospitalism – An Inquiry into Genesis of Psychiatric Conditions in Early Childhood. *Psychoanalytic Study of the Child* 1: 53–74.
Spitz, R.A. (1946) Hospitalism: A Follow-up Request. *Psychoanalytic Study of the Child* 2: 113–17.
Spurgeon, C. (1958) *Shakespeare's Imagery*. Boston: Beacon Press.
Stanescu, H. (1971) Young Freud's Letters to his Rumanian Friend Silberstein. *Israel Annals of Psychiatry and Related Disciplines* 9: 195–207.
Steiner, R. (1985) Some Thoughts about Tradition and Change Arising from the Examination of the British Psychoanalytical Society's Controversial Discussions 1943–1944. *International Journal of Psychoanalysis* 12: 27–71.
Sterba, R. (1934) The Fate of the Ego in Analytic Therapy. *International Journal of Psychoanalysis* 15: 117–126.
Stern, D.A. (1991) Technical Implications for Certain Types of Erotized Treatment Relationships. *Psychoanalytic Psychology* 8: 463–476.
Stone, L. (1954) The Widening Scope of Indications for Psychoanalysis. *Journal of the American Psychoanalytic Association* 2: 567–594.
Stone, L. (1961) *The Psychoanalytic Situation: An Examination of its Development and Essential Nature*. New York: International Universities Press.

Strachey, J. (1934) The Nature of the Therapeutic Action in Psychoanalysis. *International Journal of Psychoanalysis* 15: 127–159.
Strenger, C. (1989) The Classic and the Romantic Vision in Psychoanalysis. *International Journal of Psychoanalysis* 70: 593–610.
Swartz, J. (1969) The Erotized Transference and Other Transference Problems. *Psychoanalytic Forum*, 3: 307–318.
Ticho, E.A. (1972) Termination of Psychoanalysis: Treatment Goals, Life Goals. *Psychoanalytic Quarterly* 41: 315–333.
Troyat, H. (1967) *Tolstoy*. New York: Doubleday.
Van Der Waals, H.G. (1965) Problems of Narcissism. *Bull. Menninger Clin.* 29: 243–274.
Vermorel, M. and Vermorel, H. (1986) Was Freud a Romantic? *International Review of Psychoanalysis* 13: 15–37.
Waelder, R. (1929) The Inference of Psychoanalysis on the Outlook on Life of Modern Man. In *Psychoanalysis, Observation, Theory, Application. Selected Papers of Robert Waelder*, ed. S.A.G. Guttman. New York: International University Press, 1976.
Waelder, R. (1930) The Principle of Multiple Function: Observations on Over-Determination. In *Selected Papers of Robert Waelder*, ed. S.A.G. Guttman. New York: International Universities Press, 1976, 68–83.
Waelder, R. (1936) The Problem of the Genesis of Psychical Conflict in Earliest Infancy. In *Psychoanalysis: Observation, Theory, Application: Selected Papers of Robert Waelder*, ed. S.A.G. Guttman. New York: International Universities Press, 1976, 121–188.
Waelder, R. (1951) The Structure of Paranoid Ideas. *International Journal of Psychoanalysis* 32(3): 167–77.
Waelder, R. (1960) *Basic Theory of Psychoanalysis*. New York: International Universities Press.
Waelder, R. (1962) Psychoanalysis, Scientific Method, and Philosophy. In *Psychoanalysis, Observation, Theory, Application: Selected Papers of Robert Waelder*, ed. S.A.G. Guttman. International University Press, 1976.
Wallerstein, R.S. (1965) The Goals of Psychoanalysis: A Survey of Analytic Viewpoints. *Journal of the American Psychoanalytic Association* 13: 748–770.
Wallerstein, R.S. (1995) *The Talking Cures*. New Haven, CT: Yale University Press.
Weinshel, E.M. (1990) How Wide is the Widening Scope of Psychoanalysis and How Solid is its Structural Model? *Journal of the American Psychoanalytic Association* 38: 275–296.
Weiss, E. (1935) Todes Trieb und Masochismus. *Imago* 21: 393–411.
Whitebook, J. (1991) Perversion, Destruction, and Reparation: On the Contributions of Janine Chasseguet-Smirgel and Joyce McDougall. *American Imago* 48: 329–350.
Winnicott, D.W. (1953) Transitional Objects and Transitional Phenomena. *International Journal of Psychoanalysis* 34: 89–97.
Winnicott, D.W. (1955) Metapsychological and Clinical Aspects of Regression Within the Psychoanalytical Setup. *International Journal of Psychoanalysis* 36: 1–26.
Winnicott, D.W. (1958) The Capacity to be Alone. *International Journal of Psychoanalysis* 39: 416–420.
Winnicott. D.W. (1964) Memoirs, Dreams, Reflections. *International Journal of Psychoanalysis* 45: 450–55.
Winnicott, D.W. (1965) *The Maturational Processes and the Facilitating Environment.* New York: International University Press.
Winnicott, D.W. (1971) *Playing and Reality*. London: Tavistock.
Wittels, F. (1924) *Sigmund Freud: Der Mann, die Lehre, die Schule*. Leipzig: Tal.
Wittels, F. (1931) *Freud and His Time*. New York: Liveright.
Wrye, H.K. and Welles, J.K. (1989) The Maternal Erotic Transference. *International Journal of Psychoanalysis* 70 (4): 673–84.
Yerushalmi, Yosef H. (1991) *Freud's Moses*. New Haven: Yale University Press.
Young, M. (1989) Heinz Hartmann, M.D.: An Introduction and Appreciation. *Psychoanalytic Quarterly* 58: 521–525.
Zetzel, E.R. (1965) The Theory of Therapy in Relation to a Developmental Model of the Psychic Apparatus. *International Journal of Psychoanalysis* 46: 39–52.

INDEX